Budgeting Concepts for Nurse Managers

Budgeting Concepts for Nurse Managers

THIRD EDITION

Steven A. Finkler, PhD, CPA
Robert F. Wagner Graduate School of Public Service
New York University
New York, New York

With contributions by
Christina M. Graf, RN, MS
Massachusetts General Hospital
Boston, Massachusetts

W.B. SAUNDERS COMPANY
A Harcourt Health Sciences Company
Philadelphia   London   New York   St. Louis   Sydney   Toronto

W.B. SAUNDERS COMPANY

A Harcourt Health Sciences Company

The Curtis Center
Independence Square West
Philadelphia, Pennsylvania 19106

Library of Congress Cataloging-in-Publication Data

Finkler, Steven A.
  Budgeting concepts for nurse managers / Steven A. Finkler, with contributions
by Christina M. Graf. — 3rd ed.
      p. ; cm.
  Includes bibliographical references and index.
  ISBN 0-7216-7802-5
  1. Nursing services—Administration. 2. Health facilities—Business management.
I. Graf, Christina M. II. Title.
  [DNLM: 1. Budgets—Nurses' Instruction. 2. Nurse Administrators—Nurses'
Instruction.   WY 105 F499b 2001]
  RT89.F53 2001
  362.1'73'0681—dc21

                                                                    00-038808

Vice President and Nursing Editorial Director: Sally Schrefer
Editorial Manager: Thomas Eoyang
Editorial Assistant: Avery Roberts
Production Manager: Donna L. Morrissey

BUDGETING CONCEPTS FOR NURSE MANAGERS   ISBN 0-7216-7802-5

Printed in the United States of America

Last digit is the print number: 9   8   7   6   5   4   3   2   1

To
Lilli, David, and Gary, with love.

About the Author

STEVEN A. FINKLER, PhD, CPA

Steven Finkler is Professor of Public and Health Administration, Accounting, and Financial Management at New York University's Robert F. Wagner Graduate School of Public Service. At New York University he directs the specialization in Health Services Financial Management. Professor Finkler is a member of the National Advisory Council for Nursing Research (NACNR) at the National Institute of Nursing Research (NINR). He served as editor of *Hospital Cost Management and Accounting* from 1984 to 1997.

An award-winning teacher and author, Professor Finkler is currently engaged in a variety of research projects in the areas of health care economics and accounting. Among his current projects are a study of the cost effectiveness of using nurse practitioners to aid breast-feeding mothers of low-birth-weight infants. He is working on that project with colleagues at the University of Pennsylvania School of Nursing. He is also currently working on a new book, *Financial Management for Public, Health, and Not-for-Profit Organizations* (in press).

In addition to this book, Professor Finkler has written *Financial Management for Nurse Managers and Executives*, second edition, 2000 (with Christine Kovner), *Cost Accounting for Health Care Organizations*, second edition, 1999 (with David Ward), and *Finance and Accounting for Nonfinancial Managers*, 1996. He has also authored over two hundred articles published in many journals, including *Journal of Nursing Administration, The New England Journal of Medicine, Nursing Economic$, Journal of Neonatal Nursing, Western Journal of Nursing Research, O.R. Nurse Managers' Network, Health Services Research, Medical Care, Healthcare Financial Management, Health Care Management Review*, and other journals, and a chapter in *Strategies for Successful Nursing Management*.

He received a bachelor of science in economics and master of science in accounting from the Wharton School of the University of Pennsylvania. His master's degree in economics and doctorate in business administration were awarded by Stanford University. Professor Finkler, who is also a certified public accountant, worked for several years as an auditor with Ernst and Young and was on the faculty of the Wharton School for six years before joining New York University in 1984.

About the Contributor

CHRISTINA M. GRAF, RN, MS, PhD(Cand)

Christina Graf is the Director of Patient Care Services Management Systems at Massachusetts General Hospital (MGH) in Boston. Her professional experience includes over 16 years of progressive line management experience, from head nurse to nursing director, in hospitals in New York and Texas. She developed the position of Director of Nursing Management Information Systems at Methodist Hospitals of Dallas, with responsibility for ensuring the effective allocation and utilization of personnel resources in the departments of nursing. Since 1985, she has had similar responsibilities at MGH, expanding her scope to include not only nursing but also the health professions departments, a combined total of over 2,500 FTEs (full-time equivalents) with an annual operating budget of approximately $200 million. Ms Graf received her baccalaureate degree in nursing from Molloy College in Rockville Centre, New York, and her master's degree in maternal-child nursing from Boston University. She is currently in the doctoral program in health policy at the Heller School for Social Policy of Brandeis University, with an expected completion date of 2001.

Preface

Nurse managers face tremendous challenges in performing their administrative responsibilities. Frequently, it is clinical skill as a nurse that leads to nursing promotions into management positions. Once in a management position, administrative skills become vital. On-the-job experience provides managers with significant insights about the way that the real world functions. However, the benefits of experience have limitations. To gain additional managerial capabilities, specific knowledge about concepts, tools, and techniques must be sought from some formalized source. Budgeting is a prime example of an area where one can get by based on experience but where performance can improve considerably with some additional formalized knowledge.

This book was written to help nurses gain some valuable conceptual knowledge about budgeting. The goal of this book is to improve the budgeting skills of nurses who are currently managers or who are planning to move into management positions. The book covers a broad range of budgeting skills. It is aimed primarily at first level nurse managers and their immediate supervisors, both of whom have responsibility for planning and controlling unit budgets. However, many of the topics covered include sophisticated treatment that would be of interest to midlevel nurse managers and to top-level nursing executives. For example, the chapters on revenue budgeting and on benchmarking and productivity would be of interest to all levels of nurse managers. The conceptual budgeting issues discussed in this book are equally relevant for clinics, surgical centers, private nursing practices, hospitals, nursing homes, home care agencies, hospices, and other health care settings.

This book is not designed to create a level of expertise that will allow you to fire all the financial managers in your organization and do their jobs yourself. Rather, it should improve your ability to communicate with your organization's financial managers, improve your performance in your role in the budget process, and perhaps give you the ability to introduce some innovative uses of budgets into your organization.

Budgeting Concepts for Nurse Managers is written specifically for nursing administration students and nurse managers and, for its examples, draws upon situations in which nurse managers find themselves. It is written at a level that assumes no previous financial management experience or expertise on the part of the reader.

I would like to express my thanks to the many individuals who made this book possible. First, my thanks go to Christina Graf, RN, who wrote Chapter 8 on operating budgets. She also prepared the appendix of budget forms and instructions. Her contributions are invaluable to this book because they bridge the gap between my academic expertise about budgeting concepts and the real world specifics of budgeting in a nursing environment. Both Christina Graf and Christine Kovner reviewed the entire manuscript and made a number of helpful comments. The comments of anonymous reviewers were invaluable. Finally, my thanks go to my wife, Lilli, who once again tolerated my spending scarce leisure time working on a book.

NOTE ON CHANGES IN THE THIRD EDITION

The first edition of *Budgeting Concepts for Nurse Managers* was published in 1984. At that time, many nursing administration masters degree programs were just beginning to add courses in financial management to their curriculum. This book was a forerunner of the many nursing finance books that were written in the last half of the 1980s. The second edition was published in 1992. DRGs (diagnosis-related groups) were well-entrenched, but managed care had not yet come into its own, as it did later in the 1990s.

Much of the second edition is still as relevant today as it was in 1992. However, much has changed in the last nine years. In response to changes in the health care system, in nursing and in budgeting, each chapter of this book has been substantially rewritten, and the suggested readings at the end of each chapter have been updated. Throughout the book there is a greater emphasis on a wide variety of types of health care organizations, rather than a more limited focus on hospitals. The new edition includes examples for long-term care, home health, community health, managed care, clinics, surgery centers, and nurses in private practice, as well as the more traditional hospital-based examples. The budgeting needs of both existing organizations and new start-up ventures are addressed.

Coverage has been added or expanded in a number of areas. Some examples are the addition of a discussion of activity-based costing, expansion of the break-even analysis discussion to include break-even analysis in capitated environments, additional discussion of the development of business plans, and more in-depth discussion of strategic planning and its link to the operating budget. The operating budget chapter has new sections on computerizing the budget process, alternate workload measurement systems, the impact of required minimum staffing levels on the budget, and on implementation of the budget. A discussion of variable budgeting has also been added to the book.

A concerted effort has been made to update all numbers, forms, and references throughout the book to make it appropriate for the twenty-first century. This led to the addition of several new chapters essential for management in 2001 and beyond. Chapter 9 on revenue budgeting and managed care and Chapter 15 on benchmarking, productivity, and cost-benefit and cost-effectiveness analysis are completely new. They reflect important new focuses in nurse budgeting. The revenue chapter addresses the various sources of revenue, why revenue is often ignored in nursing budgets, why revenue is now important for nurses, and the role of managed care relative to revenues, including discussion of capitation and budgeting for risk-sharing contracts. In Chapter 13 on variances, a section has been added that looks at revenue variances. The new chapter on benchmarking, productivity, and cost-benefit and cost-effectiveness analysis addresses the growing need for health care organizations to adopt the best practices possible, to strive to be as productive as possible, and to make decisions with an understanding of whether they are likely to be cost-effective approaches. That chapter addresses the issue of unit costing as well.

Despite all the additions, this book retains its original narrow focus on issues directly related to budgeting. A number of reviewers of the book held that out as a particular strength. On the other hand, one reviewer of the second edition felt that it should cover topics such as economics, accounting, financial statements, and marketing. Those topics and others are included in a book with a broader focus on financial management but a less in-depth focus on budgeting, *Financial Management for Nurse Managers and Executives.*[1]

This third edition retains a number of features from the second edition that readers found useful. These include the chapter outlines contained in the table of contents, the statement of chapter goals at the beginning of each chapter, the summary and implications for nurse managers section at the end of each chapter, and the extensive glossary at the end of the book.

I welcome comments regarding this book. Any corrections, exercises, or other contributions that are used in the next edition will be formally acknowledged in the book.

STEVEN A. FINKLER
steven.finkler@wagner.nyu.edu
April 2000

---

[1]Steven A. Finkler and Christine T. Kovner, *Financial Management for Nurse Managers and Executives,* 2nd Edition, W.B. Saunders, Philadelphia, 2000.

Contents

3

4

5

6

7

8

11

14

15

16

1

Introduction

THE DIFFERENT TYPES OF BUDGETS

The goals of this chapter are to:
define budgeting;
describe some of the benefits of budgeting;
distinguish between budgets and budgeting;
introduce and describe the various types of budgets; and
identify the relevant time periods for budget preparation.

WHY BUDGET?

The primary role of nurses is to provide care. Why should nurses have to know about budgets? Why bother?

Health care services are costly to provide. Only health care organizations that are financially sound can provide high-quality services. Organizations that do not pay adequate attention to their finances many find themselves in a difficult position. They may suffer losses. Ultimately the losses may cause the organization to severely cut the quality of their care or even close completely.

Budgeting provides the organization with the ability to plan its activities and control its costs. It allows choices to be made that will allow it to provide the best care possible, while staying within the financial means of the organization. Budgeting provides managers with the tools needed to try to ensure that the resources benefit patients rather than being wasted.

That explains why health care organizations need to budget. But why should nurses have to get involved in an activity that seems so far removed from patient care? The answer, quite simply, is that no one knows what resources are needed to provide nursing care better than nurses. At one time financial managers tried to provide nursing departments and units with their budgets. Nurse managers were simply told how many staff members they could hire and how much they could spend.

However, such an approach to budgeting was doomed to fail. Financial managers do not have the ability to monitor the dynamic forces that affect the need for nursing care. Nurses are faced with shifts in patient demographics, illness, and changes in health care technology. Nurses know if physicians are expanding their practices or retiring. Nurses know which patients have shorter lengths of stay and where admissions are rising or falling. Only nurses working in each nursing unit or department of a health care organization can reasonably assess the nursing resource requirements.

Nurses must get involved in the budget process to make certain that they have the resources needed to provide high-quality clinical care. Budgeting is not separate from clinical caregiving. If anything, budgeting has a direct bearing on the amount of clinical care provided and the way that it is provided. Just as a blood pressure cuff or a thermometer are tools that nurses use in providing clinical care, so is a budget. Just as a nurse might prepare a patient care plan for the clinical care of one patient, developing a budget acts as a plan to determine the overall clinical care that all patients will receive. It determines whether care will be provided by a nurse or an aide. It determines what clinical supplies will be available. The elements of the budget are intertwined with the care patients receive.

In essence, for health care organizations to be efficient they must involve nurses in the budgeting process. Only then can they ensure that resources are not wasted, perhaps causing an organization-wide financial crisis, while at the same time being aware of the specific needs that nursing has in order to provide patients with quality health care services. This book provides the essential budgeting techniques that nurses need in order to determine their needs and to most effectively communicate their needs to those individuals who make the final decisions on how to allocate the organization's limited resources.

DEFINITION OF BUDGETING

A *budget** is a plan. To many individuals, budgeting is so onerous an activity that merely the word "budget" has taken on many negative connotations. A budget, however, is simply a plan. The plan is formalized (written down) and quantified (e.g., stated in dollar terms). It represents management's intentions or expectations. In financial terms, an organization-wide budget generally compares expected *revenues* to expected *expenses* in order to determine the organization's expected financial results. Revenues are the amounts of money the organization has earned by providing its services. Expenses are the costs of the services provided. Individual departments' budgets look at only a portion of the organization's overall revenue and expense information.

---

*Definitions of all words that appear in italics are provided in the Glossary at the end of the book.

Budgeting forces managers to plan ahead. The focus on the future instead of the present allows managers to anticipate problems or opportunities far enough ahead of time to respond appropriately. Budgeting can greatly enhance communication and coordination between units and departments. This can allow units or departments to work together efficiently, instead of duplicating efforts or failing to share critical information. Waste can be avoided by the knowledge developed and shared through the budget process. Budgets can be used to provide both managers and staff with the motivation to work positively for the organization. They can also show how well both management and units or departments are performing. These benefits of budgeting are discussed in greater detail in Chapter 2.

Budgeting does not happen automatically. It requires great effort and commitment from all levels of management. Often a budget committee (which should include the *Chief Nurse Executive*) is formed to insure that there is maximum cooperation and coordination throughout the budget process. Many organizations produce a budget calendar that indicates the various specific activities to be carried out in the budget process, identifies the responsible individuals (e.g., finance office, unit or department managers, Board of Trustees), and provides deadlines for completion of each budget activity. Larger organizations have budget manuals. These manuals include uniform instructions and forms to be used throughout the organization, a copy of the budget calendar, and a statement of organizational mission. They also generally include a variety of other pieces of information relevant to the process of budget preparation. For instance, inflation rates, specific measurable goals, and an environmental statement would often be included.

Budget manuals or packages are institution-specific, differing substantially from one organization to another. This book focuses primarily on concepts that are applicable to the budgeting process in a wide range of health care organizations, rather than providing a specific set of forms for the reader to fill in. The book's Appendix provides a sample set of forms, with instructions, for a unit operating and capital budget. However, understanding the budgeting process is more important than learning how to complete one specific set of forms. Managers must be able to think about budgets and budgeting in order to develop sensible, workable, efficient budgets. The focus of budgeting is not on filling in a standard set of forms.

Further, this book is about budgeting rather than just budgets. Budgets are plans. They represent an educated guess about what might be accomplished. *Budgeting* is a process whereby plans are made and then an effort is made to meet or exceed the goals of the plans. This latter effort is referred to as the *control* process. Control of costs requires a concerted effort by both managers and staff. This book will thus have its primary focus on the preparation of budgets and a second, well-emphasized focus on the topics that surround control, such as *variance analysis*, which determines how and why the actual results are varying from the budget. Such analysis uncovers problems that may have a negative financial impact on the organization and allows actions to be taken to correct those problems at an early stage.

A budget without a formal control system to ensure that actual results conform as closely as possible to the plan loses much of its managerial value. The budgeting process as a whole is of great importance because it can improve the organization's control over its use of scarce resources. This improved control can ensure that inefficiency is minimized and that the amount of dollars available for the provision of high-quality patient care is maximized.

Budgets are critical tools for the largest health care system or the smallest ambulatory care organization. Nursing entrepreneurs starting new ventures need budgets and budgeting skills every bit as much as managed care organizations, clinics, hospitals, or nursing homes. The concepts discussed in this book are relevant to nurse managers in all health care organizations.

TYPES OF BUDGETS

Many managers tend to think of the budget as simply a cap on expenses that tells them how much they may spend. This is a very limited view of just the *operating budget*. The operating budget, in turn, is only a small part of the overall budget of the organization. A well-managed organization will have a *master budget*. The master budget is a set of all the major budgets in the organization. It will generally include the operating budget, a *long-range budget*, a *program budget*, a *capital budget*, and a *cash budget* (see Fig. 1–1). Some organizations are also starting to use a new type of budget, referred to as a *performance* or *outcomes budget*, as well as a number of *product-line* budgets. From time to time the organization will also need to budget for some additional special project that is not part of its normal activities. In these cases it will prepare a *special-purpose budget*. This chapter will provide an introduction to each of these types of budgets.

The Operating Budget

Those readers who already have some budgeting experience are probably most familiar with the operating budget. It is the plan for day-in and day-out operating revenues and expenses for a period of 1 year. If the budget shows an excess of revenues over expenses, it means that the organization expects to make a *profit* from its activities for the year. If the organization is a *for-profit* company, some of the profits can be paid to the owners of the company in the form of a *dividend*. Even not-for-profit organizations need to earn profits. These profits can be used to replace worn-out equipment and old buildings or to expand the services available to the community. If any health care organization, for-profit or not-for-profit, consistently fails to earn profits, it will not be able to add new technologies and continue to provide high-quality care.

If there is a budgeted excess of expenses over revenues, it means that the

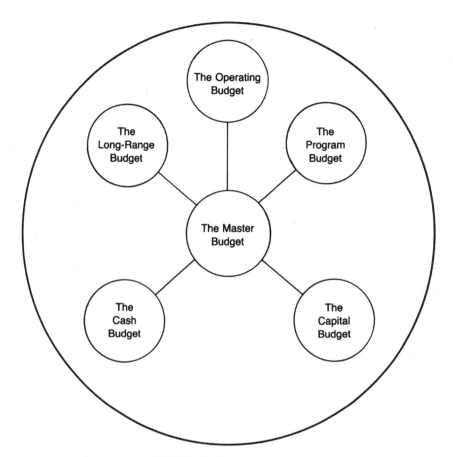

FIGURE 1–1. The master budget.

organization expects to have a loss for the budgeted year. Over time, losses mean that equipment and buildings cannot be replaced and that there are restrictions on the organization's ability to expand its quantity and quality of services. If losses occur for too many years in a row, eventually the organization would have to cease operations.

The operating budget includes the revenues that are expected to be received from *Medicare, Medicaid, managed care organizations,* other *private insurers, self-pay patients,* and contributions. In some cases, contributions are sufficient to offset losses from routine operations and to keep a health care organization in business despite losses. The operating budget also plans for the routine costs of operating each department and unit in the organization, including the purely administrative departments that do not directly provide services. The operating budget is discussed in detail in Chapter 8.

Long-Range Budgets

Budgets help managers plan for the future. Operating budgets give a detailed plan for the coming year. However, many changes in an organization require a long lead time and take a number of years to be implemented fully. To avoid suffering from shortsightedness, many organizations employ a long-range plan or budget. Such 3-, 5-, or 10-year plans allow management to ignore the trees temporarily and focus on the whole forest. Where is the organization relative to its peer group? What improvements can be made over the next 3, 5, or 10 years? What must be done each year to move toward those goals?

In many organizations, the primary focus of the budgeting process is on the development of the operating budget. Managers tend to look at what happened last year and what is happening this year. They then add an increase for inflation and produce a budget for the next year. The problem with this approach is that it contains no vision. There is no way to make a major leap forward, because what has been done in the past is simply being projected into the future. If one would like to be able to look back 5 years from now and say, "Look at how far we have come," it is necessary to have a way to make major strides forward. Otherwise, 5 years from now the organization will have made little if any advancement.

That is where long-range plans are helpful. Their focus is not on how to get through next year but rather on what major changes ought to be made over the coming years. Long-range plans frequently are not extremely detailed. When a plan is laid out for the next 5 years, it does not get into how many employees will be needed or what exact piece of equipment will be bought. It may be as general as to say that over the next 5 years three new tertiary care services will be added to the organization's services for the community. It may not even specify which ones.

Long-range plans help to give the organization a sense of commitment to the future. They provide long-term goals so that the organization is not always working only on things that can be accomplished within the arbitrary fixed time period of 1 year. Such long-range budgets serve a vital function in allowing the organization to prepare each year's detailed operating budget on the basis of an overall sense of purpose and direction. The operating budget becomes more than just next year's survival plan; it becomes a link between where the organization has been and where it is going. To develop long-range plans, we employ a strategic planning process. Strategic planning links the overall mission of the organization to its activities. Strategic planning and long-range budgets are discussed in Chapter 7.

Program Budgets

Program budgets are special budgeting efforts analyzing specific programs. Generally the orientation is toward evaluating a planned new program or closely examining an existing program, rather than merely planning the revenues and expenses for the program for the coming year. Often the program involved is in some way optional. The purpose of the program budget is to make a decision. Should the new program be undertaken or not? This question has somewhat less relevance for the types of programs and services that are considered to be essential to the organization and that are in no way optional.

Even for essential programs, however, there is the question of how the program's goals can best be accomplished. For example, a hospital must have laboratory services. This may not be seen as being optional. However, the hospital may maintain a large, fully equipped laboratory or it may have minimal equipment for tests that must be done immediately, while sending the rest of the tests to an outside laboratory service. The extent of the in-house laboratory might be the subject of a special program budgeting effort or evaluation. Once the program evaluation has been performed and the program accepted, the revenues and expenses of the program will become part of the regular operating budget.

Often, program budgets are developed for specific programs as a result of the long-range budgeting process. The long-range budget for a same-day surgery organization may determine that three additional same-day surgery locations should be added over the next 5 years. Because new locations often require a year to plan and sometimes more than a year to implement once the planning phase is complete, one result of the long-range plan may be to select one location to be added immediately. Frequently, new services involve labor and equipment from numerous departments. By setting up a program budget process for the new location, all the information related to the addition of that location can be considered and evaluated.

Since program budgets often cut across departments, they generally must be developed with committee input from at least the major departments that will be affected by the change. Program budgets also cut across years. The financial impact of the change needs to be assessed not just in the coming year but over a reasonably long period of time. Since the operating budget is a 1-year budget, this is another reason for special budget treatment for new programs or services.

In recent years, *business plans* have become a vital tool for the evaluation of new programs or projects. The elements of such plans will be discussed along with long-range budgets and other aspects of program budgeting in Chapter 7.

Capital Budgets

Many expenditures made by health care organizations are for the acquisition of items that will last for more than 1 year. Such acquisitions are defined as capital expenditures. Frequently, these purchases do not concern the introduction of an entire program and therefore do not warrant a full-scale program budget effort. Often, capital budget items will concern only one department or unit and may be part of an already existing program. Yet capital expenditures frequently concern large outlays of money that deserve special attention. The multiyear life of capital assets also creates a need for a focus on such items, separate from the operating budget.

Capital expenditures are made to purchase items that will provide benefits for a number of years into the future. If capital items are only evaluated based on their benefits for the coming year, their value to the organization will be understated. The operating budget has the capability to look at only 1 coming year's revenues and expenses. Therefore, capital items must be put into a separate budget that can evaluate their benefits over their entire useful lifetime.

For example, suppose that a nursing home were to entirely renovate one wing of its building. Patients will use the wing and the organization will receive revenues from patients in that wing for a number of years. If the entire renovation cost were charged as an expense in this year's operating budget, the project would appear financially infeasible. Patients could never be charged enough in one year to recover the full construction costs. The new wing will be available for many years, however, and patients can be charged for the renovation well into the future.

If this were treated as an operating budget expense, it might show a $1,000,000 expense for the renovation this year but only $100,000 of revenues from the patients who benefited from the renovation. The operating budget cannot match future revenues to current outlays to see if the project is feasible. It looks only at revenues and expenses for the coming year. The capital budget seeks to bridge this gap for projects or purchases with a multiyear life.

The capital budget looks at a capital investment—whether it is a renovation, a new wing for the nursing home, or a new refrigerator for a nursing station—to determine whether the expenditure is feasible economically over the lifetime of the asset. Thus, even though an item may cost only $600 or $800, by recognizing its 3-, 5-, or 10-year expected lifetime, it is more likely that a fair assessment will be made concerning whether it is reasonable to spend the money for this specific purpose.

This does not mean that all acquisitions that are not warranted on a financial basis would be rejected. The capital budget can go beyond simply dollars and cents and look at costs and benefits in a broader sense. The general benefit provided to the community can be considered. Often, capital items will be purchased even if they lose money. However, for the organization to survive, there must be an understanding of which things generate a profit and which things lose money. Enough profit-making activities must be selected to cover those expenditures that result in losses. The key thrust of capital budgeting is that the evaluation of the expenditure should be based on its impact over its full lifetime, rather than simply looking at the costs and benefits in the first year. Capital budgets are discussed in Chapter 10.

Product-Line Budgets

A product-line is a group of patients that have some commonality that allows them to be grouped together, such as a common diagnosis. Budgeting in health care organizations is largely focused on departments and units. In all hospitals, for example, radiology has a budget; dietary has a budget; nursing has a budget. However, it is becoming more and more common for there to be a budget for a specific type of patient, such as heart surgery patients or childbearing women. These budgets include the costs of surgery, recovery, delivery room, x-rays, meals, nursing care, and other costs.

In today's tight financial environment, it is often of great managerial interest to be able to budget for the planned revenues and expenses of specific patient groups, such as heart surgery patients. Such an approach has the potential to reveal the profitability of different types of patients.

The move toward product-line budgeting has also gained impetus from active pressure by *Health Maintenance Organizations* (HMOs) negotiating with health care providers for discounted rates for specific groups of patients. It is difficult to negotiate sensible revenue rates unless the related costs of the patients are known.

Health care organizations have therefore been moving in a product-line budgeting direction, while not abandoning department budgets. However, the process is a difficult one. Measuring the cost of nursing care by patients in any one category is complicated. Yet, to determine a budget, such information is essential. Product-line costing is therefore discussed in Chapter 16, along with the issue of costing out nursing services.

Cash Budgets

Cash is the lifeblood of any organization. Survival depends on the ability to maintain an adequate supply of cash to meet monetary obligations of the organization as they become due for payment. Operating budgets focus on the revenues and expenses of the organization. If the organization is expected to lose money, that will be reflected in the operating budget. It is possible, however, for the organization to have a cash crisis even if it is not losing money. Many of the expenses that an organization incurs are paid currently. Wages are typically paid at least monthly and frequently biweekly or weekly. However, revenues may take several months to collect because of the internal lags in processing patient bills and the external lags before organizations such as HMOs or Medicare make payment. Thus an organization can literally run out of cash even though it is making a profit!

Oddly enough, this problem tends to be most severe for an organization with an increasing number of patients. Although an increasing patient volume is normally thought of as a healthy development, it results in growing expenses as well as growing revenues. The revenues may well increase by a greater amount than the expenses. The expenses, however, tend to be paid much sooner than the revenues are received. Without careful management, such growing profitability can easily bankrupt an organization.

These problems tend to be particularly severe for start-up ventures. A nurse entrepreneur must carefully consider the timing of cash flows, even if a profit is made on every unit of service. Rent, phone bills, and employees have to be paid currently even if insurance companies delay payment to the health care provider. A cash budget becomes a tool critical to the survival of the organization.

Another cash problem relates to major capital expenses. Only a 1-year portion of capital outlays will show up in the operating budget as a current year expense. If the organization budgets to add a wing for $10,000,000, and it is expected to have a 20-year life, then there will typically be a charge of one-twentieth of the cost, or $500,000 per year as an expense called *depreciation* in the operating budget. However, the entire $10,000,000 will have to be paid in cash in the coming year when the wing is built. Thus there will be a cash outlay of $9,500,000 more than is shown in the operating budget as an expense.

For these reasons, a cash budget is prepared. Cash budgets plan for the monthly receipt of cash and disbursement of cash from the organization. If a shortage is predicted for any given month, appropriate plans can be made for short-term bank financing or longer-term bond financing. Cash budgets are discussed in Chapter 12.

Performance Budgets

This book introduces an approach to budgeting that is not yet widely used in health care organizations. The budget is called a performance budget, and it attempts to make plans for units, departments, and organizations that will better provide an ability to evaluate whether the unit, department, or organization is accomplishing what it wants to do.

An operating budget does a pretty good job of detailing the resources that will be needed. However, the measures in that budget, as you will see as you read this book, are fairly simplistic.

Nursing organizations or units have many objectives besides generating patient days, visits, or encounters. They want to assure quality of care and cost-effectiveness. But such goals are rarely explicit in the budget process. How much spending is budgeted to improve patient care? How much for reduction in the number of medication errors?

A performance budget attempts to determine how much money is being budgeted to provide direct care, to provide indirect care, to insure quality of care, to control costs, to provide patient satisfaction, to provide staff satisfaction and so on. One still cannot easily measure direct outcomes, such as how much health has been produced. But the nursing profession has made great strides in looking at process, such as preparing patient care and discharge plans. It is possible to create a performance budget that examines whether the prescribed process is in fact being carried out and that relates that process to its share of the costs budgeted for the unit. A look at this new approach called performance or outcomes budgeting is provided in Chapter 11.

Special-Purpose Budgets

A budget is a plan. There is not a great deal of rigidity in the definition of a budget. Therefore, there is also not a great limitation placed on the types of budgets that are possible. Any health care organization can prepare a budget for any activity for which they desire a plan.

In recent years, a number of health care organizations have offered screening for high cholesterol, colon cancer, diabetes, and HIV. In some cases, these screenings have been free, and in others there has been a charge. What will it cost to provide the service free (i.e., to help the community and at the same time get some favorable press)? How much would you have to charge just to cover the costs of such a program?

Often these programs are not part of the yearly operating budget. They are special programs, put together on the spur of the moment in response to a current need. A special-purpose budget can be prepared any time a plan is needed for some activity that is not already budgeted as part of one of the ongoing budget processes. The budget does not need any formal system or set of forms. It is desirable, however, to know the impact on staffing and on the morale of the staff. One would want to know if a profit, loss, or neither is anticipated. The key to developing a special-purpose budget is to try to consider rationally all human and financial consequences of the proposed activity.

BUDGETING METHODOLOGY

The previous discussion centered on the types of budgets. This should be contrasted with the wide variety of budgeting methodologies. Methodologies are different approaches for developing and using the types of budgets that have been discussed in this chapter. For example, these methodologies include Zero-Base Budgeting and business plans (two techniques widely used to develop program budgets). They include variable or flexible budgeting. These and other methodologies are discussed throughout this book.

RELEVANT TIME PERIODS
FOR BUDGET PREPARATION

Budgeting is often viewed as a necessary evil rather than as a labor of love. Therefore a question arises as to when and how often budgets must be prepared. The answer depends on the type of budget being considered. Some budgeting is done once and once only. Other budgets can be relegated to just several times per decade. Some budgeting must be done annually. Finally, there are proponents of performing some budgeting activities on a continuous (monthly) basis.

One-Shot Budgets

Special-purpose budgets, such as discussed earlier, only need to be prepared once. There is no particular time of the year when they are prepared. Similarly, program budgets are often prepared on a one-shot basis. Program budgets are primarily concerned with the evaluation of major new services that the organization is considering offering. Preparing a program budget is generally needed only once for any given program. However, that initial budget covers a number of years. If the project or program or service is rejected, there is no need to review it on a regular basis. If the program is approved, it is often reviewed periodically, comparing actual outcomes to the budgeted projections.

Program budgets do not have to be prepared at any specific time during the year. Generally, because the program does not currently exist, there is no experience to draw upon in making up the budget. A number of assumptions must be made. Further, numerous options and alternatives must be considered. As a result, a program budget will often take a number of months and many meetings to prepare.

Infrequently Prepared Budgets

Long-range budgets are generally prepared on an infrequent basis. Such budgets generally cover a span of 3, 5, or 10 years. Although some organizations may make annual adjustments or modification to their long-range plan, the main body of the budget typically remains unchanged over its lifetime. This provides a sense of stability and direction for the organization. Nevertheless, long-range budgets should be reviewed annually to determine if any major unexpected changes in the organization's environment require modification to the plan.

Long-range plans are much less detailed than program budgets. Therefore, they do not necessarily require the long preparation time that a program budget requires. However, rather than simply being related to one department, one program, or one part of the organization's existence, the long-range plan gets to the core of why the organization exists and where it wants to go. If the organization is having difficulty in assessing where it wants to head in the future, it may take many months before there can be agreement on a challenging yet realistic plan that meets the needs of the community, the organization, and the organization's employees.

Annual and Monthly Budgets

Most individuals are familiar with budgeting as an annual phenomenon. Operating, capital, cash, and performance budgets fall into this category. Each of these budgets must be prepared every year. However, it is necessary to divide the annual budgets into smaller time periods in order to have an adequate basis to control costs during the year. It is undesirable to have to wait until the end of the year to find out if the unit, department, or organization as a whole has been keeping to the budgeted expectations. By the end of the year it is too late to do anything about problems that arose and could have been corrected midstream. Certainly, any problems can be corrected as part of the process of budgeting for the next year—but even then one would not know if they were successful until the end of the subsequent year. Accurate monthly plans are vital to the control of operations on a timely basis.

Furthermore, the nature of the health care field makes it totally inadequate to simply take an annual budget and divide by 12 to get expectations for each month of the year. The number of days, number of weekends, type of weather, and other factors will create substantial differences in workload patterns from month to month. Normal seasonality will create some months with peak demands on the organization and other months when workload levels are lower than average. Therefore, each month must be planned for individually.

In many cases, a nursing unit or department will only be required to submit a total budget for the year. In these cases, the organization will probably provide monthly reports comparing the budget and the actual results, based on dividing the annual budget into 12 equal months (or in some cases 13 months, each with 28 days).[1] Even if this is the case, the nurse manager should take the annual budget and prepare a set of monthly budgets that take factors such as seasonality into account. In order to manage staff and supplies efficiently, the nurse manager needs to understand how unit resource consumption is likely to vary from month to month.

Continuous Budgeting

In a system that focuses on annual preparation of operating and cash budgets, there are a number of weaknesses that could be cured if budgets were prepared more frequently. Continuous budgeting is a system in which a budget is prepared each month for a month 1 year in the future. For example, once the actual results for January are known, hopefully by mid- or late February, the budget for next January can be prepared. There are four major problems with the traditional annual budgeting approach that are addressed by continuous budgeting: attitude toward budgeting, time-management concerns, accuracy of budgets, and increasing myopia regarding the future.

Attitude

Many managers find budgeting to be very disruptive to their work. Budgeting comes once a year and requires a major diversion from routine activities. Several weeks or longer of full-time effort are devoted to preparing the budget for the entire next year. It is a mammoth process that often is faced only reluctantly. On the other hand, if a much smaller effort is required on a regular monthly basis, the process may not seem so onerous. It may become a part of normal routine rather than an interruption of it. The result is a much better attitude (less antagonism), with respect to the entire budget process. This in turn leads to a better effort from managers in preparing the budget.

---

[1]Some health care providers use 13-month years. The major benefit of this is that each month has exactly 4 weeks.

Time Management

The problem of attitude goes hand in hand with the problem of time management. There are so many things to be done. Nothing else seems to get done during the most intensive period of budget preparation. With continuous budgeting, the bulk of the process is spread evenly throughout the year. One or two days of effort each and every month, instead of several weeks of full-time effort in one or two months, reduces the disruptive nature of the process.

Several days can be given up each month without important functions going undone that month. Giving up several weeks in one month is inherently so disruptive that many things get pushed off, and it takes several months of overtime effort to catch up. It is important to manage the time spent on budgets, rather than letting the budget process disrupt day-in and day-out management functions.

Accuracy

By the time the budget is prepared using the annual approach, most of the current year has passed; with it, the crises of the year have seemed to dim. The months start to run together and appear to be very much alike in the manager's memory. By preparing a budget for next July right after this July has passed, the chances are that the budget for next July will be a much more realistic and accurate reflection of what typically happens during July. It will capture peculiarities of the month with a much higher degree of precision than would be possible if next July's budget were not prepared until February or March.

In practice, the monthly budgets developed under a continuous budgeting approach do not constitute finalized, approved budgets. The negotiation and approval process would not be done more than once a year. The budget prepared each month for the month 1 year in the future will allow for compilation of a more accurate budget when the entire next year's budget is developed once a year. At the same time, as discussed previously, the time it takes to compile the budget will be substantially reduced, since it simply puts together all of the monthly budgets that have been prepared during the year.

Further, accuracy is improved because if changes occur during this year that affect some basic assumptions that were made in planning next July's budget, it is not too late to modify, adjust, or correct the budget for next July. Managers are not left with only their thoughts at one point in time. There is time before the budget is finalized to reflect on the budgets that have been prepared for the months of next year and to revise them as ways to improve operations arise.

Myopia

One of the beneficial elements of a budget is the opportunity it gives management to peer into the future. If an annual budget for the year beginning next July (assuming we use a June 30 year-end for *fiscal* purposes) is completed by April of this year, one can see 14 months into the future. Expectations regarding this May and June (i.e., the last 2 months of this year) are known, as well as those for all 12 months of next year.

This foresight allows managers to take expectations of the future into account when making current decisions. Projections of workload, inflation, future capital equipment acquisitions, and so on help managers effectively manage in the present. By the time next year begins, however, the horizon has decreased from 14 months to 12 months. Halfway into the year, the horizon is only 6 months. The resulting effect is creeping myopia. Each month one sees less far into the future. Uncertainty increases, and the efficiency of decision making decreases. Decisions that would easily be made in August must be postponed if they arise in March because the manager does not know enough about the future. Continuous budgeting assures that at any point there is a horizon of approximately 1 year.

BUDGETING BEYOND THE HOSPITAL

By the end of the twentieth century, it was clear that the hospital was no longer the be-all and end-all provider of health care services. The last few decades of the twentieth century saw hospitals lose their dominant position. Hospitals, without question, still serve a vital role as a part of the overall health care system. However, organizations providing ambulatory care such as clinics and surgi-centers, home care organizations, managed care organizations, and long-term care providers have also become important players in the health care marketplace.

All health care organizations have an important need for high-quality budgeting. The remainder of this book will at times use hospital examples. At other times the budgeting examples will focus on nonhospital health care organizations. In all cases the role of the book is to provide the reader with sound concepts of budgeting. The techniques taught in this book can then be applied in a wide variety of situations and organizations.

An alternative approach was considered. The book could have provided a chapter on budgeting for long-term care organizations, another chapter on budgeting for home care organizations, and so on. However, the fundamentals of budgeting apply across all health care organizations. A book providing a chapter on budgeting for each type of organization would basically provide a limited amount of information repeated over and over using a different specific example. Instead it was decided to integrate a variety of examples throughout a book that provides both breadth and depth in budgeting, without excessive repetition. Based on the author's experience in the field, this approach will best serve the wide readership of the book, providing the foundations that nurse managers need to prepare and control budgets in many different health care settings.

SUMMARY AND IMPLICATIONS
FOR NURSE MANAGERS

A budget is basically a plan that provides a formal, quantitative expression of what the organization's management plans to accomplish. The development of the budget helps the organization establish goals and a plan for the future.

The various types of budgets within an organization together constitute the master budget. The most familiar part of this master budget is the operating budget, which details the day-to-day operating revenues and expenses of the organization. Additionally, other budgets that are part of the master budget include a long-range plan, program budgets, capital budgets, performance budgets, and a cash budget.

Although one thinks of budgeting as an annual event, this is really a broad generalization. A budget that evaluates whether to add, expand, contract, or delete an entire program may be prepared only once. Long-range budgets providing overall organizational direction are generally prepared only every 3, 5, or 10 years. Capital, operating, performance, and cash budgets are prepared annually.

Operating and cash budgets must have detailed information regarding each month within the year, since not all months will be the same. The detailed monthly information is vital if one wishes not only to have a plan but also to use that plan for controlling operations.

Continuous budgeting, a technique with several advantages over more traditional budget approaches, calls for preparing the budget for each month nearly 1 year before that month arrives.

What implications do these basic concepts about the different types of budgets have for nurse managers? First, as one prepares any budget, whether it is a program budget or a unit operating budget, it is important to have an understanding of how that budget fits into the overall scheme of things. This chapter should have provided the reader with a sense of the different types of budgets, why they exist, and how the capital and operating budgets fit into this picture. As you read through the remainder of this book, the reader should think about each of the types of budget in terms of what information it requires from and provides to the nurse manager and the organization, and how it relates to the other types of budgets the organization prepares.

This chapter should also serve to introduce nurse managers to the fact that budgeting is a tool for planning and controlling what happens within a nursing unit, department, or organization. Budgeting is not inherently complex. A budget is a plan. After the plan is made, it must be implemented and used to try to control results.

In order to maximize the benefit of budgeting, many organizations have developed lengthy budget processes with dozens of complex forms. The budgeting process in many organizations has become complicated. But the underlying concept is not. Budgeting requires the development of a plan. It must then be determined whether the plan results in a feasible financial outcome for the organization. If it does not, the plan must be revised until there is a feasible result.

Sometimes the result will not be as good as one would like. However, it is necessary to balance the long-term financial needs of the organization, so that it can remain in business, with the short-term quality of care needs for patients and the other needs of the organization's employees. It is this balancing act that requires substantial information. Much of the rest of this book focuses on how to generate the information needed to make effective decisions on the use of scarce resources available to the organization.

SUGGESTED READINGS

Campbell, C., Schmitz, H., and Waller, L.C. (1998). *Financial Management in a Managed Care Environment (Delmar's Health Information Management Series).* Albany: Delmar.

Cleverley, W.O. (1997). *Essentials of Health Care Finance,* Fourth edition. Gaithersburg, MD: Aspen Publishers.

Gapenski, L.C. (1997). *Financial Analysis and Decision Making for Healthcare Organizations: A Guide for the Healthcare Professional.* Chicago: Irwin Professional Publishers.

Hunt, C.T. (1996, April 22). I feel totally overwhelmed in the area of budgets. What should I anticipate? *Nursing Spectrum* (D.C./Baltimore Metro Edition), 6(9), 5.

Jones, K.R. (1998, December). Introduction to budgeting. *Seminars for Nurse Managers,* 6(4), 172–173.

McLean, R.A. (1996). *Financial Management in Health Care Organizations.* Albany: Delmar.

Neumann, B.R., Clement, J.P., and Cooper, J.C. (1997). *Financial Management: Concepts and Applications for Health Care Organizations.* Dubuque, Iowa: Kendall Hunt Publishing.

Pelfrey S. (1997, March). Managing financial data. *Seminars for Nurse Managers,* 5(1), 25–30.

Ward, W.J., Jr. (1994). *Health Care Budgeting and Financial Management for Non-Financial Managers: A New England Healthcare Assembly Book.* Westport, CN: Auburn House Publishers.

Zelman, W.N., McCue, M.J., and Milikan, A.R. (1998). *Financial Management of Health Care Organizations: An Introduction to Fundamental Tools, Concepts, and Applications.* Malden, MA: Blackwell Publisher.

2

The Budgeting Process

The goals of this chapter are to:

describe the budgeting process;

discuss the elements of planning;

explain the role of communication and coordination in budgeting;

introduce the concept of a budget timetable;

describe the use of PERT and CPM scheduling tools;

emphasize the importance of controlling results;

introduce the concept of budget flexibility;

introduce the concept of organizational philosophies of fiscal affairs;

explain the role of information gathering; and

discuss the specific steps in the budgeting process, including programming; developing unit, department, and cash budgets; negotiation and revision; and feedback.

INTRODUCTION

Each organization has its own specific budget forms, timetables, and specific budget processes. Conceptually, however, there are certain elements and specific steps that should be undertaken as part of the budget process (Fig. 2–1). Four key elements exist throughout the budgeting process. These are planning, controlling, an underlying organizational philosophy of fiscal affairs, and information gathering. In addition to those four elements, this chapter also discusses specific steps in the budgeting process: programming; developing unit and departmental budgets; developing the cash budget; negotiating and revising budget proposals; budget approval and implementation; and finally feedback.

PLANNING

Preparing a budget forces the organization's managers to plan ahead. Past management experience has shown that, in general, organizations that are ac-

```
The Underlying Elements
    1. Planning
    2. Controlling Results
    3. Philosophy of Fiscal Affairs
    4. Information Gathering
Specific Steps
    1. Programming
        A. Budget Foundations
            • Environmental Scan
            • General Goals, Objectives, and Policies
            • Organization-Wide Assumptions
            • Specifying Program Priorities
            • Specific Measurable Operating Objectives
        B. Long-Range and Program Budgets
    2. Developing Unit and Department Budgets
        A. Operating
        B. Capital
    3. Developing Cash Budgets
    4. Negotiating and Revising
    5. Budget Approval and Implementation
    6. Feedback
```

FIGURE 2–1. The budgeting process.

tively managed will do better than those that just let things happen. A budget forces managers to establish goals. Without goals, organizations tend to wander aimlessly, rarely improving the results of their operations or the services they offer.

Organizations that are not serious about the budget process often move from crisis to crisis. This is basically a managerial version of fire fighting taking precedence over fire prevention. If managers push off careful attention to budget preparation because of current emergencies at hand, they are setting themselves up for the next round of emergencies. Careful planning provides an opportunity for examining options and alternatives in a calm, rational setting. The result is generally a more satisfactory outcome, with fewer crisis situations arising.

By requiring managers to prepare a budget at least annually, organizations compel their management to forecast the future. Changes in medical practice, technology, and *demographics* can be anticipated and their impact predicted. This allows managers to anticipate changes that will affect the organization and to plan actions accordingly. When one responds to changes after the fact, alternatives may be limited. By considering the impact of changes during the planning phase, the broadest possible range of alternative actions can be considered. Often the result of careful planning is that more cost-effective approaches can be found and put into place.

If management's initial plans indicate that revenues are not expected to be great enough to cover expenses, there is time during the budget planning process to consider actions that might increase revenues or reduce costs. While solutions may be difficult to find and implement, without a budget managers would not be aware of the fact that a loss is likely. By the time the organization recognizes that a loss has occurred, it may be too late to do anything about it.

Is it an important problem if the organization loses money? Many organizations that nurses work for are *not-for-profit.*[1] Does it matter if a not-for-profit organization loses money in some years? It clearly does matter. If revenues are less than expenses, then ultimately cash receipts from revenues will be less than the cash needed to pay expenses. If losses persist, a point will come when there is not enough cash to meet routine obligations, such as payroll. Lenders may not loan the organization money to pay those expenses out of fear that the organization will not be able to repay the loan. For every organization there is the question of survival. Losses a number of years in a row may lead to bankruptcy.

Nor is long-term survival the only consideration. Hospitals, nursing homes, home care agencies, and other health care organizations are providing service to their communities. If money is wasted through lax management, the quality and breadth of services offered will have to be lower than they might otherwise have been. The degree of care exercised in budgeting can make a difference in the quality of care that patients receive. It can be the difference between money spent on unneeded or wasted supplies versus money spent on hiring one additional nurse on each shift.

Communication and Coordination

An effective planning process requires a high level of communication among the managers of the organization. The managers of the organization should act as a group to develop the overall goals and directions of the organization, as well as its specific measurable goals for the coming year. Once decided upon, these goals should be communicated clearly to all managers and staff. The planning process should be based on this common set of objectives, and the managers of the various units and departments of the organization should coordinate their plans with each other.

These two managerial functions of communication and coordination go hand in hand. Many managers feel that they know their objectives, so they have no need to formalize those goals as part of the budget process. Yet the fact that a given manager has certain goals and objectives does not mean that everyone in the organization knows what those goals are. The budget provides a document for systematically informing all managers and staff of exactly what they and their

---

[1]Not-for-profit or nonprofit health care organizations are formed primarily to provide service to the community. For-profit health care organizations have a goal of providing service but have a primary goal of earning a profit for their owners. Both types of organizations generally do make profits. However, while for-profits may distribute some of their profits to their owners, not-for-profits must reinvest all their profits back in the organization (for expansion of services and replacement of plant and equipment).

units or departments are expected to accomplish. It also provides a basis for discussion if some of those expectations appear to be unreasonable.

Communication among various levels of management should be more than simply a statement of overall goals. Organizational policies, constraints, and assumptions must be communicated to all managers working on the budget. Staffing cannot be planned efficiently without an assumption about patient-load expectations. Nursing salary costs cannot be planned without assumptions about anticipated pay raises. Overtime and part-time employee needs cannot be calculated without assumptions about staff availability. All this information has little value in budget preparation unless it is communicated to the managers who are preparing the detailed elements of the budget. The budget preparation process should bring together information in a formalized manner and disseminate it to the individuals who need that information to operate their units or departments.

Communication is also a requirement for employee motivation and evaluation. Using budgets for motivation and evaluation is discussed in Chapter 3. Budgets can be an effective motivational tool if they have been communicated to the individuals that they are aimed at motivating. One can only hope to get individuals to work toward accomplishing the organization's objectives if they have been informed as to what those objectives are. A sense of equity requires that individuals be told what is expected of them if they are going to be subsequently evaluated based on how well they met those expectations. The budget lays out in black and white the organization's goals and expectations. The budget can communicate the organization's expectations directly to its managers.

Budget Timetable

It is important to have a plan for the planning process. Managers should have a road map that tells them what steps must be taken in the planning process and when they should be undertaken. Figure 2–2 presents a sample budget timetable.

ACTIVITY	RESPONSIBILITY	DEADLINES
1. Appointment of the Budget Committee	CEO	December
2. First Meeting of Budget Committee	Budget Committee Chair	January
3. Complete Budget Foundations Activities and Communicate to Department Heads	Budget Committee	February 28
4. Complete Long-Range and Program Budgets	Budget Committee and Subcommittees	March 31
5. Unit Capital and Operating Budgets	Unit Managers	April 15
6. Negotiation between Nursing Units and Nursing Administration	Chief Nurse Exec.	April 22
7. Compilation of All Nursing Unit Budgets	Chief Nurse Exec.	April 30
8. Development of Cash Budget	Chief Financial Officer	May 15
9. Negotiation and Revision Process	All Managers	June 15
10. Approval and Implementation	Board of Trustees; All Managers	June 16

FIGURE 2–2. Sample budget timetable.

Each organization will have its own timetable. In small organizations, the entire process described by the timetable may take only a few months. In large health care systems, the budgeting process often takes more than 6 months from start to finish.

Just as the length of time to complete the budget process varies from organization to organization, so do the specific elements of the budget timetable. Figure 2–2 assumes a budget process for an organization with a July 1 through June 30 fiscal year. As one reviews this sample timetable, it becomes clear why budgeting is a complex task and one that is constantly subject to deadlines.

The first step is appointing the supervisory Budget Committee. This committee is usually selected by the CEO but may be appointed by the Board. This selection process should take place as early as feasible, and the committee should meet promptly. In this example, it is assumed that the committee first meets no later than January, a full 6 months before the next fiscal year. The committee must go through all the steps of *budget foundations* (discussed later in this chapter) to assure that department heads will have the information needed to prepare their budgets. In this example, 2 months are allowed for that process.

The long-range plan and program budgets cannot be completed without having at least information about the organization's environment, as well as its goals, objectives, and policies. This information is prepared by the Budget Committee as part of the foundations activities. During the month of March, the long-range plan must be formulated (or reviewed) and specific programs considered. The decisions regarding these programs must be known early in the budget process so that all department heads can take the impact of new programs or program changes into account in preparing their operating and capital budgets. In actuality, the long-range plan and new programs are generally considered at some length even before the budget process begins, and the month of March in this example is used to finalize decisions based on months of consideration and data collection and analysis.

Each organization creates its unique set of budget forms to meet its particular needs and situation. Before departmental or unit managers can begin to prepare their operating and capital budgets, these documents must be reviewed, modified, and distributed to all managers involved with budget preparation. Unit managers will have started preparing their budgets in early March. However, the long-range and program budgets may cause some changes to be made. This leaves just a 2-week period for unit nurse managers to finish preparing a first draft of their unit's budget. This is followed by a brief but intense period of negotiation between the nursing administration and its units. In this example, only one week is available for this negotiation process. If this time could be expanded, there would be less likelihood of an atmosphere of crisis and more time for reasoned discussions.

The nursing department has one week in this timetable to compile all the unit budgets into a final nursing department budget. Finance has two weeks to take the information from all the budgets of the organization and develop a unified cash budget. One month is then allowed for organization-wide negotiation and budget revision. If all goes well, the budget can be approved by the Board at its June meeting so that it can be put into effect July 1. Even with this 7-month process, it would not be unusual for there to be delays (especially in negotiation and revision) that prevent an acceptable budget from being developed by July 1. To avoid such a situation, the process could be started earlier. However, to start the process any earlier would mean that the information collected at the very start of the budget process would be outdated by the start of the year.

Since many aspects of the budgeting process cannot be undertaken without information generated by one of the previous activities, the budget timetable becomes a crucial guide in the budget process. Failure to meet one deadline may impact on all remaining deadlines.

PERT and CPM

The budget timetable provides an indication of the complexity of the budgeting process. In fact, the timetable gives information about just the major events in the process. As one works on preparing the budget, there are many other elements of the planning process that must be worked into that time frame. Unit managers must receive information such as admissions or patient day projections, as well as planned changes in services offered. Communication must take place concerning recruiting efforts planned by the personnel department (or nurse recruiting office). Many other pieces of the process must come together at just the right time in order for each phase of the budget to be completed by its deadline. *CPM* and *PERT* are two techniques that can be used to aid in this process.

CPM, or *Critical Path Method,* and PERT, or *Program Evaluation and Review Technique,* are two industrial engineering approaches to scheduling that are widely used in industry. The two approaches are similar in many respects. Both were developed in the 1950s. Both techniques use an arrow diagram to indicate the various events or activities that must take place in a complex project. They both identify a critical path that represents the shortest time to complete the project. And both use time estimates for each activity. Based on those activity time estimates, a project schedule is developed. Such techniques could be used to determine the most efficient budget timetable. They could also be helpful to managers who are working on specific projects, such as getting a new program or system from the planning stage to the active patient care stage.

In developing these systems, there is a planning phase in which the activities are identified. Then there is a scheduling phase in which the length of time for each activity is estimated and a determination is made regarding which activities must be completed before others can be started. A control phase is sometimes used that monitors progress along the path and makes schedule revisions as needed.

In most projects, certain activities can take place concurrently with each other. These form different parallel branches in the diagram (see Fig. 2–3 for a

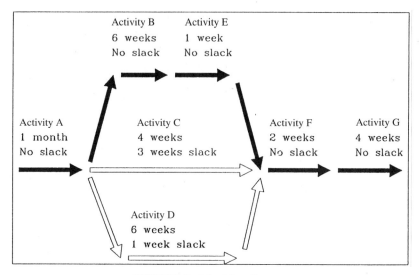

FIGURE 2–3. Scheduling diagram.

simplified example). Some activities must precede other activities. For example, suppose that activity A provides basic foundations information that all departments need to begin their budgets. Once activity A is completed, activities B, C, and D can all start at the same time and continue on parallel courses.

Suppose further that there is a department that needs information from activity B before it can complete its budget. For instance, the dietary department might need to wait for the nursing department budget to be complete, in order to know the total number of patient days in the budget, so that its workload can be predicted. Activity E (dietary budget) will follow activity B (nursing budget) on the same path.

All department budgets will have to be completed before a cash budget (activity F) can be completed. Therefore, all parallel paths will have to come together. Then activities F and G can be completed. Activities B and E together require 7 weeks. This is more than activity C or activity D. Activity C has 3 weeks of slack. A delay of up to 3 weeks would have no impact on the overall process. Activity D has 1 week of slack. It can be delayed 1 week with no negative impact. Activities B and E are critical. A delay of even 1 day in that path will create a delay in the entire process. Therefore, the path from A to B to E to F to G (bold on Fig. 2–3) is said to be the critical path. One of the major benefits of CPM and PERT is the identification of where delays are critical and where they are not.

In recent years, a number of software programs have been developed to enable a manager to do project planning more efficiently on a personal computer. Programs such as Microsoft Project incorporate the essentials of PERT and CPM, while making the computational aspects substantially easier for the manager.

In order to get everything done most efficiently, it is useful to have a system to track how much time is available for each activity and to determine which activities will create roadblocks in the process if they are not completed in time. Both these methods provide such systems, and both are useful not only for scheduling the budgeting process but also for a wide variety of other time-dependent projects. A more detailed discussion of CPM and PERT is contained in most industrial engineering and operations research texts.

CONTROLLING RESULTS

Just as planning is a critical element of the budgeting process, so is the control of the organization's financial results (Fig. 2–1). Control is an attempt to keep the organization functioning in accordance with its plan. It is desirable for all employees to act in an efficient manner, within the constraints of the budget. If the agreed-upon budget calls for a 10% reduction in staffing, then that reduction should take place.

The budget itself should be arrived at based on the best overall interests of the organization and the community it serves. The development of the budget should be a give-and-take process that results in the elimination of only nonessential costs. In extremely hard financial times, the final budget may even cut essential items. In this case, top management would choose to eliminate the least essential of the essential items. Prioritization is crucial. Once a budget is agreed upon, managers are obligated to do their best to follow it, even if it calls for undesirable cuts. How can management insure that the reduction will take place? This is the role of the control process. Through the use of motivational tools, management can give the employees of the organization incentives to try to carry out the budget (see Chapter 3). Through the use of variance reports, managers can examine how well they are succeeding and can assess where and why the organization is not meeting its budgeted expectations (see Chapter 13).

Budget Flexibility

The control process can do more than give incentives to follow the budget and assess whether the budget is being met or not. If actual results start to vary substantially from the budget, the control process will alert the manager that there may be a need to make midstream corrections. For example, if the state government were suddenly to cut Medicaid payment levels, what should the organization do? Even though patient workload may remain the same, the cut in revenue may be significant enough to require layoffs or some other belt-tightening actions.

As painful as such actions are, it may be foolhardy to simply ignore the implications of the revenue change until the next budget year. This would allow the organization to be out of control. By year-end, the accumulated losses could be devastating to the organization. By alerting managers to the problem, the control process has given the organization a choice: make no cost changes now or make an immediate budget response. In some cases, no immediate action may be an appropriate choice. However, it is desirable to avoid the chance of being in a situation in which an immediate budget response is required but in which managers are unaware of that fact because of the lack of a working control system. The role of the control process is to make managers aware so that they can decide whether or not some action is in fact needed immediately.

Many budgeting experts believe that once in place, budgets should not be revised. They are the original plan, and all results should be compared to that plan. Certainly, if budget revisions were allowed on an unlimited basis, an enormous amount of time might be spent developing new budgets and getting them approved throughout the year. Even if the budget is not revised, however, that does not mean that actions must remain as planned. If census drops sharply, it may be necessary to reduce staffing to be financially prudent. The fact that a certain staffing level has been budgeted does not mean that a unit is entitled to that staffing level no matter what else happens.

On the other hand, a great rise in patient census may require more staffing to ensure provision of quality care. The budget should not be viewed as an arbitrary dictator. A budget should be a flexible guide to actions. When some uncontrollable events occur that were not considered in the budgeted expectations, actual actions should contain appropriate responses to actual events. Such responses will sometimes justify additional spending above budget. In other cases, spending the amount called for in the budget may be excessive, based on what the actual events would dictate.

The key is not whether or not the budget is revised. The budget is simply the plan. The essential issue is what actions are taken throughout the year. If the budget is ignored, the value of the plan is largely lost. But by revising actions from those called for in the budget in response to actual occurrences, the original budget is not being ignored. Rather, it becomes a base that is built upon. The revised actions should produce a better result than even strict adherence to the budget would obtain.

Figure 2–4 provides a summary of the elements of planning and control.

PHILOSOPHY OF FISCAL AFFAIRS

The budgeting process in any organization will depend as much on the specific individuals working in that organization as it will on the formalized mechanical steps involved in budget preparation and use. The role of individual human beings in the budget process cannot be overemphasized. Not only do organizations have their own forms and procedures, they also tend to have specific philosophies of fiscal affairs. The philosophical underpinnings of the budget process constitute the third key element in the budget process (Fig. 2–1). The amount of participation that any individual manager has in the budget process depends on the approach or philosophy of the organization's top management. Some organizations are top-down—allowing unit managers limited control over their budget. Other organizations delegate substantially all budget preparation

FIGURE 2–4. Planning and control.

BUDGETING

PLANNING

Think Ahead
Anticipate Change
Establish Goals
Forecast Future
Examine Alternatives
Communicate Goals
Coordinate Plans

CONTROLLING

Keep to Plan
Motivate Employees
Evaluate Performance
Alert Management to
    Variations
Take Corrective Action

and control duties. While many managers have to suffer with unrealistic budgets imposed upon them from above, other managers are given full responsibility but little guidance.

Teachers of budgeting often stress the importance of participation in the budget process by individuals at all levels in the organization. The further basic budget preparation is removed from the top management, the more likely the budget will reflect a full understanding of why the cost structure is as it is. If the budget is expected to be a useful tool for managing, it must be realistic. It is hard for managers high up in the organization to make correct determinations of what is realistic minimal spending, while maintaining efficiency and high-quality care. It is often not possible for top-level managers to be aware of all the specific circumstances and conditions that exist in the day-to-day operations throughout the organization. Unit managers work for years to gain their insight and understanding. They have the experience, judgment, and specific information about their units that lets them put together a sensible budget. They are in the best position to be able to plan for that unit for the coming year.

GATHERING INFORMATION

The fourth critical element in preparing budgets (Fig. 2–1) is gathering key information. One type of information needed is cost information. Whether one is preparing a program budget, capital budget, or operating budget, an understanding of how costs relate to the item being budgeted is needed. One needs to be able to collect and use information about costs in order to prepare the budget. A second major area of data collection concerns personnel issues. Given a history of alternating periods of nursing surpluses and shortages, managers must plan their budgets with an understanding of issues related to recruiting and retaining nurses. Finally, budget preparation requires managers to peer into the future. To do so, they need to be armed with adequate forecasting techniques.

Cost Information

Cost behavior is a particularly complicated area. If patient workload rises by 10%, can costs be expected to rise by 10% as well? This relationship would imply that costs are directly proportional to patient volume. However, this assumption is generally a poor one. Some costs do not change at all as volume changes. For example, the salary of the top nurse administrator in a community health center will not vary if the average number of patient visits rises or falls by 5% or 10%. Other costs do, of course, vary as there are more or fewer patients. Understanding how and why costs vary and being able to predict costs are critical parts of the budgeting process.

Additionally, when budgets are prepared, it would be helpful to be able to predict the patient volume necessary for the service not to lose money. The so-called break-even point at which one neither makes nor loses money requires a costing technique commonly referred to as *break-even analysis.*

Cost behavior, cost estimation, and break-even analysis are discussed in Chapter 4.

Personnel Issues

In the area of nursing, the single greatest cost relates to personnel. During nursing shortages, issues of nursing recruitment and retention became critical to most health care organizations. Operating budgets in many health care organizations lose much of their effectiveness if they do not fully take into account the costs and difficulty of attracting and keeping nurses.

During nursing shortages it is not at all uncommon for positions to remain unfilled. In place of the new staff members, agency nurses and overtime are often used. Frequently, these stopgap measures are more costly than filling the position would be if it were possible to attract a nurse to take the job. Chapter 5 looks at issues of personnel and staff recruitment and retention. A thorough understanding of this topic is necessary to be able to prepare an operating budget that allows (1) sufficient resources for recruitment and retention costs to keep all positions filled or (2) a realistic personnel portion of the operating budget that considers the costs related to temporary staffing of vacant positions. This personnel information is important not only to operating budgets but also as a consideration when preparing long-range and program budgets as well.

Forecasting

In order to determine the amount of staff needed (which is calculated as part of the operating budget process in Chapter 8), it is first necessary to have some idea of how many patients there will be and how sick they will be. Therefore, a critical step in gathering information for the budgeting process is *forecasting*. This can provide many pieces of information needed to design a budget to carry out programs and services.

Will there be the same number of patients next year as this year? How do you forecast the number of patient days? These are critical questions for the preparation of the budget. If more patients are expected, it will be necessary to budget for more staff. How do you forecast the number of discharges by *case-mix*? Under *DRGs*, this becomes vital to the organization. How do you forecast the level of patient acuity? How do you know how many chest tubes to order for inventory? Forecasting allows prediction of any items that will help in the planning process. Chapter 6 looks at several forecasting techniques.

Integration of Information

Although costs, personnel, and forecasting have been discussed as distinct topics, they are in fact interrelated. A nurse manager is unlikely to predict a unit or department's costs for the coming year without introducing some knowledge of recruiting and retention plans and without the use of forecasting techniques. Chapters 4 through 6 work together to provide a conceptual foundation and specific workable techniques to allow the reader to generate information that is needed for preparing the different types of budgets.

It should also be noted that the budget process does not require a manager to gather all the information needed for all types of budgets before preparing any of the budgets. Some cost information and forecasts may be developed as a guide to the managers who are preparing the organization's long-range plan. That plan may well be completely finished before any cost information, personnel calculations, or forecasts are prepared for the operating budget.

In fact, in many cases managers will begin to prepare a particular type of budget and then realize that they need certain background information that has not been gathered. A nurse manager creating an operating budget for a unit might start to put together the operating budget described in Chapter 8. However, before staffing could be determined, the unit would need a forecast of patient workload. At this point, the manager would have to forecast next year's workload, if this has not already been done.

The budgeting process does not have a rigid path that first requires that costs are conceptualized, then recruitment issues considered, then forecasts made, and then a given type of budget prepared. To the contrary, the process is highly integrated. However, in this book the chapters related to gathering information (Chapters 4 through 6) precede the chapters on preparation of each type of budget. This is because, at a minimum, managers should be aware of these concepts and the availability of the techniques as budgets are prepared.

PROGRAMMING

Up until this point, this chapter has focused on essential elements that are integral to all aspects of budgeting. These elements are planning, controlling, organizational philosophy, and information gathering. The remainder of this chapter is concerned with specific steps in the process of budgeting. These steps are listed in Figure 2–1.

A common approach to budgeting is to start initially on the compilation of the operating budget. However, a bit of preliminary thought and background work will improve the budget outcome substantially. The first part of the budget process is *programming*. It should be started well before the actual operating budget is started. Programming includes a total organizational review with a focus on where the organization is headed. Programming also includes determining which specific programs should be undertaken. The programming process can be viewed as consisting of two major phases. The first phase provides the foundations for all budget preparation. Essentially, these foundations are established by determining the organization's goals and its relative strengths and weaknesses within its environment. The second phase is concerned with strategic planning.

Budget Foundations

The foundations of the budgeting process consist of a scan of environmental position; a statement of general goals, objectives, and policies; a list of organization-wide assumptions; specification of program priorities; and finally, a set of specific, measurable operating objectives (Fig. 2–5).

Environmental Scan

No organization exists in a vacuum. The community, its economy, shifting demographics, inflation, the roll of a key employer, the socioeconomic setting, and other external factors play a vital role in the organization's success or failure. Each organization must understand its position within the community and its relative strengths and weaknesses. Once this has been determined, the organization can move forward to fulfill a particular role or mission.

The environmental scan must analyze the needs of the community. It must also assess the competition that exists. Based on knowledge of the needs of the community, the characteristics of the population, the existing competition, and other similar factors, the organization can determine its relative strengths and weaknesses and set its overall goals and objectives.

The potential dangers of not examining the environment cannot be stressed too much. If a community hospital opens an open-heart surgery facility in spite of

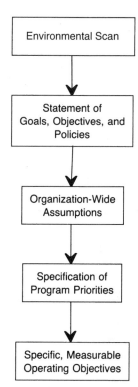

FIGURE 2–5. Programming foundations.

the existence of several high-quality, high-volume open-heart surgery facilities at nearby tertiary care centers, there is the potential for a medical disaster (if high mortality rates are associated with low volume) as well as an economic disaster (due to the inability to recover all the high equipment costs associated with the open-heart surgery program) at the new facility. The fact that several thoracic surgeons want the hospital to offer open-heart surgery does not mean that it is in the best interests of the organization.

It is only through carefully reviewing the needs of the community and examining its own relative strengths and weaknesses that a health care organization can establish a set of goals, objectives, and policies that will serve to enhance the comparative strengths of the organization and to minimize its weaknesses. Reviewing the environment may result in eliminating weaknesses. For example, a relatively weak maternity service can be improved and expanded if the community needs that type of care, or it can be totally eliminated.

If there is adequate maternity care in the community, then providing maternity services at the hospital may simply deprive other services at the hospital from having adequate resources. Sometimes the choice is between doing two things very well or doing three things only adequately. If the community urgently needs all three things, it may well be better to do all three than to eliminate any one of them. If one of the three is readily available elsewhere, however, then the long-run interests of both the community and the organization may best be served by eliminating one of the three services and devoting greater attention and resources to the remaining two.

What data can a nurse manager collect to contribute to the organization's environmental review? Although much of the demographic data will be collected by the marketing and other nonclinical staff, nurse managers can contribute some critical information. For example, they can get a sense about changing physician attitudes toward the use of the organization's facilities as opposed to a competitor's. Based on their industry contacts, they may be aware of changes taking place at other organizations that will affect the competitiveness of their facilities. This information forms part of the overall picture that the organization requires to assess its position in the community correctly.

Many health care organizations would benefit by getting all levels of nursing management more actively involved in the environmental review process. The starting point for this activity would be for the Chief Nurse Executive (CNE) to solicit this type of information from the various nurse managers well before the operating budget is prepared. The CNE could then use this information when participating in the major planning sessions that precede the specific preparation of the operating and capital budgets.

The environmental review serves as the guiding force for determining the organization's long-run direction. The total environmental statement need not be prepared annually. Hopefully, the major direction of the organization will not change each year. However, the environmental statement should be reviewed annually, for two major reasons.

First, an annual review of the environmental statement is necessary so that it can be modified as significant changes in the environment occur. While some changes may occur only rarely, such as the addition of a major new competitor, other elements of the environment are much more subject to change. For example, the overall state of the economy is one environmental element subject to frequent change. Some health care organizations tend to be relatively immune to the impact of economic change, but others must seriously consider economic fluctuations in preparing their various budgets.

The second reason for an annual review of the environmental statement is that it serves as a good review of where the organization is and where it wants to be going. Having done that review, it is more likely that a budget will be prepared that takes the organization's desired long-term direction into account in the coming year's plan.

General Goals, Objectives, and Policies

Once the organization's position in the environment is understood, the overall goals of the organization can be established. These goals are broad, long-term objectives, established in light of the organization's strengths and weaknesses.

For example, based on the environmental review, a home health agency may decide that the adjacent communities are underserved and may decide to institute a 5-year period of geographic expansion. A nursing home may set a goal of substantially increasing its occupancy. A hospital may decide to phase out its maternity service.

The key to long-run objective setting is that it is basically more of a qualitative direction-setting process than a quantitative exercise with specific numerical goals. The detailed numbers can be worked out later. First, the overall direction must be set.

Objectives need not always point to growth. Maintaining a current high level of care is a possible objective. Contraction is also a possible direction—an organization may have a goal of retreating from areas of care where losses are occurring in order to ensure financial survival. As was the case with the environmental statement, the overall goals, objectives, and policies of the organization may not change each year. They should be reviewed annually, however, if only to place in the minds of budget preparers the picture of the forest before they start to plan for the individual trees.

Organization-Wide Assumptions

Throughout the budget process it will be necessary for all managers to work on the basis of some explicit assumptions. How large will salary increases be during the next year? What will be the impact of inflation on the purchase price of supplies? Will the government change its policies with respect to reimbursing Medicare and Medicaid patients? Probably the most crucial of assumptions concerns workload. What will be the occupancy or patient volume in the coming year? How about for the next 5 or 10 years?

These critical questions are sometimes ignored at the organizational level, but when they are each manager has to make independent assumptions when preparing the portion of the budget for the department or unit. It is highly likely that the various individual managers will come up with different assumptions in many areas. For purposes of coordination, it makes more sense if the managers in the organization agree upon an entire set of assumptions for all managers to use when the budgets are prepared. In this way, the assumptions can be questioned, corrected, adjusted, improved, or, at the very least, made uniform before they are employed in actual budget preparation.

Specifying Program Priorities

The next foundations step is to establish a set of priorities for the entire organization. It is not unusual for the long-range plan, program budget, and capital budget to contain proposed spending for more things than the organization will be able to afford. There is a tendency to want to achieve all elements of a long-range plan immediately. When it becomes clear that the organization cannot do everything, how can a choice be made between what is done and what is postponed?

If the setting of priorities takes place after long-range plans, program budgets, and capital budgets have already been prepared, a ferocious battle may ensue. In preparing detailed budgets, special interest groups are formed that take on a vested interest in the projects they help plan. Trying to make rational choices at this stage becomes quite difficult. Politics may make more of a difference than common sense.

Therefore, it is advisable to try to set a generalized hierarchy of priorities at an early stage—before detailed program budgets are developed. When it is necessary to make choices, top management can use the formalized guidelines that have been developed from the perspective of long-term growth and development, as opposed to letting power politics rule the budgeting process.

Specific, Measurable Operating Objectives

One of the most frustrating elements of budgeting for unit and department managers occurs when they are expected to develop a budget, totally unaided by any communicated goals or guidelines, and then find the budget rejected because it does not provide for adequately achieving goals, such as improved efficiency or reduced cost per patient day.

Organizations should provide a set of specific, measurable goals that the budget should accomplish. This set of goals should be communicated before the units and departments prepare their budgets. Managers can then attempt to prepare a budget that achieves these goals. If the goals are unattainable, managers can be prepared to explain why they feel that is the case.

The established goals should be consistent with the overall general policies and goals of the organization, but they should be much more specific. For example, staffing reductions of 5% or ceilings on spending increases of 3% provide firm, specific goals. After individual budgets are prepared, a negotiation process will occur. Some units and departments may successfully argue for increases in excess of the specific guidelines. If the financial position of the organization is tight, this may mean that other units and departments will have to accept less than the specific guidelines. However, at least everyone will have a common starting point and a reasonable knowledge of what is expected from their budget.

Strategic Planning

Programming represents a total organizational review. This includes reviewing the programs the organization uses to carry out its mission. It requires establishing certain foundations for the budget process, as described above. Once these foundations have been laid, the organization can employ a strategic planning process to establish a long-range plan or budget, deciding upon the direction that the organization should be taking over the next 3, 5, or 10 years. This long-range plan will focus on the types of major programmatic changes the organization must undertake to continue to meet its mission.

One outcome of the long-range plan is the decision to prepare specific program budgets. Program budgets are used primarily to evaluate new programs being considered to help the organization attain its long-range plan. Strategic planning and long-range and program budgets are discussed in Chapter 7.

UNIT AND DEPARTMENT BUDGETS

Once the programming process is completed, the next step is preparing unit or departmental budgets (Fig. 2–1). There are two different types of budgets that are generally prepared at this level of the organization. These are the operating budget and the capital budget, which were introduced in Chapter 1 and are discussed more fully in Chapters 8 and 10 respectively.

The operating and capital budgets are generally prepared at the same time. Decisions concerning one budget are also likely to affect the other. For example, if the capital budget includes computer equipment for the nursing station, there may be some impact on staffing. Perhaps less overtime from the clerical staff is expected to be needed because of efficiencies created by having a computer. Therefore, it is not appropriate to create either the operating budget or the capital budget without reference to the other.

Once a decision is made to purchase a capital asset, a calculation must be made to allocate its cost into the various years that it will provide useful benefits. The amount allocated to each year is called the *depreciation*. The operating budget of an organization must reflect all costs of providing services for the coming year. The entire purchase price of a capital asset is not a cost of the coming year, since only a portion of the capital asset will be used up during the year. However, one year's share, the annual depreciation, is treated as a cost for the budgeted year. This depreciation becomes one element in the operating budget.

THE CASH BUDGET

Having completed an operating and capital budget, the next step in the budget process would be preparing a cash budget (Fig. 2–1). Most nurse managers will not be directly involved in the annual cash budgeting for their organization. However, there will be times that nurse managers will be preparing a business plan for a new venture or service and will need to prepare a cash budget in conjunction with that plan. Whether nurse managers are directly involved in the preparing of cash budgets or not, it is vital to understand the cash budgeting process, since it does impact on nursing services.

Chapter 12 will give the reader some understanding of how the financial manager handles the organization's cash resources.

BUDGET NEGOTIATION AND REVISION

The fourth specific step in the budgeting process is negotiation and revision (Fig. 2–1). Conceptually, most yearly budgets are prepared based on one of three basic approaches: (1) annual increments; (2) negotiation; or (3) detailed evaluation. All these approaches result in at least some negotiation and revision of proposed budgets.

The first approach assumes that initially each department or unit is assigned a percentage increase that will be allowable for the coming year. For example, a nursing home might indicate that all departments can plan to spend 4% more in the coming year than was allocated in the current year. The second approach is based on the fact that political power rules and that each unit or department can request whatever it wants and then negotiate the best deal it can manage. The third approach follows the rule of reason. A unit or department should request what it actually needs to provide its services in a high-quality, cost-effective manner. The budget will be evaluated to check that all expenses proposed are in fact essential.

In actuality, the third, and on the surface most sensible, approach often tends to be too time-consuming and costly to use. Top-level managers cannot review in detail each budget each year to evaluate whether each element is indeed justified. The negotiation approach does not seem to be an equitable approach. Therefore, the use of a flat percent increase is the most common approach to budgeting. However, preparing budgets based on a flat percentage increase represents just a starting point in the budget negotiation, revision, and approval process.

As a result of limitations on the resources available to health care organizations, budgets often cannot be accepted as submitted. Even if everyone is told to assume a certain percentage increase, some needs will be so critical that they will have to receive more than the flat percentage. Often, approval of a larger increase in one department results in adjustment downward in other departments. This results in a series of negotiations, with managers having to defend why their proposed budget should not be cut. This creates substantial complexity because most of the budgets that comprise the organization's master budget are interrelated. Changes in one type of budget can have direct ramifications on the other budgets of the organization.

For example, the capital budget for the various units and departments of the organization cannot be finalized until all program budgets have been prepared, because a new program may require departments to purchase additional capital items. This is why program budgets are prepared earlier in the budget process than are unit and department budgets.

The operating budget, in turn, must contain revenues and expenses related to capital items to be purchased during the coming year. And the cash budget cannot be prepared until after the operating budget is established. Since the cash budget must be prepared in time for the financial officers to arrange any necessary short-term borrowing to start the year, the operating budget preparation and the subsequent cash budgeting cannot be left until the last minute. Therefore, first make the long-range plan. Then make decisions regarding program budgets, and follow up with the necessary capital and the operating budgets. Finally, prepare the cash budget. This represents a first round of budget preparations.

However, the master budget is prepared in a series of repeating rounds, as seen in Figure 2–6. Since most managers are not involved in preparing all the different types of budgets, they do not observe this cycling process. Instead, they observe only a back-and-forth process in which their budget is submitted and comes back for either cuts or additional justifications. The manager revises and resubmits the

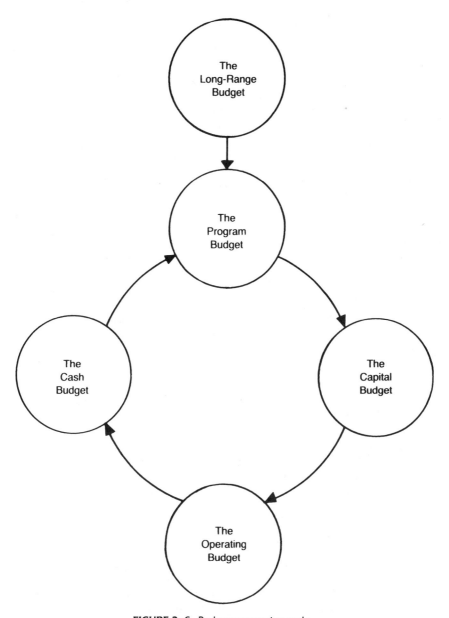

FIGURE 2–6. Budget preparation cycle.

budgets with explanations for why the requested expenses should be allowed. This process of negotiation over the operating and capital budgets may occur several times.

From the organizational point of view, the back-and-forth negotiations are part of a larger effort to gain consistency and feasibility across all parts of the *master budget*. Often, the outcome of the first attempt at preparing the master budget is not feasible. For example, the cash budget may show that there will not be enough cash for all the proposed capital expenditures and new programs. The operating budget may have an excess of expenses over revenues that is deemed to be unacceptable. The next step might be to ask various departments to tighten up on their operating costs so that the organization will at least break even. A revised operating budget will be prepared. That operating budget can be used to project a new cash budget.

Even with cuts in the operating budget, the cash budget may still show an unacceptable cash shortfall. This will necessitate reevaluating which programs and capital budget items provide the most benefit and which can be postponed or disapproved. Some capital expenditures may be put off until the future or scrapped. This may result in an acceptable set of budgets that comprise the master budget.

On the other hand, there may be so many vital capital expenditures that it is preferable to go back and increase revenues or cut the operating budget expenses again, rather than cut enough capital items to make the cash budget balance. Or perhaps more borrowing will be planned. The repetitive process must continue until the program and capital expenditures contained as part of the master budget can be paid for within the structure of the operating and cash budgets. Note in Figure 2–6 how this results in a clockwise cycling until all of the budgets are compatible.

BUDGET APPROVAL AND IMPLEMENTATION

Once all budget negotiation and revision is completed, the budget must be approved. For most organizations, management must take the budget to a board of trustees or directors, who formally vote on whether to adopt it. Even after extensive revisions by management, the board may change the budget before finally approving it. The final approved budget must then be implemented. Management must actively take steps to carry out the budget as approved and achieve all its revenue and expense targets.

FEEDBACK

The last step in the budget process is *feedback* (Fig. 2–1). Information about actual results that is used to improve future plans is called feedback. A critical element of the budget process is to provide such information or feedback. During the year, many things will not happen according to budgeted plans. Some variations from the budget will be due to random uncontrollable events that establish no pattern. A particularly cold winter may cause the census to rise unexpectedly.

At the very least, the unusual nature of the winter must be recognized. When planning for next year's budget commences, should it be based on the most recent year or on prior years? It is known that this past winter was unusual. Therefore, the patient volume from this winter should be discounted as next year's budget is prepared. This is called a feedback process. The information generated by the control system allows for more effective planning for the coming year.

In some cases, such as the example just given, the feedback information will lead managers to ignore this year's actual results when preparing next year's budget. In other cases, feedback information may stress this year's results for preparing next year's budget. In all cases, this feedback approach can be used when the following year's budget is prepared, to improve its accuracy.

SUMMARY AND IMPLICATIONS FOR NURSE MANAGERS

Budgeting consists of planning and controlling. The planning phase of the budget process requires that managers think ahead, anticipate changes, establish goals, forecast the future, examine alternatives, communicate goals, and coordinate plans. The controlling phase of budgeting requires that managers work to keep actual results close to the plan, motivate employees, evaluate performance of staff and units, alert the organization to major variances, take corrective actions, and provide feedback for future planning.

Each organization has its own approach to budgeting and its own philosophies regarding the budget process. Some health care organizations treat budgeting as a highly centralized process. This approach tends to generate frustration by the managers asked to carry out the budget. Other organizations call for more participation by managers throughout the organization. Such budgets tend to gain more support by the staff and are more likely to result in targets that are achieved.

The actual budgeting process requires that the organization consider its environment, define goals and policies, make assumptions for use throughout the organization, specify priorities, and define specific, measurable objectives. Managers within the organization must collect information on costs and personnel and must prepare forecasts of items into the future. Each of the various types of budgets in the master budget must be prepared, and they are generally not approved without a process of review, justification, and revision. Finally, once budgets have been approved and are in place, a system must be created to control the results of operations.

Some of the concepts discussed in this book are not used in all organizations. That is a simple reality. Some of the budgeting concepts and techniques that are not already being widely used are new advanced techniques. You have the opportunity to be one of the first nurse managers to employ them. This will require that you act as an innovator. Trying to innovate is often the most frustrating—and rewarding—part of being a manager.

Many nurse managers are frustrated because they find that real-life health care organizations have a variety of budgeting weaknesses. Often, these are not even in areas that require particularly high levels of sophistication. Instead of becoming frustrated by the lack of a perfect system, managers should act to improve the system. If this book is successful, readers not only will learn from it but also will begin to use the knowledge to improve the budget process in their respective organizations. Such use will lead to a personal sense of accomplishment (for both the nurse manager and the author). In addition, health care organizations will be placed in a better position to meet the financial challenges of the future.

In reading this book, one should consider the following questions: Why must a nurse manager understand the budget process? How will such an understanding affect a nurse manager's performance and the performance of the manager's subordinates? Finally, how will such knowledge affect the performance and evaluation of the nursing unit and/or nursing department?

This chapter has provided no more than an overview of the budgeting process. Each of the chapters in the remainder of this book will provide more detail about the process of budgeting. Even when the reader has completed the book, many specific details of the budget process will have gone without discussion. These details tend to be elements of the process that are specific to each institution. As a manager works within an organization, many specific details will have to be learned about the budget system in place in order to supplement the information contained in this book. The author recognizes that there is an inherent limitation on what one can learn from a book. He hopes, however, that having read this book, the nurse manager will find that the details that must be learned on the job will make more sense and be substantially easier to grasp.

SUGGESTED READINGS

Gapenski, L.C. (1997). *Financial Analysis and Decision Making for Healthcare Organizations: A Guide for the Healthcare Professional.* Chicago: Irwin.

McLean, R.A. (1996). *Financial Management in Health Care Organizations.* Albany: Delmar.

Neumann, B.R., Clement, J.P., and Cooper, J.C. (1997). *Financial Management: Concepts and Applications for Health Care Organizations.* Dubuque, Iowa: Kendall Hunt Publishing.

Nowicki, M. (1999). *The Financial Management of Hospitals and Healthcare Organizations.* Chicago: Health Administration Press.

Samuels, D.I. (1997). *The Healthcare Financial Management & Budgeting Toolkit.* Chicago: Irwin.

Swansburg, R.C. (1997). *Budgeting and Financial Management for Nurse Managers.* Boston: Jones & Bartlett.

Valentine, P.E., Richardson, S., Wood, M.J., and Godkin, M.D. (1998, September–October). Nurse educators'/administrators' ways of handling conflict. *Journal of Professional Nursing.* 14(5), 288–297.

Ward, W.J., Jr. (1994). *Health Care Budgeting and Financial Management for Non-Financial Managers: A New England Healthcare Assembly Book.* Westport, CN: Auburn House.

3

Motivation and Incentives

The goals of this chapter are to:

explain the role of budgets in employee motivation;

identify the issues of goal divergence and goal congruency;

explore alternative incentive systems, including their strengths and
weaknesses;

consider the negative implications of unrealistic expectations;

reiterate the role of communication in the control process; and

clarify the importance of using budgets for interim evaluation.

INTRODUCTION

The planning process and the resulting budget lay the groundwork for
motivating managers and other staff members and in providing a yardstick for
their evaluation. Managers can tell from the budget exactly what is expected of
them. Actual results are compared to the budget. If managerial performance is
evaluated based on that comparison, the budget can be an effective motivational
tool. This assumes that pay raises and promotions depend, at least in part, on the
evaluation of the manager's performance in the budgeting area.

However, the effectiveness of budgeting in motivating managers and staff
depends largely on the organization's approach to budgeting. If a budget is so
tight as to be impossible to meet, it can discourage managers and cause a negative
result. On the other hand, a challenging but attainable budget can draw out the
best effort from individuals. By setting goals, managers tend to be more efficient
because they are striving to reach a specific end. This is especially true if there is
some reward structure for meeting or surpassing budget requirements. In
addition to raises and promotions, budget performance can be tied to bonuses.

THE BUDGET AS A TOOL FOR MOTIVATION

The budgeting process primarily concerns individuals, not numbers. If the
employees of an organization do not work to make the organization succeed, the
numbers constituting a budget will have little relevance. Motivating staff and

managers cannot be overemphasized. If people are not motivated to carry out the budget, it is likely to fail. This is why budgets that are arbitrarily imposed from above without fair consideration of input from those expected to carry out the budget tend to do so poorly. It is why such a sense of frustration exists when managers are denied the needed authority to go along with their responsibility. It is why there is a need to have budget flexibility in the face of changing realities. Motivation is the critical underlying key to budget success.

One of the attractive motivational features of budgets is that they present a specific, measurable goal. When there is a clearly stated goal, or set of expectations, managers and staff can work toward meeting that goal. Individuals are much more likely to work efficiently if they have a target to shoot for, assuming that the target is not unrealistic. People like to be motivated. They want to feel a sense of accomplishment.

Compare the likely progress of a dieter with specific weight-loss goals to one who simply wants to lose a lot of weight, or compare an athlete with measurable objectives to one who wants to be strong or run fast. Setting specific goals and working toward them is a tremendous self-motivator. This holds true in the workplace as well.

Motivation is also related to the problems of nurse retention. Turnover is a costly problem in the nursing profession. It costs money to recruit and train new nurses. Why do nurses leave? It is probably not solely because of money. Nurses are clearly motivated by other factors in addition to money. Nurses do not enter the profession as a way to get rich quick. Individuals who seek out professions for reasons other than solely the monetary return are particularly likely to be looking for self-satisfaction in their jobs.

A feeling of helping the patients is probably of predominant importance in generating nurse job satisfaction. However, helping the organization stay within its financial constraints can also add to the nurse's job satisfaction. Most employees want their organization to do well. Nevertheless, a goal of "staying within financial constraints" is no better than the dieter's hope to "lose weight." A more specific goal, such as "Let's use less than 100 rolls of 1-inch bandage tape this month, because that's all we're budgeted for," is likely to be a better motivator. Then if the nurses spend the month being careful not to waste bandage tape, they can see at the end of the month that they have reached the goal and helped the organization. To control results, there must be clearly defined goals.

Control is complicated by the fact that even when the primary goal of the nursing staff is to help patients, it is the basic nature of individuals that their own personal goals will often be different from the goals of the organization they work for (Fig. 3–1). This does not mean that human nature is bad—just that there is such a thing as human nature and one is foolish to refuse to recognize it.

For example, other things being equal, most employees of a hospital would prefer a salary that is substantially larger than they are currently receiving. Most would be quite content if the hospital were to double their salary overnight. There

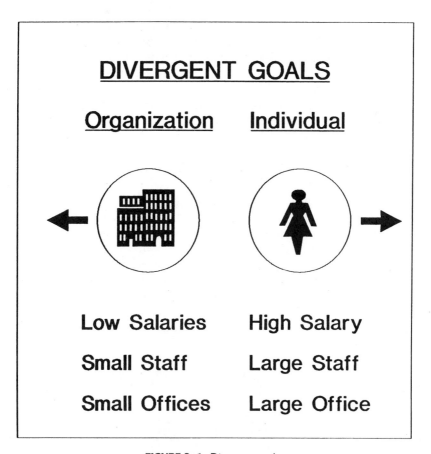

FIGURE 3–1. Divergent goals.

is nothing particularly wrong in their wanting more money. In fact, ambition is probably a desirable trait among staff.

On the other hand, hospitals will not provide employees with 100% raises, because they lack the revenues to pay for those raises. While the nursing staff is not wrong to desire the raises, the hospital is not wrong to deny such raises. Inherently, a tension or conflict exists as a result.

Most nurse managers would like more office space. They would like nicer offices with new furniture and remodeled facilities. They would certainly like more staff to carry out their existing functions. Introductory economics books clearly indicate that society simply has limited resources. All organizations must make choices concerning how to spend their limited resources.

Thus the fact must be faced that even where morale is generally excellent and is not considered to be a problem, an underlying tension will naturally exist. Even though the employees may want to achieve the mission of the organization in providing care, their personal desires will be for things the organization will choose not to provide. This is referred to as *goal divergence.*

The organization must bring together the interests of the individual with its own interests so that they can work together. In the budgeting process, the manager is attempting to control the amount the organization spends. But it is not the organization that controls costs; it is the human beings involved in the process. There must be some motivation for the human beings to want to control costs. Bringing the individuals' desires and the organization's needs together is referred to as *goal congruence* (Fig. 3–2).

In order to be sure that the human beings will in fact want to control organizational costs, the manager needs to make sure that it is somehow in their direct best interests for costs to be controlled. The key is to establish some way that the normally divergent desires of the health care organizations and their employees become convergent or congruent. The goal is for both the organization and the employee to want the same thing.

Management by Objectives (MBO) is one approach that can help accomplish this end. The superior and subordinate (supervisor and manager; manager and staff) sit down and develop a set of objectives that form the basis for performance evaluation. By allowing participation in the process of determining the objectives to be achieved, people are likely to work harder to achieve them. (MBO is discussed further in Chapter 11.)

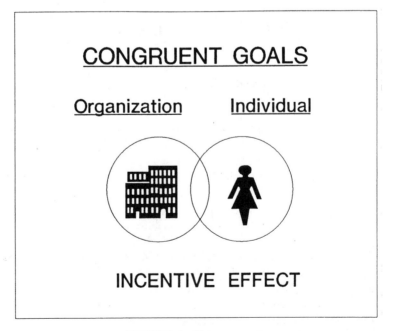

FIGURE 3–2. Congruent goals.

Since congruent goals are not always the norm, and since divergent goals frequently exist, it is necessary to formally address how convergence is to be obtained. Organizations generally achieve such convergence or congruence by setting up a system of incentives that make it serve the best interests of the employees to serve the best interests of the organization.

MOTIVATION AND INCENTIVES

Although nurses are motivated by factors other than money, it would be foolish to ignore the potential of monetary rewards to influence behavior. Health care organizations are searching for the proper mix of incentives that will motivate managers and staff to control costs. Financial incentives are frequently employed. The most basic financial incentives are the ability to retain your job and get a good raise.

In industry, another common motivating tool is a bonus system. Since managers have many desires that relate to spending money (e.g., larger offices, fancier furniture, larger staffs), formalized approaches need to be developed that will provide incentives to spend less money. For example, one can tell a nurse manager that last year her department spent $2,000,000 and that next year her budget is $2,080,000 (a 4% increase). However, for any amount that her department spends below $2,080,000, she and her staff can keep 10% of the savings. If the department spends only $1,950,000 next year, the nurse manager and the staff will get a bonus of $13,000 (i.e., $2,080,000 less $1,950,000, multiplied by 10%) to share. The total cost to the organization is $1,963,000, including the bonus, as opposed to the $2,080,000 budgeted. The nurses benefit and the organization benefits. In this case, goal congruence is likely to be achieved.

Many health care organizations have in fact added bonus systems. The use of bonus systems has both positives and negatives. The positives relate primarily to the strong motivation employees have to reduce costs. The negatives relate to the potential detriment to quality of patient care and to the potential negative effect on employee morale.

Incentive approaches such as bonuses have complex implications. When an incentive is given to accomplish one end, sometimes the responses to that incentive are unexpected. In the case of Medicare, it has been found that DRGs, intended to reduce hospital spending, increase spending on nursing homes and home care agencies. In the case of a 10% bonus on spending reductions from budget, a nurse manager may have an incentive to provide less staff nurse time per patient day. The organization must be concerned about the impact their incentives will have on the quality of patient care. If incentives cause nurse managers to reduce staff to save money, this may unexpectedly reduce quality of care as well.

These are not insurmountable problems. However, managers must try to anticipate unintended consequences when developing an incentive system. The quality issue requires that a strong internal quality assurance program be in place.

Part of the bonus process would have to place restrictions on bonuses when quality of care has declined.

An incentive to treat fewer patients can be solved by making the incentive depend on patient volume, adjusting automatically for changes in volume. This adjustment is important even if volume is totally outside the control of the manager and the unit. If patient volume and revenues are falling, costs should naturally decline. The bonus system should not reward a manager simply because there are fewer patients. On the other hand, increasing costs resulting from rises in patient volume should not cause bonuses to be lost.

For example, suppose that a department has a budget of $2,080,000. Suppose further that half of that represents costs that remain constant regardless of volume and that half represent costs that vary in direct proportion with volume. If the volume of patients drops by 10%, one would expect costs to fall by $104,000 (i.e., 10% of the half of the $2,080,000 that varies with volume). Therefore, costs should have been $2,080,000 less $104,000, or a total of $1,976,000. If actual costs were $1,950,000, the bonus would be based on the $26,000 difference between the adjusted budget of $1,976,000 and the actual cost, rather than being based on the full difference between the original budget and the actual result. In this case, the bonus would be only $2,600, rather than the $13,000 calculated earlier.

A volume adjustment such as this would be appealing to managers if workload is rising. It is hard to convince managers that a bonus based on reduced costs will help them, if each year the patient volume increases and costs rise with patient load. No matter how hard the manager and staff work to reduce costs, a large increase in workload will undoubtedly keep them from spending less than was budgeted. A bonus based on a fixed budget will never yield a payoff to hard work. On the other hand, if the budget basis for the bonus adjusts with patient volume, then as workload increases, the allowed spending would increase. It would become possible to earn a bonus even if more money was spent than had been budgeted originally.

This does not mean that bonuses are the solution to all motivational problems. Bonus systems have a variety of other problems. Some bonus systems reward all employees if spending is reduced. But, if everyone gets a bonus, then no one feels that their individual actions have much impact. As long as everyone else holds costs in check, individuals may feel that they do not have to work particularly hard to reap the benefits of the bonus. In that case, probably very few will work hard to control costs.

On the other hand, bonuses given only to some employees may create jealousy and discontent. It is also possible that bonuses may create a competitive environment in a situation in which teamwork is needed to provide quality care.

There are incentive alternatives to bonuses. For example, one underused managerial tool is a letter from supervisor to subordinate. All individuals responsible for controlling costs should be evaluated explicitly with respect to how well they do in fact control costs. That evaluation should be communicated in writing. This approach, which is both the carrot and the stick, costs little to implement but can have a dramatic impact.

Telling managers that they did a good job and that their boss knows they did a good job can be an effective way to get the manager to try to do a good job the next year. In the real world, praise is both cheap and in many cases effective. On the other hand, criticism, especially in writing, can have a stinging effect that managers and staff will work hard to avoid in the future.

MOTIVATION AND UNREALISTIC EXPECTATIONS

While motivational devices can work wonders at getting an organization's staff to work hard for the organization and its goals, they can also backfire and have negative results. This occurs primarily when expectations are placed at unreasonably high levels.

There is no question that many people do attempt to *satisfice*—to do just enough to get by. One thing incentives are used to accomplish is to motivate those individuals to work harder. A target that requires hard work and stretching, but that is achievable, can be a useful motivating tool. If the target is reached, there might be a bonus, or there should be at least some formal recognition of the achievement, such as a letter. At a minimum, the worker will have the self-satisfaction of having worked hard and reached the target.

But all those positive outcomes can only occur if the target is reachable. Some health care organizations have taken the philosophy that if a high target makes people work hard, a higher target will make them work harder. This may not be the case. If targets are placed out of reach, this will probably *not* result in people reaching to their utmost limits to come as close to the target as possible.

It may seem like the organization is shortchanging itself whenever someone achieves a target. The executive may think, "We set the target too low. Perhaps if the target were higher, this manager would have achieved the higher target. Since the target we set was achieved, we really do not know just how far this person can go. We haven't yet realized all of his or her potential." The problem with that logic is that there are risks associated with it.

If a nurse manager fails to meet a target because of incompetence or because of not enough hard work, the signal of failure that is sent is warranted. In fact, repeated failure may be grounds for replacing that individual in that job. But if a manager is both competent and hard working, failure is not a message that should be sent. Even though it is desirable to encourage the individual to achieve even more, the signal of failure will be discouraging.

When people work extremely hard and fail, they often question why they bothered to work so hard. If hard work results in failure to achieve the target, then why not ease off. If you are going to fail anyway, why must it be so painful? Thus managers must be extremely careful to ensure that all goals assigned are reasonable or results may be less favorable than they otherwise would be.

THE BUDGET AS A TOOL FOR COMMUNICATION

Of course, for motivation to really exist, the budget goals must be communicated. This concept was introduced in Chapter 2. It is important enough to warrant a few additional comments. The earlier examples should make it clear that this discussion does not relate to motivating only the managers of the organization. Costs are incurred because of the actions of all individuals in an organization. A nurse manager will have little success in controlling costs without the cooperation of all the nurses and other staff on the floor.

A good practice is to sit down once a year and review all aspects of the budget on which the staff nurses have some impact. However, communication should also be an ongoing process. When a manager has a once-a-year meeting with the staff concerning the budget, it is quickly forgotten. In order to reinforce that meeting, a short weekly or monthly meeting should be held to discuss the budget for one or several items, such as bandage tape, diapers, chest tubes, disposable gloves, or sponges. It does not even have to be a separate meeting; it can be a 2-minute note made at any regularly scheduled meeting. The key is to make the staff aware of specific, definite, attainable goals that they can work toward. Further, by having the budget mentioned every week, an awareness is created, and it becomes second nature to conserve the organization's resources.

Note that in no way does this imply reducing quality of care. The focus is on reducing inefficient use of resources. To the staff nurse, this means, for example, taking care not to rip off 2 feet of tape when 6 inches would do the trick. For the nurse manager, it means setting a staffing schedule that minimizes overtime and agency nurse costs. Conservation of resources is the key, and it should become second nature. The benefits of once-a-year meetings wear off in a few weeks. If the manager does not mention the budget again until a month of excessive use has occurred, a strong admonition at that time will tend to create budget antagonism rather than cost control. When a nurse manager conveys specific, measurable goals in a routine manner, then cost control can become a routine part of the way nurses function. The best control of resource use requires that the staff view controlling resource use to be a key part of their job.

USING BUDGETS FOR INTERIM EVALUATION

Evaluation is a necessary element of controlling costs. The organization must evaluate how well managers are keeping to their budgets. In this respect, interim evaluations are of particular importance.

If the manager simply prepares a budget, tells everyone what it is, and then puts it in a drawer until it is needed to help prepare next year's budget, an important element of motivation and control is lost. Even if the manager takes the budget out of the drawer each month and tells the unit's staff, "This is how much we have budgeted for bandage tape for this month, that's your goal," the last major step toward controlling costs has not been taken. The budget has not been used to evaluate how well the unit, staff, and manager are doing.

Many organizations would argue that at the end of each year they compare the budgeted amounts to the actual results to see how well they did. The problem is that by then it is too late to do anything about it. The budget should be a living document; it should be used as a motivational and control tool throughout the year.

Each month there should be comparisons between what was expected and what has been accomplished. First, this will allow managers to give feedback to the staff nurses, their supervisors, and themselves as to whether or not the budget's goals are being attained. The person attempting to lose 10 pounds quickly gives up if there is no scale available on which progress can be observed. Telling the nurses the goals without giving timely reports on whether or not they are being attained will weaken their motivation.

Second, these monthly evaluations help to bring any unanticipated results to the manager's attention. Then the manager may be able to make adjustments in staffing or correct behavior so that the budget will be met in the future months. When one examines the actual results just once a year, it is possible to cry a lot over the spilt milk. If the actual results are evaluated monthly, there is still time to save most of the milk before it spills.

This, of course, assumes that the situation is under the manager's control. Perhaps the manager will watch month after month as the unit fails to meet the budget because something outside the unit or manager's control is affecting the results. Since the unit and manager will likely be blamed if the budget goals are not met, monthly information allows a manager to serve early notice that a problem outside of the manager's control exists.

In evaluating any individual in an organization, there is one primary rule that must be followed: responsibility should equal control. If managers are held responsible for things they have no control over, the organization will reward and punish the wrong individuals. The result is invariably an unhappy group of individuals.

SUMMARY AND IMPLICATIONS FOR NURSE MANAGERS

Budgets can help control costs if they are used to motivate all staff members, not just managers. This requires communication of specific, measurable goals on a regular, frequent basis. Such a process will improve results as individuals make a self-motivated effort to achieve specified, attainable goals.

However, one must try to understand what incentives are needed to cause individuals to work toward the overall well-being of the organization. When a health care organization asks a nurse to accomplish something, it is necessary to be concerned with why that person would want to do it. Perhaps to benefit patient care. But that motive provides little incentive for cost control. Perhaps the nurse will control costs out of loyalty to the organization or out of fear of losing a job. Or perhaps it will be done in hopes of earning a promotion.

Getting an understanding of what people will want to do and what they will not want to do is important. And once a manager knows what they will not want to do, a careful attempt should be made to develop some clear motivational device that will give them an incentive to do what they otherwise might not want to. After all, how many people would work if they did not get paid at all? Some psychologists view paychecks as a bribe to get people to come to work. Once they are at work, additional incentives should be provided to make sure that the organization benefits from their efforts to the greatest extent possible.

SUGGESTED READINGS

Adams, D. (1995, December). Teaching the Process of Delegation. *Seminars for Nurse Managers*. 2(4), 171–174.

Appelbaum, S.H., and Mackenzie, L. (1996). Compensation in the year 2000: Pay for performance? *Health Manpower Management*. 22(3), 31–39.

Avigne, G., Guin, P., Pittman, L., and Surdez, M. (1998, September). Moving from an hourly pay model to a professional salary model. *AORN Journal*. 68(3), 400–402, 405–408.

Brady, D.J., Cornett, E., and DeLetter, M. (1998, September–October). Cost reduction: What a staff nurse can do. *Nursing Economic$*. 16(5), 273–274, 276.

Brown, B. (1999, March). How can I create a more collaborative practice environment in the unit? *Nursing Management*. 30(3), 17.

Caroselli, C. (1996, September–October). Economic awareness of nurses: Relationship to budgetary control. *Nursing Economic$*. 14(5), 292–298.

Cronin, S.N., and Becherer, D. (1999, January). Recognition of staff nurse job performance and achievements: Staff and manager perceptions. *Journal of Nursing Administration*. 29(1), 26–31.

Crowell, D.M. (1998, May). Organizations *are* relationships: A new view of management. *Nursing Management*, 29(5), 28–29.

Elliott, M.A., and Turrell, A.R. (1996, September). Dilemmas for the empowering nurse. *Journal of Nursing Management*. 4(5), 273–279.

Evan, K., Aubry, K., Hawkins, M., Curley, T.A., and Porter-O'Grady, T. (1995, May). Whole systems shared governance: A model for the integrated health system. *Journal of Nursing Administration*. 25(5), 18–27.

Havens, D. (1998, January–February). An update on nursing involvement in hospital governance: 1990–1996. *Nursing Economic$*. 16(1), 6–11.

Girvins, J. (1998, July). Satisfaction and motivation. *Nursing Management*. 5(4), 11–15.

Laschinger, H.K., and Havens, D.S. (1997, June). The effect of workplace empowerment on staff nurses' occupational mental health and work effectiveness. *Journal of Nursing Administration*. 27(6), 42–50.

Lehmann, D.M. (1997, March). Is there a conflict between management, leadership, and empowerment? *Seminars for Nurse Managers*. 5(1), 7.

Lookinland, S., and Crenshaw, J. (1996, July–August). Rewarding clinical competence in the ICU: Using outcomes to reward performance. *Dimensions of Critical Care Nursing*. 15(4), 206–215.

MacDonald, G. (1995, September). Shared governance—A unit based concept. *Axone*. 17(1), 3–5.

Prince, S.B. (1997, March). Shared governance. Sharing power and opportunity. *Journal of Nursing Administration.* 27(3), 28–35.

Proch, M.L. (1995, October). Creating a climate to promote internal motivation in employees. *Journal of Nursing Administration.* 25(10), 5.

Sabiston, J.A., and Laschinger, H.K. (1995, September). Staff nurse work empowerment and perceived autonomy. Testing Kanter's theory of structural power in organizations. *Journal of Nursing Administration.* 25(9), 42–50.

Schweitzer, J. (1997, Summer). Staff nurses vs. nurse managers—no winners here. *Revolution.* 7(2), 38–40.

Wilson, T.B. (1995, Fall). Utilizing reward systems to mobilize change. *Quality Management in Health Care.* 4(1), 13–26.

Yingling, S., and Bolster, C.J. (1998, September 5). Banking on bonuses. *Hospitals & Health Networks.* 72(17), 24–26, 28–36.

4

Cost Concepts

The goals of this chapter are to:

define service units;

define basic cost terms;

explain the underlying behavior of costs and the importance of that behavior;

provide tools for cost estimation;

explain how costs can be adjusted for the impact of inflation;

provide tools for break-even analysis; and

explain the activity based costing technique.

BASIC COST CONCEPTS

To prepare a budget that can provide a good plan of expenses for the coming year, it is necessary to have an understanding of the nature of costs. Revenues are also important. Revenues are discussed in Chapter 9.

Service Units

Costs are generally collected for *service units* or units of service. A service unit is a basic measure of the item being produced by the organization, such as discharged patients, patient days, home care visits, or hours of operations. Most measurements of cost relate to the volume of service units. Within one health care organization, a number of different types of service units may exist.

Fixed versus Variable Costs

A critical basic cost issue is the distinction between fixed and variable costs. The total costs of running a unit or department can be divided into those costs that are fixed and those costs that are variable.

Fixed costs are those costs that do not change in total as the volume of service units changes. For instance, the salary of the Chief Nurse Executive (CNE) does

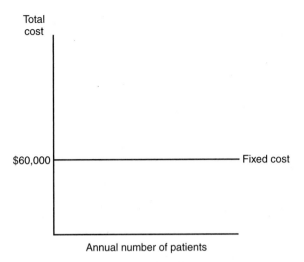

FIGURE 4–1. Fixed costs: Cost for a nurse manager.

not change day by day as the census changes. *Variable costs,* on the other hand, vary directly with the volume of service units. The definition of the service unit measure is crucial in defining fixed and variable costs. Most clinical supplies used in a hospital vary with the number of patient days. However, surgical supplies are more likely to vary with the number of surgical procedures, and clinic supplies will likely vary with the number of clinic visits.

The concepts of fixed and variable costs are often conceptualized with the use of graphs. Figure 4–1 gives an example of fixed costs. Specifically, the graph shows the annual salary for a unit nurse manager for the coming year. The salary is 60,000.[1] That salary is a fixed cost for the organization. The salary paid to a nurse manager is not dependent on any patient-volume statistic. In Figure 4–1, the vertical axis shows the cost to the institution. As you go up this axis, costs increase. On the horizontal axis are the number of patients. The further to the right you move, the more patients the institution has.

Note that the fixed costs appear as a horizontal line. This is because, regardless of the volume, the salary for the nurse manager will remain the same. Thus the cost is the same for 8,000 patients, or for 10,000, or for 12,000.

Variable costs, on the other hand, vary with the volume of service units. Suppose that each hospital patient's temperature is taken twice a day. If the hospital's thermometers use disposable thermometer covers, then one would expect use of disposable covers to vary directly with patient volume. Assuming that each thermometer cover costs $.50 and that two a day are used for each

---

[1]This is a hypothetical number. Nurse manager salaries vary with geographic region, institution size, and institution type.

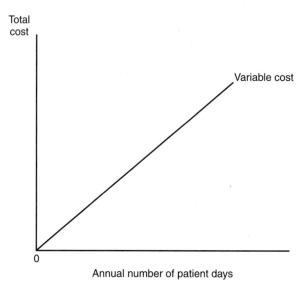

FIGURE 4–2. Variable costs: The costs of a disposable supply.

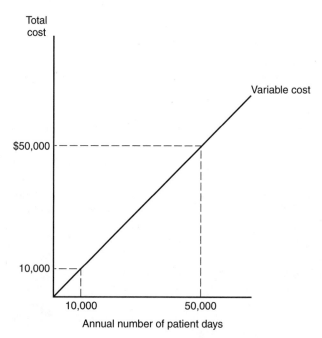

FIGURE 4–3. Variable costs: The costs of a disposable supply at volumes of 10,000 and 50,000 patient days.

patient, then the cost of these items would be $1 for each patient each day. The more patient days, the more the cost for that disposable item in the total nursing unit budget.

Consider Figure 4–2. This graph plots the cost for disposable thermometer covers as they vary with patient volume. As in Figure 4–1, the vertical axis represents the cost, and the horizontal axis represents the patient volume. Since the thermometer cover example relates to inpatients, the label on the horizontal axis has been changed from "Annual number of patients" in Figure 4–1 to "Annual number of patient days" in Figure 4–2. Unlike Figure 4–1, which showed some positive amount of cost even at a volume of zero, Figure 4–2 shows zero cost at a volume of zero, since zero patient days implies that none of this particular supply will be used. The total variable cost increases by $1 for each extra patient day.

For instance, in Figure 4–3 dotted lines have been inserted to show the cost when there are 10,000 patient days and the cost when there are 50,000 patient days. As you can see, $10,000 would be spent on the disposable item if there were 10,000 patient days and $50,000 if there were 50,000 patient days.

The total of the fixed and variable costs is shown in Figure 4–4. This figure combines the fixed costs from Figure 4–1 with the variable costs from Figure 4–2.

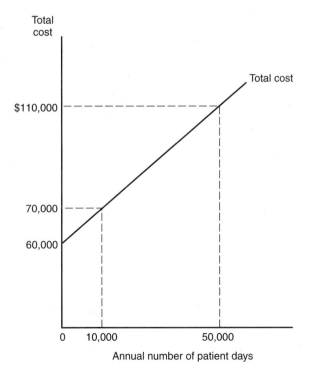

FIGURE 4–4. Total costs for the unit.

Note that the total costs start at $60,000, even if volume is zero, because of the fixed costs of the nurse manager.

The Relevant Range

One potential problem exists with this type of graphical analysis of fixed and variable costs. This concerns an issue accountants refer to as the *relevant range*. The relevant range represents the likely range of activity covered by a budget. For example, a unit might expect 80% occupancy. However, a range from 75% to 85% occupancy is possible. In that case, the relevant range is the number of patient days from a 75% occupancy for the unit to an 85% occupancy level.

Variable costs increase proportionately over the relevant range. It is unlikely that a health care organization would pay $.50 for each disposable thermometer cover at *any* volume level. If purchases increase substantially, there probably will be a price reduction per unit. On the other hand, if purchases were to decrease substantially, the hospital possibly would have to pay more per unit. However, the variable costs may reasonably be considered to increase proportionately over the relevant range.

Fixed costs are not fixed over any range of activity. If a nursing unit had zero patient days, the hospital would close the unit and would not have any fixed cost for a nurse manager. If patient volume rose substantially and exceeded the capacity of the unit, the hospital might need to open a second unit and have the additional cost of a second nurse manager. The costs are, however, fixed over the relevant range.

Essentially, variable costs do not increase by exactly the same amount per unit over *any* range of volume, and fixed costs do not remain fixed over *any* range of volume. However, for most budgets, volume expectations for the coming year do not assume drastic changes in volume.

When fixed and variable costs are graphed, the relevant range issue is often ignored (e.g., costs appear fixed over all ranges of activity in the graph). However, the user of the graph should bear in mind that the graph's information is only accurate within the relevant range.

Other Complications

In health care, there are several additional problems related to applying the concepts of fixed and variable costs. These problems generally concern issues of step-fixed costs, mixed costs, and relevant costs.

Many costs are *step-fixed* (sometimes called *step-variable*). Such costs do vary within the relevant range, but not smoothly. They are fixed over intervals that are shorter than the relevant range (Fig. 4–5).

For example, staffing patterns may be such that a nursing unit will use five nurses over a range of workload. If that range is exceeded, the unit would have to use six nurses. Clearly, more patient days or greater average acuity requires more

Total
cost

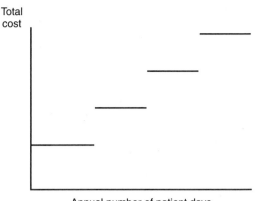

Annual number of patient days

FIGURE 4–5. Example of step-fixed costs.

nursing care hours. However, if the staffing pattern is about 4.2 hours of nursing time per patient day, the unit would not expect to hire a nurse for an additional 4.2 hours every time the patient-day census increases by one.

As long as there is a staffing chart that tells how many full-time equivalent (FTE) nurses are needed for any volume of patient days, the presence of step-variable costs do not present a major budgeting problem. Generally, because of the use of overtime and agency nurses, a step-fixed pattern of cost is estimated by treating the staffing costs as if they were variable. While this will not give a perfectly precise result, it is usually a reasonable approximation.

A more difficult problem is posed by *mixed costs.* A mixed cost is one that contains some fixed cost and some variable cost. For instance, electricity is a mixed cost. A hospital or nursing home spends some basic amount to light the hallways and public areas of a building regardless of volume, but patient rooms will have lights on only if there is a patient in the room. Therefore, the more patient days, the higher the electricity cost—even though part of the overall cost is fixed. Most units and departments have some mixed costs.

For example, suppose that a home care agency pays some staff every day regardless of the amount of work and some staff by the visit. This creates a mixed-cost situation. Or, suppose that the intensive care unit of a hospital has highly variable patient volume. The nurse manager of the unit knows that this year the unit will have a total of 10,000 patient days, and for next year 12,000 patient days are predicted. Because the unit is busy at some times and slow at others, it is difficult to use a staffing chart based on step-fixed costs. The patient days are not incurred evenly throughout the year. Can a nurse manager simply assume that a 20% increase in patient days from 10,000 to 12,000 will cause a need for 20% higher staffing costs than the unit had in the year with 10,000 patient days?

Probably not. There is likely to be some minimum staffing level as long as the unit is open. The cost for that minimum staffing level represents a fixed cost, since it does not change with volume. Then as volume increases, there will be additional staff requirements. If the nurse manager wishes to determine how much staff to budget for in the coming year, it is necessary to be able to separate the mixed cost into fixed-cost and variable-cost components. As volume increases, the fixed cost will not change and the variable costs will increase in direct proportion to the volume change.

There are several ways to separate mixed costs into their fixed-cost and variable-cost components so that future costs can be predicted. Later, this chapter will examine the high-low approach and regression analysis techniques of *cost estimation* to solve that problem.

The Impact of Volume on Cost per Patient

If a nurse manager were to ask what it costs to treat patients in the unit, accountants would probably answer that it depends. Costs are not unique numbers that are always the same. The cost to treat a patient depends on several critical factors. One of these is the volume of patients for whom care is being provided.

Suppose that an outpatient cardiology center has fixed costs of $200,000 and variable costs of $200 per patient. Using this hypothetical data, what is the total cost per patient? If there are 3,000 patients for the year, the total costs will be the fixed cost of $200,000 plus $200 per patient for each of the 3,000 patients. The variable costs would be $600,000 (i.e., $200 per patient times 3,000 patients). The total cost would be $800,000 (i.e., $200,000 fixed cost plus $600,000 variable cost). The cost per patient would be $267 (i.e., $800,000 total cost divided by 3,000 patients) per patient.

However, what if there were only 2,500 patients? Then the variable costs, at $200 per patient, would be $500,000, and the total cost would be $700,000. In that case, the cost per patient would be $280. The cost is higher because there are fewer patients sharing the fixed costs. Each patient causes the center to spend another $200. The $200,000 fixed cost remains the same regardless of the number of patients. If there are more patients, each one shares less of the $200,000 fixed cost. If there are fewer patients, the fixed cost assigned to each would rise.

Suppose there were only 500 patients. The variable costs of $200 per patient would total $100,000, and the total cost would be $300,000. The cost per patient would be $600—more than double the previous results from 2,500 and 3,000 patients.

In trying to understand costs, it is critical to grasp the concept that because fixed costs do not change in total, the cost per patient or per patient day does change as volume changes. The greater the volume, the more patients that are available to share the fixed costs. There is no one unique answer to the question. "What does it cost the unit per patient?" That question can only be answered by giving the cost per patient, assuming a specific volume of patients. The volume of patients is critical.

One implication of this result is that health care organizations almost always find higher volume preferable to lower volume. As volume increases, the average cost per patient declines. If prices can be maintained at the original level, the declining cost will result in lower losses or higher profits.

Relevant Costs

Another costing concern is the issue accountants refer to as *relevant costs.* Relevant costs are those costs that change as a result of a decision. Costs that remain the same regardless of the decision made are not "relevant" costs for making the decision.

If someone were to ask the nurse manager the cost of treating a particular type of patient, the answer should be, "It depends." The previous section has pointed out that it depends on the number of patients. It also depends on what the answer will be used for. If the question is just one of historical curiosity, the average cost is an adequate response. The average cost is the total cost divided by the volume. In the above example, the total cost at a volume of 2,500 patients was $700,000 and the average cost (i.e., the total $700,000 divided by the volume of 2,500 patients) was $280 per patient. However, if the information will be used for decision making, that response may well be incorrect.

Suppose that the center was trying to decide whether to negotiate with an HMO to accept additional patients of the same average acuity and mix as the 2,500 patients it currently has. The HMO has offered $250 per patient for 500 patients. From the earlier calculations, the cost per patient for 500 patients is $600! However, the center would not be providing only 500 patients with care. It already has 2,500 patients. From the earlier calculations, the average cost is $280 per patient at 2,500 patients. At 3,000 patients the average cost would be $267. Given that information, would it pay to accept the additional patients at a price of only $250?

It definitely would. Why should the center accept $250, if the additional patients will cost at least $267? Actually, the additional patients will not cost at least $267. All the patients, on average, will cost that amount. The $267 includes a share of both fixed and variable costs. If the center is going to treat at least 2,500 patients regardless of the HMO negotiation outcome, then the fixed costs of $200,000 will be incurred. The fixed costs will not change if the center has the extra 500 patients.

Decisions such as this one rely on *marginal analysis.* The margin refers to a change from current conditions by even a minor amount. A patient on the margin refers to adding one more patient or reducing volume by one patient. Marginal costs are the costs for treating one more patient.

On the *margin,* if the center were to take the additional HMO patients, it would have more variable costs but would not have any additional fixed costs (assuming that 3,000 patients is within the relevant range). Each extra patient causes the center to spend only the variable costs of $200 per patient. That is less than the $250 the HMO has offered to pay. The center will be better off by $50 for each additional patient.

The additional costs incurred for additional patients are often referred to as the *marginal,* or *out-of-pocket,* or *incremental* costs. If fixed costs were to rise because the relevant range was exceeded, those costs would appropriately be included in the incremental costs along with the variable costs. The key element in relevant costing is that the only costs relevant to a decision are those that change as a result of the decision.

The decision may be to add a new service or to close down an existing one. It may be to expand volume (as shown in the above HMO example), or it may be to contract volume. In any case, where a decision is being made that contemplates changing patient load, the essential information to be considered are the revenues and costs that change. Effective managerial decisions require that the manager know the amount by which total costs will increase and the amount by which the total revenues will increase or, alternatively, the amount by which both will decrease. Costs that do not change in total for the organization are not relevant to the decision. Fixed costs generally do not increase when additional patients are added (within the relevant range), and therefore they are not relevant.

In the cardiology center–HMO example, suppose that prior to the HMO negotiation, the center was receiving $275 for each of its 2,500 patients. Total revenue ($275 times 2,500) was $687,500. Total costs were $700,000 (calculated earlier). The center was losing $12,500 (the amount that the cost of $700,000 exceeds the revenues of $687,500). If the HMO business is accepted, the additional revenue would be $250 times 500 patient days, or $125,000. The total cost for 3,000 patients (calculated earlier) is $800,000. The cost increase of going from 2,500 patients to 3,000 patients is only $100,000 (i.e., $800,000 total cost for 3,000 patients versus $700,000 total cost for 2,500 patients).

The total costs with the HMO patients are $800,000, and the total revenues are $812,500 (i.e., the original $687,500 plus $125,000 revenue from the HMO). The unit has gone from a loss of $12,500 to a profit of $12,500. The costs have increased by $100,000 while the revenues have increased by $125,000. The amount by which the extra revenues exceed the extra costs for the 500 HMO patients accounts for the turnaround from a loss to a profit. This should not be surprising. The extra revenue per patient is $250. The additional cost per patient day is $200. The difference between incremental revenue of $250 per patient and incremental cost of $200 per patient is a profit of $50 per patient. This extra profit of $50 for each of the 500 HMO patients accounts for exactly the $25,000 profit from the HMO patients.

Had the center used average cost for its decision, since the $250 revenue per extra patient is less than the $267 average cost, it would have turned away the extra business and lost the chance to gain a $25,000 profit. The average cost is not relevant because it incorrectly assumes that each extra patient will cause the center to have additional variable and fixed costs. The incremental cost is relevant because it considers only the additional revenues and additional costs that the center will have as a result of the proposed change.

COST ESTIMATION

One of the most difficult parts of the budget process is predicting the individual elements of the budget. Trying to predict how much will be spent on each type of expenditure in the coming year presents great problems for both inexperienced and experienced managers.

One approach is simply to look to what happened this year and predict that it will occur again next year, with an increment for inflation. At the other extreme is an approach that says it is desirable to do better next year than this year, so it is appropriate to budget a certain percentage less than was spent this year. In each case, the approach is far too simplistic. A priori, there is no reason to believe that next year will be just like this year, and simply wishing to spend less than this year will not make it so.

Some sort of clear methodology is needed that will allow prediction of what will happen next year based on the past. Some way to consider formally why that prediction may not come true is also needed. Finally, if costs are to be reduced below the predicted outcome, there must be a specific plan of action that the nurse manager believes can accomplish the cost cutback.

This section will consider several methods of cost estimation. Not all elements of the budget are simply costs. Items such as the number of patient days must be predicted as well. A discussion of general forecasting is presented in Chapter 6. Here the focus will be solely on prediction of costs. Often, historical information about costs incurred in the past can be a great aid in predicting what costs will be in the future. This is especially true in the case of mixed costs, which have both fixed and variable cost elements. Cost estimation techniques exist that look at historical information and compare the change in cost over time with the change in volume over time, in order to isolate fixed and variable costs.

If costs rise as volume rises, what could account for the increase in costs? Fixed costs, by definition, do not change as volume changes. Therefore, any change in cost as volume changes must be attributable to the variable cost. By seeing how much costs change for each unit change in volume, it is possible to calculate the variable cost per unit. In turn, the fixed cost can be determined. The fixed and variable costs can then be used to estimate costs for the coming year, based on a forecast of the volume in the coming year.

There is one critical problem in the flow of logic that allows cost estimation to take place. Changes in cost over time are assumed to be the result of changes in volume. To some extent, changes in cost over time are the result of inflation. If inflation was a constant percent that was the same each year, one could argue that past inflation can be ignored and inflation will automatically be built into predictions for the future. However, inflation rates tend to fluctuate from year to year. Over a period of years the fluctuations can be substantial. Therefore, in order to be able to predict fixed and variable costs, the data being used should be free from the impact of inflation.

Adjusting Costs for Inflation

Suppose that a nurse manager is interested in determining how much the total RN staff cost of a unit will be for the coming fiscal year, 2002.[2] The unit is staffed with a minimum of 10 FTE RNs for any volume up to 9,000 patient days at a certain acuity level. The cost of those 10 FTEs is a fixed cost, because the unit will always have at least that cost. As volume increases above 9,000 patient days, additional nursing time will be needed. In 2000, patient days numbered 9,800 and the cost, including fringe benefits, was $500,000. In 2001, the patient days totaled 11,000 and the cost was $580,000. The cost increase of $80,000 was attributable to the increased volume and due to inflation.

Most readers are probably familiar with the consumer price index (CPI). This is the most widely used measure of inflation. The CPI and many other indexes of inflation, such as the hospital market basket index, were developed by or for the federal government. The CPI measures the relative cost of a typical basket of consumer goods. Whatever the basket of goods cost in the base year is considered to be 100% of the cost in that year, or simply 100. The index is revised and a new base year established from time to time. If it costs twice as much to buy the same goods in a year subsequent to the base year, then the index would be 200% of the base year costs, or simply 200.

The U.S. Department of Commerce, Bureau of the Census annually publishes the *Statistical Abstract of the United States.* Included in this book are Indexes of Medical Care Prices. There are several useful indexes under that heading, including the index of Medical Care Services and the Hospital Daily Room Rate index.

Recall that in this example the nurse manager wants to find the variable cost per patient day of nursing labor for 2002, using current dollars as of the end of 2001. If information from 1997 through 2001 is used, the nurse manager would have to find the value of an appropriate index in each of those years. The financial managers in most health care institutions can provide nurse managers with appropriate indices adjusted for labor costs in the specific geographic area. Failing that, most library reference sections can be of assistance with current index information. Assume that an appropriate index for those years has values as follows:

1997: 258
1998: 287

---

[2]A fiscal year may have a starting point at any convenient date, not necessarily January 1. For example, a fiscal year could begin on July 1 and end on June 30. In that case, fiscal year 2002 would refer to the year from July 1, 2001 to June 30, 2002.

1999: 318
2000: 357
2001: 395

Suppose also that the following cost and volume information is available:

Year	Patient Days	Cost
1997	8,000	$328,000
1998	8,700	364,000
1999	8,850	404,000
2000	9,800	500,000
2001	11,000	580,000

It appears that costs have risen from 1997 to 1999 even though volume is below 9,000 patient days in each of those years. Because the staffing is fixed at 10 FTEs for any volume below 9,000 patient days, the cost is expected to be about the same in each of those 3 years and to only increase as volume increases above 9,000 patient days, thus requiring more nursing staff. The cost information, however, is not comparable because of the impact of inflation. In order to make the numbers reasonable for comparison purposes, they must be restated in *constant dollars* (i.e., amounts that have been adjusted for the impact of inflation).

This adjustment can be done by multiplying the cost in any given year by a fraction that represents the current value of the index divided by the value of the index in the year the cost was incurred. This is not a complicated procedure. For example, in 1997 the cost was $328,000. The hypothetical index value is currently 395. In 1997 it was 258. Multiply $328,000 by the fraction 395/258. The result is $502,171, which is the 1997 cost adjusted to 2001 dollars. Now the $580,000 spent when there were 11,000 patient days in 2001 can be compared to $502,171, the constant-dollar cost of 8,000 patient days in 1997.

In a similar fashion all of the data can be restated into 2001 dollars as follows:

Year	Patient Days	Original Cost		Index Fraction		Adjusted Cost
1997	8,000	$328,000	×	395/258	=	$502,171
1998	8,700	364,000	×	395/287	=	500,976
1999	8,850	404,000	×	395/318	=	501,824
2000	9,800	500,000	×	395/357	=	553,221
2001	11,000	580,000	×	395/395	=	580,000

Note that, adjusted for inflation, there was little change in costs from 1997 to 1999, the period during which the staffing was fixed because patient days were less than 9,000.

High-Low Cost Estimation

The high-low approach is a relatively simple, quick-and-dirty approach to cost estimation. It is unsophisticated and therefore not terribly accurate, but in many cases it may be good enough. It certainly is better than simply taking a guess.

The key to the high-low method is the fact that fixed costs do not change at all in response to changes in volume. The way the method works is to look at the organization's cost for a specific area over the last 5 years. When you do this, remember to use costs after adjusting the original amounts spent for inflation, as described above.

The use of 5 years is arbitrary. It might be more appropriate to use a longer period of time, but you would not want to use data from much fewer than 5 years. Less than 5 years should be used only if there have been substantial changes in the unit that would make earlier data no longer relevant. For the period of time chosen, find the highest volume and the lowest volume and compare the costs at these two volumes. These costs are readily obtained from *variance reports* of prior years.

The amount by which the costs changed should be compared to the amount by which the volume changed. In this example, the highest volume in the last 5 years was 11,000 patient days, and the cost for nursing labor that year for the department was $580,000. The lowest volume in the last 5 years was 8,000 patient days, and the constant dollar inflation adjusted cost in that year was $502,171. In this case, inflation adjusted cost increased by $77,829, while volume increased by 3,000 patient days. If $77,829 is divided by 3,000 patient days, the result is $25.943 per patient day. Although it is certainly likely that nursing labor is a step-fixed cost and therefore will not go up by $25.943 for *each* additional patient day, this volume provides a reasonable measure of the amount of additional nursing services needed per patient day when there are significant changes in volume.

If the variable cost per patient day is $25.943, then what is the fixed cost? The yearly total variable cost is first found by multiplying the variable cost per patient day by the number of patient days ($25.943 × 8,000 = $207,544). The total nursing labor cost for 8,000 patient days was $502,171 in 1997; if $207,544 is the variable cost, then the remainder, $294,627, represents the fixed cost. Similarly, for 11,000 patient days at $25.943 per patient day, the variable cost is $285,373; and given a total cost of $580,000 in 2001, the fixed cost would be $294,627. The fixed cost is expected to be the same at either volume level, since by definition it is fixed.

This fixed and variable cost information can be used in preparing next year's budget. If 12,000 patient days are expected, then costs would be expected to rise by $25.943 times 1,000 patient days, or $25,943. The fixed cost portion will not change. Since this information has been calculated using 2001 constant dollars, both the fixed and variable costs would have to be adjusted upward for the expected 2002 salary increases or, more generally, for the expected impact of inflation during the next year.

The high-low method is not terribly accurate because it only considers the experience of 2 years. One or both of the 2 years chosen may have had some unusual circumstance that would skew the costs in that year. A superior prediction is possible if some method is used that takes more experience into account. *Regression analysis* is a method that can provide such a prediction.

Regression Analysis

The volume of patient days and the total cost for those days for a number of years can be plotted on a graph. The horizontal axis would represent the volume, and the vertical axis would represent the cost. The result would be a scatter diagram. The series of points on the graph would each represent a volume and the cost at that volume. If a line were drawn through the points, it could be used for future predictions. By selecting any expected volume on the horizontal axis, it is possible to go vertically up to the line and then from the line move horizontally across to a point on a vertical cost axis. That point would represent the prediction of cost. For example, Figure 4–6 shows a scatter diagram with a line drawn through the points.

The difficulty in drawing the diagonal line connecting those points is placing it properly so that it will give accurate predictions. Regression analysis is a technique that applies mathematical precision to a scatter diagram. Regression technique can select the one line that is effectively closest to all the individual points on the scatter diagram and that will therefore give the best predictions of cost for the future. This can fairly accurately break costs down into their fixed-cost and variable-cost components.

Simple linear regression analysis can take all available past information into account in estimating that portion of any cost that is fixed and that portion that is variable. The phrase "simple linear regression" refers to several issues. First, it is simple in the sense that there is only one *dependent* variable and one *independent* variable. Cost is the dependent variable that is being estimated. Cost depends on the value of the independent variable.

An independent variable is a causal factor. For example, the most significant causal factor for nursing costs in a hospital might be patient days. The more patient days, the greater the costs for nursing. For the admissions department of

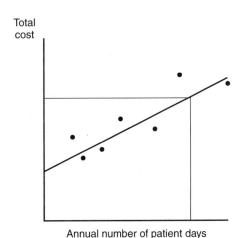

FIGURE 4–6. Predicting costs from a scatter diagram.

the hospital, it would not be patient days but rather the number of patients that is important, since admission time is the same for each patient regardless of their ultimate length of stay. For a home health agency, the most significant causal factor might be the number of home visits.

The second part of the phrase "simple linear regression" refers to the presumption that cost behavior can be shown in a linear fashion (i.e., using a straight line). What if a slightly lower price per disposable supply unit was paid for every increase in volume (e.g., $.75 for one unit, $.7499 per unit for two units, $.7498 per unit for three units, and so on)? In that case, Figure 4–2 would not be an accurate reflection of how variable costs change. It would be necessary to draw a curved line in the graph—but the mathematics involved with curved lines instead of straight lines are far more complicated. Variable costs are generally treated as if they were linear even if that is only an approximation of their true behavior.

Finally, the term regression refers to trying to regress or bring all the points from the scatter diagram as close as possible to the estimated line.

For example, suppose that the Chief Nurse Executive wanted to make a rough starting prediction for the total cost of all nursing units in a hospital for the coming year. If last year there were 50,000 patient days and this coming year patient days are expected to be 52,000, then there is a 4% expected increase in the number of patient days. However, it cannot be assumed that all nursing costs will go up by 4% because some costs, like the salary of the Chief Nurse Executive, are fixed and will not rise in proportion to the number of patient days.

The high-low method discussed above would be one way to make the prediction, but the high-low method relies on only two data points. Far greater accuracy in breaking out fixed and variable costs is possible if the past years' costs were examined on a detailed basis, cost item by cost item, to determine which were fixed and which were variable. This would be a time-consuming procedure. Gathering information costs money, and even if that information were gathered, there are always some costs that cannot be separated into fixed and variable components without some estimating methodology because they are mixed costs. For example, nonmedical supplies such as paper, pens, and forms will be needed to some extent regardless of patient volume. On the other hand, the more patients, the more nonmedical supplies used. How can you separate that cost into the fixed portion and the variable portion? Even looking at past cost records cost item by cost item will not allow you to determine how much of the cost was fixed and how much was variable. In this case, how can costs be divided into their fixed and variable components and less money spent on gathering information than by examining each line item from past years? Regression analysis can help to separate these mixed costs.

Mixed Costs and Regression Analysis

Suppose it is known that last year the combined cost of the salary of the nurse manager and the disposable supplies was $110,000 and that the number of patient days was 50,000. This uses the information represented in the graphs presented in Figures 4–1 through 4–3. The volume of patient days is expected to go up to 52,000 next year. Should the $110,000 cost be increased by 4% because volume is increasing by 4%? No, it should not. Some costs are fixed. Only variable costs would increase as volume increases.

One would expect costs to increase by $2,000, or $1 for each extra patient day, because it is known in this example that variable costs for the disposable thermometer covers were described in this simple example as being $1 per patient day. However, dealing with a more realistic example with many different fixed, variable, and mixed costs, the variable costs per patient day would not necessarily be known. Suppose that the following historical information were available (already adjusted for inflation using the indexing techniques):

Year	Patient Days	Cost
1992	40,000	101,000
1993	42,000	102,000
1994	43,000	103,000
1995	44,000	104,000
1996	45,000	105,000
1997	46,000	106,000
1998	47,000	107,000
1999	48,000	108,000
2000	49,000	109,000
2001	50,000	110,000

If the high-low technique were used to evaluate the fixed and variable costs, there would be a strange result. The highest cost is $110,000, and the lowest cost is $101,000; costs have risen by $9,000. At the same time, volume has increased from 40,000 patient days to 50,000 patient days, or an increase of 10,000. When $9,000 is divided by 10,000 patient days, a variable cost of $.90 per patient day results. Is this an accurate estimate? No, because it is known that the variable cost is $1 per patient day. What might be the cause of the discrepancy?

It is possible that 1992 was the first year that disposable thermometer covers were used. Perhaps many of them were defective and were thrown away, or perhaps some were wasted because of lack of familiarity with using them. In any case, if more than $1 per patient day was spent on disposables in the low-volume year, then the costs were unduly high in that year. Therefore, the change in cost from 1992 to 2001 looks unrealistically low, and the variable cost measure is unrealistically low.

At the other extreme, had there been unusual waste (perhaps the fault of the nurses, but possibly due to quality problems with a large batch of the disposable item) in the most recent, high-cost year, the change in cost would look especially high and the variable cost per unit would have come out to more than $1. As has been stated before, if you rely on just two data points, as the high-low method does, your results are subject to the whims of unusual events in either one of those years.

In reality, one would not expect to use exactly $1 per patient day on disposable supplies in any year. For one reason or another, some patients will have their temperature taken only once on a given day. This might be caused by admission to the hospital late in the day, for instance. On the other hand, patients running a fever will undoubtedly have their temperature taken more often. A pattern of costs that is more likely to be observed is as follows:

Year	Patient Days	Cost
1992	40,000	101,000
1993	42,000	101,800
1994	43,000	103,600
1995	44,000	103,800
1996	45,000	105,300
1997	46,000	106,700
1998	47,000	106,900
1999	48,000	108,800
2000	49,000	108,900
2001	50,000	110,000

Simply looking at this list does not provide a lot of insight about fixed and variable costs. Figure 4–7 shows a scatter diagram for these points. By looking at this diagram, one can roughly see how the costs are increasing as volume increases. A straight line cannot go through all the points on this scatter diagram.

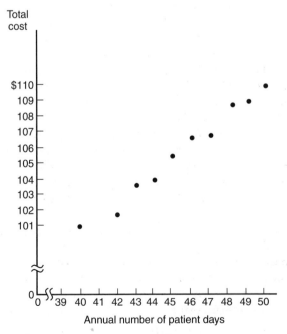

FIGURE 4–7. Scatter diagram of total costs for nursing (costs and patient days in thousands).

However, the regression technique uses all the available information to select a line that will provide the best estimate, in the absence of any other information.

Regression analysis uses information about the dependent and independent variables in the past to develop an equation for a straight line. As part of that process, it calculates a constant value and a coefficient for the independent variable. If the dependent variable is the cost, then the constant represents the fixed cost, and the coefficient of the independent variable represents the variable cost.

Regression analysis is a statistical technique. A detailed discussion of statistics is beyond the scope of this book. However, there are many mechanical approaches to regression that have made it a workable tool for use in health care institutions. Regression can be performed on many handheld calculators. There are also a wide variety of statistical programs and spreadsheet programs for personal computers that have regression capability.

Turning back now to the scatter diagram in Figure 4–7, it is possible to use regression analysis to predict what the costs will be for the nursing unit next year if there are 52,000 patient days. Regression analysis will determine a specific line to plot through this scatter diagram that will give the best possible estimate of fixed and variable costs and therefore allow prediction of the cost next year.

Basically, the process requires several simple steps. First determine the cost associated with each volume of patient days. For instance, when there were 40,000 patient days, the cost was $101,000. The independent variable, patient days, is often referred to as the X variable because it is plotted on the horizontal axis. The dependent variable, cost, is often referred to as the Y variable, because cost is plotted on the vertical axis.

Any computer program used will require that you provide the X values and the Y values for each year. Having provided that information, it is generally only necessary to give a command to compute the regression in order to complete the process. It is important not to let the extremely quantitative nature of regression theory learned in a statistics course discourage you from attempting to use this tool. In practice, little mathematics is required of the user. Regression is a tool to help you manage better. The major difficulty in using regression is simply a fear of the process (and this relates not only to nurses but also to most managers throughout most industries).

In the example, regression analysis predicts that the fixed cost is $62,255 and the variable cost is $.96 per unit. Figure 4–8 shows the resulting line. If extended to the left, the line would have its intercept at $62,255, increasing with a slope of .96. These figures are not exactly the expected variable cost of $1 per patient day and fixed cost of $60,000 for the salary of the nurse manager. They are, however, better estimates than the ones the high-low method would give us. The high-low approach predicts a fixed cost of $50,000 and a variable cost of $.90 per patient day. Regression analysis is an inexpensive, potentially very useful, and relatively simple way of estimating fixed and variable costs and helping to predict the future.

For any number of patient days predicted, it is now possible to multiply by

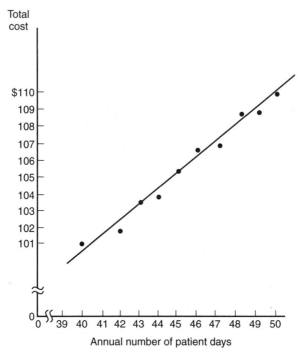

FIGURE 4–8. Simple linear regression of total costs for nursing (costs and patient days in thousands).

.96 and then add $62,225 to get a forecast of future costs. In many of the computer regression packages, the process is made even simpler by just requiring that the forecast volume be entered into the computer along with the historical data. The computer will then generate the estimated cost for the coming year automatically, based on the forecast volume. Remember, however, that it is necessary to adjust upward the resulting cost for expected increases due to inflation for the coming year.

While you will soon find this approach to be quite simple, it is useful only as a tool to aid you in managing. It should not be allowed to take over the role of your judgment. The mathematical model is accurate in predicting the future if nothing has changed. It is your role as a manager to know if there are reasons that costs would be likely to change from their past patterns.

For instance, if you knew that 1992 was the first year disposable thermometer covers were used and that there was an awful lot of waste that year, you might want to eliminate that year from the analysis. If you did, your regression results would have shown fixed costs of $59,970 and variable costs of $1.005. Recall that the fixed costs were actually $60,000 and the variable costs were $1.00. As you can see, the input of judgment into the process can substantially improve the resulting estimates.

When a regression analysis is performed, one statistic that is generally provided by the calculator or the computer is the R-squared (R^2). This value can range from a low of zero to a high of 1.0. If the value is close to zero, it means that the independent variable does not do a good job of explaining the changes in the dependent variable. An R-squared of .20, for example, might indicate that patient days are not a good predictor of nursing cost. On the other hand, an R-squared of .80 would indicate that it is a very good predictor. However, it is possible to become even more exact in estimating costs, by using multiple regression analysis.

Multiple Regression Analysis

There is a type of regression analysis that is more sophisticated than simple linear regression. It is called multiple regression because it allows for use of multiple independent, or causal, variables. The use of simple linear regression can be a substantial aid in estimating future costs because it is so efficient at predicting the fixed cost and the variable cost per unit when there is one major independent variable. Sometimes, however, there will be several key variables. For instance, suppose that the nursing costs vary with the number of patient days but also with the number of patients. That is most probably the case.

Certainly the costs vary with the number of patient days. The more patient days, the more temperatures to be taken, pulses to be checked, medications to be administered, and so on. Yet for each patient there is a medical history to be recorded, a chart to be set up, a patient care plan to be established, valuables to be stored, orientation to be given, discharge planning to be done, discharge education, and so on. These costs are not fixed—the more patients, the more time spent on these activities—but they do not vary directly with the number of patient days. Several patients with a long length of stay will cost less than many patients with a short length of stay, even if the total patient days are the same. So it is likely that the cost of a nursing unit varies with both the number of patient days and the number of patients.

Most handheld business calculators will not perform multiple regression, although some will. However, most spreadsheet and statistical programs for personal computers can handle this easily. Instead of simply entering the X and Y values for each year into the calculator or computer, you now enter an X value for the historical information for each of the independent variables, as well as the Y value. Then when you want to predict a future cost, you provide the computer with, for example, the expected number of patient days and the expected number of patients, in order to predict the expected costs.

Sometimes, the multiple regression level of sophistication adds extra work and complexity without substantially changing the results. Recall that when all is said and done, the result is just an estimate; all types of events can happen in the future that will throw off the estimate, no matter how finely tuned it is. It is not necessary to add complexity for its own sake. At times, however, multiple regression can produce information that would not otherwise be available.

For example, there has been more and more attention placed on measures of patient acuity or the level of intensity of required nursing services. It certainly is clear that the amount of nursing services vary not just with the number of patient days but also with the severity of the patients' illnesses. If data about the number of patient days and the average acuity level are used as independent variables, the accuracy of estimated costs might improve substantially.

For a home care agency, costs might vary with the number of visits. However, the nurse manager might be able to better predict costs if the number of visits by nurses were used as one variable and the number of aide visits as another variable. We might even divide nurse visits into two variables—one for short visits and one for longer visits.

Another use for multiple regression is in investigatory work with respect to costs. Suppose that there is a strong feeling by the nursing staff that the way a particular physician practices medicine is extremely costly. This is common in the operating room, where particular surgeons often exhibit out-of-the-ordinary behavior. The number of operations by that specific physician each year can be used as an independent variable. If costs do increase as a result of more cases by that physician, it would show up as a positive coefficient for that independent variable. The nurse manager would then have evidence to support the more general feelings of the staff that the physician is an unusually high resource consumer.

The reader of this book is encouraged to pursue the topic of regression analysis further. This should be done on both a conceptual basis, reviewing the underlying principles and theories of regression analysis, and on a practical basis, using a computer software package to perform some regression analyses.

BREAK-EVEN ANALYSIS

To this point the general behavior of costs (fixed vs. variable) has been discussed, as well as the techniques for cost estimation (high-low and regression). Attention will now be focused on using cost information for understanding whether a particular unit or service will lose money, make money, or just break even. This technique is useful for the evaluation of both new and continuing projects or services. It is often used in developing a business plan. Business plans are discussed in Chapter 7.

Nurse managers in many instances find it necessary to be able to determine whether a program or service will be profitable. One key to profitability is volume. Prices are often fixed. Average cost, however, is not fixed. As the number of patients rises, the cost per patient falls because of the sharing of fixed costs. One cannot make a simple comparison of price and average cost and determine that a program or unit will make a profit or a loss. To determine whether something will be profitable, it is critical to know the volume of patients. Break-even analysis is a technique that is used to find the specific volume at which a program or service neither makes nor loses money. Forecast information about the likely volume of the service can be compared to the break-even volume to predict whether there will be profits or losses.

Break-even analysis is based on the following formula:

$$\text{The Break-Even Quantity (Q)} = \frac{\text{Fixed Costs (FC)}}{\text{Price (P)} - \text{Variable Cost per Patient (VC)}}$$

or

$$Q = \frac{FC}{P - VC}$$

where Q is the number of patients needed to just break even, FC is the total fixed cost, P is the price for each patient, and VC is the variable cost per patient. At a quantity lower than Q there would be a loss; at a quantity higher than Q there would be a profit. The P is assumed to be the average amount collected per patient. Often health care organizations give discounts or have bad debts or charity care. This analysis is not based on a P equal to the charge for the service but instead considers P to be the average amount of revenue the organization ultimately receives per patient.

The basis for the formula is the underlying relationship between revenues and expenses. If total revenues are greater than expenses, there is a profit. If total revenues are less than expenses, there is a loss. If revenues are just equal to expenses, there is neither profit nor loss, and the service is said to just break even. Expenses are the sum of the total fixed costs and total variable costs.

A Break-Even Analysis Example

For example, suppose that an integrated health care delivery system opens a new home health agency that charges, on average, $50 per visit. The agency has fixed costs of $10,000 and variable costs of $30 per patient visit. If there are no patients at all, there is no revenue, but there are fixed costs of $10,000, and there is a $10,000 loss. If there were 100 patients, there would be $5,000 of revenue ($50 times 100 patients), $10,000 of fixed cost, and $3,000 of variable cost ($30 times 100 patients). Total costs would be $13,000 ($10,000 of fixed cost plus $3,000 of variable cost), while revenues are $5,000, and the loss is $8,000. This data is hypothetical.

Each additional patient brings in $50 of revenue but causes the agency to spend only $30 more. The difference between the $50 price and the $30 variable cost, $20, is called the *contribution margin*. If the contribution margin is positive, it means that each extra unit of activity makes the organization better off by that amount. The contribution margin from each patient can be used to cover fixed costs, or if all fixed costs have been covered, it represents a profit.

In this example, when there are 100 patients, there is $20 of contribution margin for each of the 100 patients, or a total contribution margin of $2,000.

Note that the loss with zero patients was $10,000, while it was only $8,000 when there were 100 patients. The loss decreased by $2,000—exactly the amount of the total contribution margin for those 100 patients.

How many visits would the agency need to have to break even? The answer is 500. If each additional patient generates $20 of contribution margin, then 500 patients would generate $10,000 of contribution margin (500 patients × $20 = $10,000), exactly enough to cover the fixed costs of $10,000. If the agency has 500 patients, it will just break even.

This could have been calculated using the formula:

$$Q = \frac{FC}{P - VC}$$

or

$$Q = \frac{\$10,000}{\$50 - \$30} = \frac{\$10,000}{\$20} = 500 \text{ visits}$$

Break-even analysis can also be viewed from a graphical perspective (Fig. 4–9). The total cost line starts at a level of $10,000 because of the fixed costs. The total revenue line starts at zero, because there is no revenue if there are zero patients. Where the revenue line and the total cost line intersect, they are equal, and the agency just breaks even. Note that at quantities of patients less than the break-even point, the cost line is higher than the revenue line. This means that for

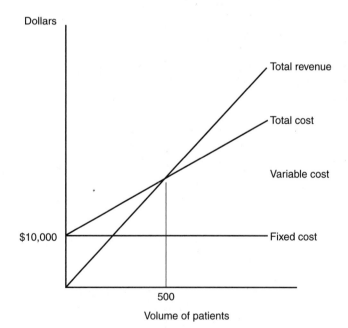

FIGURE 4–9. Break-even analysis.

that volume the total costs are more than the total revenues. The organization will lose money. At quantities of patients above the break-even point, the revenue line is higher than the costs and a profit is made.

Break-even analyses can focus on the number of patient days needed to break even or on the total number of patients, surgeries, clinic visits, or other appropriate volume measure.

When there are different types of patients, break-even becomes more complicated. The formula presented at the beginning of this section assumes that there is only one price and one variable cost, and therefore one contribution margin. If there are different types of patients with different prices and different variable costs, it is necessary to find a weighted average contribution margin. This weighted average can be divided into the fixed costs to find the break-even volume for all patients.

For example, suppose that there are three classes of home care visits, which will be referred to here as complex, moderate, and simple. The price for the visits is $80, $50, and $30, and the variable costs for the visits are $55, $30, and $20, respectively. The contribution margin for each type of patient can be calculated by subtracting the variable cost from the price, as follows:

	Price		Variable Cost		Contribution Margin
Complex	$80	−	$55	=	$25
Moderate	50	−	30	=	20
Simple	30	−	20	=	10

The crucial piece of information for calculating the break-even point is the relative proportion of each type of visit. Management of the home health agency expect that 20% of all visits are complex, 30% are moderate, and 50% are simple. This information can be used to determine a weighted average contribution margin. This requires multiplying each type of visit's individual contribution margin by the percentage of patients that type of visit makes up. The results are added together to get an overall weighted contribution margin, as follows:

Visit Type	Percentage of Visits		Contribution Margin		Weighted Average Contribution Margin
Complex	20%	×	$25	=	$ 5
Moderate	30%	×	20	=	6
Simple	50%	×	10	=	5
TOTAL WEIGHTED AVERAGE CONTRIBUTION MARGIN					$16

This $16 weighted contribution margin (CM) represents the average contribution margin for all types of visits. It can be used to calculate the break-even quantity. Assume that fixed costs are $10,000. The break-even quantity of visits is:

$$Q = \frac{FC}{P - VC} = \frac{FC}{CM}$$

or

$$Q = \frac{\$10,000}{\$16} = 625 \text{ visits}$$

Of the total of 625 visits needed to break even, 20% or 125 would be expected to be complex, 30% or 188 would be moderate, and 50% or 312 would be simple.

This method works for three different kinds of patients. What if there were more than three kinds? The same weighted average approach that can be used to find the break-even volume when there are three different types of patients could be used even if there were hundreds of different types of patients, as is the case with the Medicare DRG system. Similarly, for outpatient care, patients can fall into a number of different categories.

What if there is more than one price for each type of patient? Medicaid pays one price, Medicare another, HMOs another, and self-pay yet another. This still can work within the same framework that has been presented. It would be necessary to calculate a weighted average contribution margin treating each payer for each type of patient as a separate group. For example, if Medicaid pays $40 per visit regardless of the type of visit, and the other payment rates are the same as indicated earlier, the contribution margin by type of patient by payer would be as follows:

	Price	Variable Cost	Contribution Margin
Complex Medicaid	$40	$55	($15)
Complex Other	80	55	25
Moderate Medicaid	40	30	10
Moderate Other	50	30	20
Simple Medicaid	40	20	20
Simple Other	30	20	10

If it is possible to anticipate the percentage of patients that will be Medicaid, a weighted average contribution margin can be estimated. Assume that 10% of all patients are Medicaid complex patients and 10% are other complex patients. Assume that 20% of all patients are Medicaid moderate patients and 10% of all patients are other moderate patients. Assume that 30% of all patients are Medicaid simple patients and 20% of all patients are other simple patients. The weighted contribution margin would be:

Visit Type	Percentage of Visits		Contribution Margin		Weighted Average Contribution Margin
Complex Medicaid	10%	×	($15)	=	($ 1.5)
Complex Other	10%	×	25	=	2.5
Moderate Medicaid	20%	×	10	=	2.0
Moderate Other	10%	×	20	=	2.0
Simple Medicaid	30%	×	20	=	6.0
Simple Other	20%	×	10	=	2.0
TOTAL WEIGHTED AVERAGE CONTRIBUTION MARGIN					$13.0

The break-even volume could then be calculated as follows:

$$Q = \frac{FC}{P - VC} = \frac{FC}{CM}$$

or

$$Q = \frac{\$10,000}{\$13} = 769 \text{ visits}$$

The number of visits of any type could be determined by multiplying the 769 break-even volume times the percent of patients in any given class. For example, since 30% of the patients are Medicaid simple, 30% of 769, or 231 Medicaid simple patients would be expected at the break-even level.

Using Break-Even Analysis for Decision Making

If a particular service is expected to have a volume of activity well in excess of the break-even point, managers have a clear-cut decision to start or continue the service. If the volume is too low to break even, several options exist.

One approach is to lower the volume needed to break even. There are three ways to reduce the required break-even level. One approach is to lower the fixed costs. In some cases, it might be possible to do that. Another alternative would be to increase prices. Price increases would increase the contribution margin per patient. This would also have the effect of lowering the break-even point. However, price increases might reduce the expected volume. In that case, the price increases would be defeating their purpose. Also, prices are sometimes regulated and beyond the control of the organization. Finally, one could try to reduce the variable cost per unit. This might be accomplished by increased efforts toward improved efficiency.

If it is not feasible to change the fixed costs, price, or variable costs, an organization can try to attract more patients so that the volume will rise above the break-even point. In the example presented, what type of patients would be desirable? The most desirable type of visit is a complex, non-Medicaid patient. That patient yields a contribution margin of $25 per patient. The least desirable is a Medicaid complex patient. The contribution margin is negative. For each additional complex Medicaid patient, the agency loses money. In this particular example, the most attractive patient has the highest revenue. However, the focus should not be on revenue. If the highest revenue patient also had extremely high variable costs, it might not be as attractive as a patient with lower revenue and much lower variable costs. The attractiveness of additional patients is determined by how much contribution margin they provide to the organization.

Break-Even and Capitation

As managed care has become more and more prevalent, many negotiated contracts call for capitated payments. In such an arrangement, the managed care organization pays the health care provider a set amount for each member for each month. This is called the PMPM (per member per month) payment. Under capitation, an increase in the amount of services provided to patients will not cause revenues to increase. On the other hand, an increase in the number of members will increase revenues.

Suppose that an HMO were to offer a home health agency $1 per member per month to provide all home care services for all its members. Over the course of a year revenue would be $12 per member ($1 PMPM time twelve months = $12). Assume that the agency's variable costs are $30 per visit. Furthermore, the agency will have increased fixed costs of $20,000 if it takes the HMO members. How many members would the HMO need to have for the home health agency to break even on the contract?

We can use break-even analysis to calculate the break-even number of members. The fixed costs are $20,000. The variable costs are $30 per visit. The price is $12 per member per year. However, we do not have enough information to calculate the break-even point. This is because we only know the variable cost per visit. We need to know the variable cost per member per year. In order to find the break-even volume of members, it is necessary to predict the utilization levels—that is, the number of home visits each member will have.

Most individuals will not need any visits in a typical year. Suppose that the average person consumes .3 visits in a given year.* The variable cost for .3 visits per year is $9 (the $30 variable cost per visit multiplied by .3 visits per year). That $9 represents the variable cost per member per year. We can now calculate the break-even point as follows:

$$Q = \frac{FC}{P - VC}$$

$$Q = \frac{\$10,000}{\$12 - \$9} = 3,333 \text{ members}$$

Both the price and the variable costs in the calculation are per member per year. The quantity calculated represents the number of members needed to break even. If the HMO guarantees 5,000 members, the agency will likely make a profit. If there are only 2,000 members, it will lose money.

What if the agency has other fixed costs as well. Are they needed for the calculation? No. The determination of whether the HMO contract is profitable depends only on the marginal costs of the contract. Fixed costs that exist whether the agency contracts with the HMO or not are not relevant to the decision or calculation. What if the HMO contract did not cause fixed costs to rise? Then the contract would be profitable for the agency as long as the revenue per member per year exceeded the variable cost per member per year.

---

*To avoid using fractions, HMOs often perform their analyses per thousand members. They would say they expect 300 visits per year per thousand members. That approach would not have an effect on the number of members needed to break even.

Break-Even Analysis Cautions

A few words of caution are advisable when working with break-even analysis. First of all, once a break-even point is calculated, one must decide whether it is likely that actual volume will be sufficient to exceed that point. This will require a volume forecast, such as those shown in Chapter 6. To the extent that the forecast of volume is incorrect, the decision to go ahead with a new service may turn out to be a bad one, even if the break-even analysis is perfect.

Another potential problem is that break-even analysis assumes that prices and costs are constant. If it can be reasonably expected that prices will fall over time, then a higher volume would be needed to keep a service viable, unless variable or fixed costs would be falling as well. On the other hand, if prices are expected to rise faster than costs, then a marginal service today may become profitable over time, even without an increase in volume.

Another consideration is that there is an assumption that the mix of patients will stay constant. Suppose that in the above example, over time there are more and more Medicaid complex patients. The contribution margin for such patients is negative. If the demographics of the population are such that a shift in mix in that direction is likely, then the results of the break-even analysis require very close scrutiny. Will there be enough of those patients to shift a profitable service over to a loss?

As with all budgeting tools, judgment is essential. The nurse manager must, through experience, insight, and thought, examine the assumptions of any modeling technique and also consider the reasonableness of the results. If a result does not seem to make sense, this is often because it does not make sense. However, break-even analysis is a tool that can help give a manager a firm starting point in understanding whether or not a project or service is likely to be financially viable.

ACTIVITY BASED COSTING

Activity based costing (ABC) is a relatively new approach to determining costs. In the last half of the 1990s, ABC started to become used widely in health care organizations. The approach is based on the observation that costs are incurred because of specific activities. In most costing methods, costs are assigned to cost centers and patients based on some measure of volume, such as patient days, visits, or hours. For example, operating room (OR) costs are assigned to patients based on minutes in the OR. From an ABC perspective, it is not necessarily the amount of time but rather the specific activities that generate costs. Based on this notion, managers need to focus on the actions that drive costs higher. The activities of an organization that cause it to incur costs are referred to as *cost drivers*.

The use of cost drivers to assign costs has the impact of improving accuracy by focusing cost measurement more on a cause-and-effect basis. For example, suppose that a health care organization has a purchasing department that orders many items on a routine basis and some items on a special-order basis. The activity is placing orders. However, it is quite possible that a special order will be more costly than a routine order.

The costs of the purchasing departments must be allocated to patients if the organization is to recover its full costs. One common approach to such allocation is based on the number of purchase orders. Departments that generate a lot of purchase orders are assigned a greater share of the cost of the purchasing department. In turn, those costs are allocated to patients that use the department. This seems to be quite reasonable.

However, if a rush order is an activity that causes purchasing to spend extra money (on the time of the personnel in the department, express freight costs, etc.), then from an ABC perspective one would argue that the departments that generate a large number of rush orders should be charged more than departments that don't, all other things being equal. In other words, costs should not be assigned simply based on the number of purchase orders generated by each department. Within purchasing, the activity of placing a rush order is more costly than the activity of placing a regular order. Rush orders drive costs higher.

The ABC approach requires the manager to analyze the activities of each cost center or department in an organization. The various activities that are cost drivers must be identified. Then costs are assigned to departments and ultimately to patients based on the amount of cost-driving activities they require.

For example, suppose that an operating room has traditionally assigned its costs based on minutes of surgery. A patient with a 2-hour surgery is charged twice as much as a patient with a 1-hour surgery. However, one of the costs of surgery is cleaning and preparing the room after every surgery. Suppose that those costs are the same for each surgery, regardless of the length of the surgery. The activity of cleaning and preparing the room should then be charged equally to each surgical patient, rather than being based on the length of the surgical procedure.

This probably means that more allocation bases will be needed. The depreciation cost of the surgical suite may be charged to patients based on the length of the procedure. The cost of cleaning the room may be charged equally per patient. The cost of supplies consumed during the surgery should include the extra cost of any rush orders that were required for the procedure. This will complicate the costing process but will produce substantially more accurate information. ABC proponents argue that most industries really do not have a good sense of which of their products or services are profitable and which lose money. Further, employees may be more cost conscious if they use ABC information.

Consider the purchasing department/operating room examples discussed in this section. The surgical patients who require special-order items are being subsidized under the old costing system. The costs of the rush orders are being spread over all departments that order supplies. This could cause a particular type of surgery to appear more profitable than it is, because the true costs of the rush orders are not assigned to the departments and patients that caused the special orders.

However, once the ABC system is in place, that will change. The OR will be charged directly for each special order. It can then assign the order to specific patients who required the rush-order items. This in turn will provide more accurate information about the cost of care for each type of patient. Further, seeing the higher costs resulting from rush orders, the manager of the OR may plan more carefully, thus avoiding the need for many of the rush orders. This will reduce the total costs for the patient, department, and organization.

In terms of routine medical or surgical nursing, using ABC requires an examination of what nurses do and why they do it. ABC works well with the concept of value-added costs. By examining everything we do to determine the cost drivers, we can also assess whether each activity adds value to the patient. If it doesn't, perhaps it can be eliminated. If it does add value, then the cost of the activity should be assigned to the patient who directly benefits from it.

One problem with ABC is deciding how minutely to define activities. Is taking a pulse or blood pressure an activity? Certainly. However, should we determine the cost of that activity and then track how many times each is done for each patient? This is not an easy question. From a clinical perspective, we already track such activities in the patient chart. However, until costing and clinical systems are fully linked, it would require additional data input to track the activity for costing purposes. And what about activities that are necessary but never enter the clinical chart? With ABC, as with any approach to costing, we must always balance the value of more accurate information against the extra cost of collecting that information.

SUMMARY AND IMPLICATIONS FOR NURSE MANAGERS

Assessing costs is a complex topic. In general, costs do not increase in proportion with volume. The implications of this are that, while money might be lost on a particular program, higher volume may be desired. More patients do not necessarily mean greater losses. It is possible that volume increases can turn a loss into a profit. Understanding how that can happen requires an understanding of cost behavior. Some costs are fixed, while other costs are variable. The result of that basic nature of costs is that the cost per patient will decline as there is increasing volume. The greater the number of patients that share the fixed costs, the lower the average cost per patient. Costing is further complicated by the fact that, since not all costs vary with volume, there are times when decisions must be based solely on the costs that do vary. This is referred to as relevant costing.

An important part of the budgeting process is the prediction of costs. Estimated costs for the future can be based upon historical cost information. Some estimation relies upon using the historical information to isolate variable costs from fixed costs. In order to make such calculations, it is first necessary to convert historical cost information into common or constant dollars. This requires *indexation* of costs for the impact of inflation. Indexation is a process that adjusts a dollar value for the impact of inflation over a period of time by using a *price index,* such as the Consumer Price Index (CPI). A price index is a tool that indicates year-to-year changes in prices. Using indexed historical costs, the results of the cost-estimation process will be in constant dollars. In preparing next year's budget, the cost estimate has to be adjusted upward by the anticipated inflation rate over the next year.

Once constant-dollar information is available, cost can be estimated using the high-low method, simple linear regression, or multiple regression analysis. Being able to estimate fixed and variable costs is potentially a valuable tool. In order to apply the results, however, projections of the estimated number of patients, patient days, acuity level, and so forth are needed. Chapter 6 focuses on the process of forecasting such data.

Break-even analysis is a tool that allows one to focus specifically on the quantity of patients needed for a program, project, or service to be financially viable. Its foundations are in fixed and variable costs. At low volumes of patients, the average cost may surpass the revenue per patient. As the number of patients increases, the cost per patient falls as fixed costs are shared. Eventually the cost per patient falls below the revenue. Break-even analysis allows the manager to determine what the break-even quantity is, so that a reasonable decision can be made about the financial viability of a program, project, or service.

From the nurse manager's standpoint, the topics of this chapter have critical implications. At the most basic levels, falling volume will mean rising cost per patient. In such cases it is likely that a revenue crisis will exist, and actions to restrain costs should be immediately contemplated. On the other hand, rising volumes represent an opportunity. They not only bring in more revenue but also decrease the average cost per patient. Therefore, there is the opportunity for profit from more patients and for more profit from each patient. Profits ultimately allow the organization to replace buildings and equipment, add services, add staff, improve quality, and raise salaries.

Additionally, in preparing budgets, nurse managers should take into account the behavior of costs. The fact that certain costs vary in proportion while others are fixed may reorient your thinking from the notion that a 10% increase in volume requires 10% more resources. This in turn can allow a manager to prepare budgets in a more sophisticated and exact manner.

Similarly, the use of ABC can assist the manager in obtaining a more accurate measure of costs. Accuracy in turn leads to better decisions and ultimately to improved financial results.

SUGGESTED READINGS

Anderson, L., and Clancy, D. (1998). *Cost Accounting*, Second edition. Houston: Dame Publications.

Baker, J.J. (1998). *Activity-based Costing and Activity-based Management for Health Care*. Gaithersburg, MD: Aspen Publishers.

Baker, J.J., and Boyd, G.F. (1997, Fall). Activity based costing in the operating room at Valley View Hospital. *Journal of Health Care Finance*. 24(1), 1–9.

Bruttomesso, K.A. (1995, January). Variable hospital accounting practices: Are they fair for the nursing department? *Journal of Nursing Administration*. 25(1), 6.

Cleverley, W.O. (1997). *Essentials of Health Care Finance*, Fourth edition. Gaithersburg, MD: Aspen Publishers.

Crockett, M.J., et al. (1997, November). Activity-based resource allocation: A system for predicting nursing costs. *Rehabilitation Nursing*. 22(6), 293–298, 302.

Dodson, G.M., Sinclair, V.G., Miller, M., et al. (1998, September–October). Determining cost drivers for pediatric home health services. *Nursing Economic$*. 16(5), 263–271.

Finkler, S.A. (1995, February). Breakeven analysis for capitated arrangements. *Hospital Cost Management & Accounting*. 6(11), 1–2.

Finkler, S.A., and Ward, D.R. (1999). *Cost Accounting for Health Care Organizations: Concepts and Applications*, Second edition. Gaithersburg, MD: Aspen Publishers.

Garber, A.M., and Phelps, C.E. (1997, February). Economic foundations of cost-effectiveness analysis. *Journal of Health Economics*. 16(1), 1–31.

Hansen, D., and Mowen, M. (1997). *Cost Management*, Second edition. Cincinnati: South-Western Publishing.

Heshmat, S. (1997, Winter). Managed care and the relevant costs for pricing. *Health Care Management Review*. 22(1), 82–85.

Jones, K.R. (1995, September). Standard cost accounting. *Seminars for Nurse Managers*. 3(3), 111–112.

McKeon, T. (1996, January). Activity-based management: A tool to complement and quantify continuous quality improvement efforts. *Journal of Nursing Care Quality*. 10(2), 17–24.

Neumann, B.R., Clement, J.P., and Cooper, J.C. (1997). *Financial Management: Concepts and Applications for Health Care Organizations*. Dubuque, Iowa: Kendall Hunt Publishing.

Pelfrey, S. (1995, December). Cost-accounting techniques for health care providers. *Health Care Supervisor*. 14(2), 33–42.

Storfjell, J.L., and Jessup, S. (1996, December). Bridging the gap between finance and clinical operations with activity-based cost management. *Journal of Nursing Administration*. 36:13, 12–17.

Swindle, R.W., et al. (1996, March). The quality of cost data: A caution from the Department of Veterans Affairs experience. *Medical Care*. 34(3), 83–90.

West, D.A., West, T.D., Balas, E.A., and Micks, L.L. (1996, May–June). Profitable capitation requires accurate costing. *Nursing Economic$*. 14(3), 162–170, 150.

Wodchis, W.P. (1998, Winter). Applying activity-based costing in long-term care. *Healthcare Management Forum*. 11(4), 25–32.

5

Personnel Issues*

The goals of this chapter are to:

explain the relationship between nursing shortages and budgeting;

explain how to lessen the impact of nursing shortages;

provide some insights on how an organization can work to limit its own nursing shortages through retention and recruitment;

describe causes of nursing shortages;

outline the various costs associated with nurse recruitment; and

identify some alternative solutions when staff nurses are in short supply.

BUDGETING AND NURSING SHORTAGES

The largest part of most operating budgets for nursing units, departments, and organizations consists of *personnel* costs. Getting an operating budget approved is sometimes difficult. Justifying the need for a given level of staff requires careful calculations and a lucid argument. However, in preparing an operating budget, it is often assumed that hiring the amount of labor approved in the final budget is not a problem. This is not necessarily the case in nursing. Nursing shortages occurred on and off throughout the last half of the twentieth century. The existence of budgeted but vacant positions is a common occurrence. It also creates a great deal of budgeting difficulty.

At the time the reader uses this book, there may or may not be a nursing shortage. However, issues related to recruitment, retention, and the impact of nursing shortages on the budget preparation process are a critical part of budgeting. History has shown that nursing shortages occur from time to time. Nurse managers should be prepared to work through the budget process to lessen

---

*Note: This chapter focuses primarily on issues of nursing shortages, nurse recruitment, and nurse retention. Readers familiar with the literature in this area may choose to skip this chapter. It is included in this book because it is critical that all nurse managers with budget responsibility have at least some exposure to these issues.

the impact of such shortages on their organization when they occur. Therefore, this chapter represents a topic that is essential reading whether a critical shortage of nursing currently exists or not.

If vacant positions are left unstaffed throughout the year, two potentially serious side effects occur. The first is that the nurses working on a unit begin to suffer burnout from being overburdened. Shortages of staff lead to overwork, poor morale, increased sick leave, and other stress-related problems. This in turn tends to lead to loss of staff, exacerbating the shortage on the unit.

The second side effect is that the health care organization starts to assume that less money will be spent than has been put into the budget. Positions are approved with the expectation that they will never be filled. Eventually, if staff is finally available to be hired, the organization may resist filling the positions because it has made its overall plans based on the expectation that the money allocated for those positions would never be spent. The approved but vacant positions provide top management with a cushion to ease the impact of other unexpected financial problems throughout the year. Essentially, the budgeted but unfilled positions may be permanently lost. This effectively lowers the nursing care hours per patient day, procedure, or visit on a permanent basis.

Both of these side effects are offset at least partially if the money budgeted for the vacant positions is spent on some combination of overtime and per diem agency nurse use. This creates additional budgeting difficulties because it is rare that the cost of overtime and agency nurses will match the budgeted cost for the vacant positions. On a per hour basis, both overtime and agency nurses are more expensive than the cost of a full-time staff member being paid on a straight-time basis. This excess hourly cost is partially offset by the fact that the position may not need to be staffed every day. However, it may be difficult to determine whether the net effect will be greater or less spending, as compared to filling the vacant position(s).

An attempt must be made to budget based on the expected *actual* staffing pattern. If 12 FTEs are authorized in a budget, the dollars in the budget should be based on the best expectation of how those 12 FTEs will be staffed. If the most likely event is that the unit will be able to have 11 regular full-time staff members, but that the 12th position will be covered with 1,200 hours of agency nurse time, then the budget should replace the cost of the 12th staff member with the cost of 1,200 agency nurse hours. In order for such a calculation to be made, it is critical to have some idea as to whether the 12th position will be staffed by hiring a staff member or using agency nurses. Alternatively, the 12th position could be covered by regular staff overtime.

Another approach is to revise the manner in which nursing care is offered. Nursing units can be reorganized to make greater use of alternative types of personnel. Or computers could be acquired in an effort to reduce the number of nursing hours needed for documentation. It is likely that attempts to introduce shared governance, case management, alternative manpower, or computers will have an impact on the actual spending of a nursing unit. These expected changes and their costs should be built into the budget.

Some health care organizations will attempt to "stretch" their available staff over the existing number of patients when an adequate number of nurses cannot be recruited. Such stretching can only mean fewer nursing hours per patient day and a lower quality of care. It is the obligation of the organization and its employees to be explicit in addressing both the problem and its ultimate impact on care. Such explicit recognition is not only ethically correct but also likely to push the organization to work harder to resolve its nursing shortages.

Therefore, before the development of operating budgets can be discussed fully in Chapter 8, it is important to address issues that are related to nursing recruitment and retention as well as to alternative models of providing patient care. This is the topic of the remainder of this chapter.

THE NURSING SHORTAGE AND ITS CAUSES

Has there really been a nursing shortage? The answer to this question would clearly be yes. There have been unfilled positions. Many health care organizations have not been able to hire as many RNs as they have wanted to. Has this shortage been caused by drastic reductions in the number of nurses? Perhaps surprisingly, the answer to that question would clearly be no. There are more nurses working as nurses today than ever before.

Part of this increase may be accounted for by increasing levels of patient acuity. As DRGs began to take effect in the 1980s, hospital lengths of stay dropped, and the average acuity level for the remaining inpatient days rose. On average, patients were sicker each day they were in the hospital. This trend increased under pressure from managed care organizations in the 1990s. Therefore, the average inpatient day requires more nursing care. At the same time, demand for nurses for home care and other types of ambulatory care has also grown at a rapid rate.

The long-term trends for availability of adequate numbers of RNs do not appear to be favorable. The aging of the American population constantly increases the demand for nurses. At the other end of the spectrum, there has been a declining number of people in the college-age group. Thus, as the need for nurses will probably continue to increase, the pool of people available to become nurses will not keep pace.

The shortage of nurses is also at least partly the result of the feminist movement, which has seen proportionately more women move away from traditionally female jobs than the number of men moving into such jobs. As growing numbers of women seek out employment as physicians, engineers, accountants, and lawyers, there are fewer women who are becoming nurses.

Nor has the nursing profession managed to overcome many serious image problems perpetuated by a wide variety of stereotypes that do not accurately reflect the profession. The actual degree of responsibility and autonomy of nursing is often not fairly depicted.

At times when a national shortage of nurses occurs, solutions have to be national in scope. They may involve major media campaigns by nursing associations to change nursing's image. They may involve federal infusions of cash to schools of nursing in the form of scholarship money. Many other national approaches have been suggested. Increases in the rate of pay for nurses may have a strong enough impact to eliminate shortages, but it takes time before wage increases can have much overall impact because of the years of education required once someone decides to go into nursing. To the extent that pay raises eliminate shortages, they fail to resolve many long-range problems, and shortages may occur again in the future as raises for nurses begin to lag when there is no existing shortage.

The remainder of this chapter will confine itself to the actions that individual nurse managers can take or should be aware of in their management of nursing within their organizations. A given organization may be relatively helpless when it comes to overcoming the entire industry nursing shortage. However, organizations have a great degree of control over the availability of their own nursing staff.

RETENTION OF STAFF

The most effective personnel strategy a health care organization can take is to work at retaining the staff it already has. Since national shortages of nurses mean that every nurse you hire must be hired away from somebody else, it is clear that recruiting nurses requires a costly level of competition. Therefore, major efforts should be made in an attempt to reduce undesired turnover. One key to staff retention is to have a high level of nurse satisfaction.

Nursing Satisfaction

Surprisingly, very little is known definitively about what leads to nurse satisfaction. There are many factors that are believed to be relevant to keeping a nursing staff happy. Studies have not consistently shown any one factor or any unique set of factors that are always present in satisfied staffs or whose absence will necessarily lead to a dissatisfied staff. Nevertheless, there are a number of elements that are generally accepted as being related to nursing satisfaction. These elements are discussed here.

One primary element of nursing satisfaction is the development of professionalism in the delivery of health care services through a combination of increased autonomy and the availability of resource personnel for consultation. Nurses must feel like professionals and be treated like professionals in order to be happy in their employment. Time cards, for example, are often thought to be demeaning for nurses and can lead to dissatisfaction. Similarly, working as hourly workers does not generally result in the same level of satisfaction as working as salaried employees.

A positive attitude toward nursing and professional treatment by the physician staff and the administration can be critical factors in having a satisfied staff. Negative attitudes by these groups can cause significant unhappiness on the part of the staff. This ties in with the overall issue of nursing image. The institution has little control over the national image of nursing. However, it can take strides toward creating a positive image internally. The way nurses are treated and the way nursing is presented to patients can make a substantial difference in the attitudes of nurses as well as the rest of the organization's staff. Image building begins with actions taken by nursing to create a positive image. Programs with physicians and administration can be suggested by nursing administration, if they are not forthcoming otherwise.

The issue of financial payment is, of course, relevant. High salaries and good benefits will help keep staff from wanting to look elsewhere. This also requires that there be ample opportunity for advancement, either into management or on a clinical track.

Flexible hours have also become a key to retaining staff. A wide variety of alternative working hours have been developed by organizations attempting to recruit new nurses. These flexible arrangements must be made available to existing staff as well or they may become dissatisfied and move to an organization that will offer such hours.

From a budgeting perspective, this can become complex. The use of four 10-hour shifts to create a 4-day work week is not a major budgeting problem. Although it may create a complicated staffing pattern for coverage, it still results in 40 hours of pay for 40 hours of work, the same as 5 days, 8 hours each. On the other hand, innovations such as three 12-hour shifts, or two 12-hour weekend shifts, for 40 hours of pay can create a variety of budgeting complications. Clear decisions must be made concerning whether a full-time equivalent (FTE) employee represents 40 hours of work or 40 hours of pay. (See Chapter 8 for further discussion.)

Fringe Benefits

Clearly, one of the elements of nursing satisfaction will be related to the organization's employee benefits, commonly referred to as *fringe benefits*. How many weeks of vacation do staff get each year? How many paid holidays are there? Is free life insurance provided to employees? Those are several of the most obvious employee benefits. Some benefits are required by law. For example, the employer must pay for FICA, a tax for social security, which will eventually provide the employee with a social security pension. Most benefits, however, are voluntary or the result of labor negotiations.

Other critical benefits concern the quality of the health insurance package offered to employees. Do nurses have to contribute to the cost of their health insurance? If so, how much? Are their family members covered? If so, is there additional cost to the nurse? Are staff members subject to *co-payments* and *deductibles* on their health insurance? A co-payment means that the insurer bears a portion of the cost (often 70% or 80%) and the employee bears the remainder (usually 20% or 30%). A deductible means that 100% of some amount must first be paid by the employee before there are any health benefits (usually $200 to $2,000 per year).

Most employers also offer a variety of other benefits that are somewhat less obvious and are more responsible for the term "fringe benefits" as opposed to employee benefits. For example, if the CEO belongs to a golf club and the membership is paid for by the organization, that is a fringe benefit. If the CEO drives a company-owned car, that is another example of fringe benefits.

In terms of the budget, the fringe benefits referred to above really represent several different types of cost. The vacation and holiday time for each employee is already built into the annual salary cost for that individual. There is no need to budget for that fringe benefit, except for making sure that there is adequate staff coverage for all days off. This is accounted for by budgeting additional personnel (see Chapter 8). On the other hand, the cost of life insurance, pension payments, social security taxes, health insurance, and other fringe benefits that require cash outlays must be budgeted for explicitly.

In most organizations, the specific costs of the fringe benefits are calculated by the finance office and are assigned to departments based on salaries, usually as a percentage. For example, a nursing unit might be charged 28% for fringe benefits for every dollar of salary paid to any staff member. Certainly, not all employees have the same cost to the organization per dollar of salary. This is simply an average. Is it fair? It might well be that certain fringe benefits are worth more to employees of some departments than employees of other departments. However, over the years it has been decided that it is not worth the effort to get a more refined measure of costs. Therefore, budgeting for fringe benefits generally requires only the addition of a set percentage (provided by the finance office) to the budgeted salary amounts.

The Burnout Problem

One key reason for the failure to retain nurses is burnout. This issue is not based primarily on competition. A higher salary or more flexible hours at another institution may serve to cause staff to move from one organization to another. Burnout is more likely to cause nurses to leave nursing completely. Nurses suffering from burnout tend to be less productive, to be more error-prone, to have low morale, and to accrue a high number of sick days.

Burnout can be caused by a variety of factors. Unrealistic expectations, the excessive use of agency nurses who depend heavily on the regular staff, lack of a good working relationship with physicians, and inconsistent organizational policies are among the various causes. However, the most obvious cause of burnout is short-staffing. When there are simply not enough nurses to get the job done on a given day or week, the existing staff can push themselves. When 9 nurses are doing the work of 10, each of the 9 is very tired at the end of the shift.

Hopefully, they can relax a bit before their shift the next day. When some of those 9 are asked to follow the shift with an immediate second shift, the problem increases. However, over their days off, they can hopefully relax and recuperate from the stress of trying to do more than one person's work on their regular shift, as well as working a few second shifts. On a short-term basis, such a situation may be unpleasant but bearable.

The problems in nursing can and sometimes do become much worse, however. The general financial difficulties faced by many health care organizations already cause staffing levels to be cut to the bone. A fully staffed unit may be staffed with so few nurses as to push each nurse to the limit on a regular basis. When a vacancy occurs on top of that tight staffing situation, the extra stress caused by trying to do more than one can do on a continuous basis can become unbearable. Effectively, lack of adequate staff causes nurses to leave the organization, resulting in even greater stress on those that remain.

What can be done to help reduce burnout? Staff are more content if they believe that they have a caring manager, who is interested in their development. Managers should be supportive and fair. Managers should be seen as using staff time wisely. The overall attitude and management approach of unit managers and higher level nursing administrators can, at least to some extent, offset the problems of burnout.

Flexible hours are another measure aimed at reducing burnout. Allowing nurses to take four 10-hour shifts and have 3 days off is one approach to reduce the draining effect of the constant day-in and day-out stress related with a nurse's job. Having 3 days off may not only reduce burnout but may also be seen by nursing staff as quite desirable, thus increasing nurse satisfaction. Care must be exercised, however. A nurse may take three 12-hour shifts at one hospital and four 10-hour shifts at another. The financial rewards to the individual nurse are great, but the physical and emotional stress may be overwhelming. The impact on patient care may be negative.

The most direct approach to reducing burnout is to increase the overall staffing level. However, this may be nearly impossible, given both the financial constraints of the organization and the overall shortage of available staff. Using alternative personnel (so-called nurse extenders) for providing care presents a potential option to reduce the amount of work per staff nurse. The use of alternative providers of care is discussed later in this chapter.

RETENTION PROGRAMS

The problem of turnover is significant enough to warrant specific attention and direct programs aimed at staff retention. This should go beyond the basic notions of having competent managers, physicians who work on a collegial professional basis with nurses, autonomy in work, and the other elements of nurse satisfaction. Such programs should work toward making the institution one that shows caring for its staff and creates a loyalty bond that is hard to break.

Some such programs involve significant financial investment, while others take relatively little.

First of all, employees should have a way of being recognized. There should be a formal mechanism that allows a pattern of exemplary work, or even one good deed, to gain recognition. There are a variety of ways that employee behavior can be recognized. The first is in the form of performance evaluations with interviews. Such evaluations are a two-edged sword. They need to be firm enough to make clear that poor performance will not be ignored or rewarded. However, there should be a strong focus on positive aspects. This may be in terms of recognizing good performance or even in terms of offering training in areas where performance could be improved. Rather than dwelling on poor past performance, a greater amount of time should be spent on discussing ways to accomplish more and to improve future performance.

Performance evaluation meetings are often uncomfortable for both the evaluator and the one being evaluated. However, such meetings should not be given short shrift. Employees should leave the meeting with a feeling that they understand what is expected of them, with a sense that their individual efforts make a difference in the overall performance of the unit, and with a clear sense that their positive contributions have been noted and specifically recognized by the organization.

Another key element of performance conferences should be to elicit input. What is going on that the employee likes, and what is going on that the employee objects to? Open lines of communication—with honest follow-up on suggestions and complaints—is likely to win over support and loyalty. A refusal to budge from the way things are is more likely to result in resentment and in some cases resignations.

In addition to meetings, specific actions may warrant letters of commendation. Such letters could be the result of favorable patient comments on a form supplied to patients for that purpose. Or they could be based on recommendations from other staff. Commendations should be presented in appropriate ceremonies and noted in organizational newsletters so that as many people as possible are made aware of them. This provides further psychic benefit to the recipient and perhaps serves notice to other workers of the possibility of gaining such recognition. Achievement of such recognition should be within the reach of most staff members.

In providing motivation, the carrot can be used or the stick can be used. There are some schools of thought that argue that the stick is more appropriate than the carrot. Poor performance is unacceptable, and that fact should be conveyed to workers. Other schools of thought argue that in the long run the carrot will have more positive results. By accentuating the positive and decentuating the negative, a happier and psychologically healthier work environment results. In many cases, a combination of the carrot and the stick is probably optimal.

Another program for retention involves financial remuneration. Money is not a solution to all problems. One study has shown that having adequate numbers of staff, nursing management support, alternate weekends off, support of administration, and permanent shift assignments all rank ahead of benefits and salary in terms of importance to nurses. On the other hand, benefits and salary ranked ahead of general staffing patterns, support of physicians, opportunity for advancement, location, and staff development programs.[1] Nursing departments should attempt to deal with all these factors. However, while money is not the solution to all problems, financial incentives have become a major competitive factor.

Higher salaries are one type of financial incentive. They can be costly to health care organizations. Other types of financial incentives can be achieved without substantially higher cost to the institution. One example is the use of salaries instead of hourly wages. This approach may make nurses feel better about themselves and their institutions. Another financial approach is the use of bonuses. Bonuses generally are paid only out of cost savings. Thus, the institution can afford to pay for them because the payment is only part of a larger amount that would otherwise have been spent anyway. Bonuses are becoming more and more widespread. Bonuses were discussed in Chapter 3.

Innovative employee benefits are another area that can be used to help retain nurses. For example, the use of child care centers located at the health care organization (perhaps with discounted or subsidized rates) can help retention significantly. Additionally, such centers have the capacity to reduce sick leave substantially. Much sick leave is the result of a nurse staying home to take care of a sick child. Sick leave can therefore be reduced if the child care center has facilities for mildly ill children.

The above approaches to retention are already in the nursing literature. However, to be truly competitive, an organization must be innovative. For example, suppose that a nurses' dramatics group were formed and it were to stage a dramatic or musical play with performances for the staff and patients every six months. A club of this type provides an excellent release from the routine work pressures. In this way it reduces the burnout syndrome. Over the years such a club develops intense loyalties. Nurses might not leave the organization because they don't want to be left out of the show. Bridge clubs and other organization-sponsored activities (annual picnics and trips to the ballpark) result in the development of a sense of family and community, rather than strictly a workplace. And when times get tough, families and communities hang together.

Career Ladders

A frequent complaint of staff nurses is that there is little room for advancement within the clinical ranks. Nurses can go into management. However, if they chose to pursue a bedside, hands-on, clinical career, there is little

---

[1]"What Nurses Want Most from a Job," *Nursing 88,* Springhouse Corp., Vol. 18, No. 2, February 1988, p. 38.

difference in reward for a nurse with 30 years of experience as compared to one with 5 years. The concept of career ladders or clinical ladders is one suggestion for overcoming this deterrent to nurse retention.

There are a wide variety of career ladder models. Some are completely distinct from administrative career paths (clinical ladders). Others allow for branching off from a clinical ladder into an administrative path after a certain point. Some clinical ladders simply require on-the-job experience for promotions, while others require additional education, including advanced degrees. In some models, moving up the ladder requires community and/or professional service and publications. Another distinction among models is the amount of additional responsibility that must be assumed as one moves up the ladder.

There is a widespread belief that clinical ladders do improve nurse retention. Such an approach improves the professional identity of the nurse and generates loyalty. Another perspective is that if nurses with more experience with a given institution earn substantially more than those with fewer years at the specific organization, it becomes more costly to move. It becomes expensive to give up seniority. If this is the case, then retention of the more experienced/expensive personnel becomes easier, but higher turnover rates may occur among the nurses at the lower (and less expensive) rungs of the ladder. Over time this may lead to an organization with a large proportion of its staff near the higher compensation end of the career ladder.

The Hawthorne Effect

With all attempts to improve retention, it is necessary to be wary of the Hawthorne Effect, which is widely discussed in the general management literature. The Hawthorne Effect is based on a study in which a number of changes were made in a factory to examine their impact on worker productivity. With each change productivity improved. However, it turned out that the specific changes were not directly responsible for the improvement. Improvement occurred as a result of the attention the workers were receiving.

Consider researchers making factory lighting brighter, to see if more light improves worker productivity. Productivity in fact increases after the lighting is changed. Then the researchers add music, and productivity goes up again. If the lighting and music are responsible, then taking them away should reduce productivity to the earlier levels. However, removing the better lighting and the music causes productivity to go up even further. It is the *attention*, rather than the lighting or the music, that makes productivity improve.

All the efforts to improve nurse retention risk falling subject to the Hawthorne Effect. Put a career ladder in place and turnover decreases. Have joint awareness seminars with nurses, administrators, and physicians. Institute a bonus system. Have performance evaluations twice a year. Declare a new era of nursing autonomy. The one thing not known about any of the changes is whether it is the specific nature of the change that is significant or simply the response of nurses in recognition of the fact that the organization finally seems to care about them.

This does not mean that the changes in themselves have no impact. There has been enough literature reporting results to indicate that certain factors are in fact likely to improve nurse satisfaction and hopefully retention. Open communication, greater participation in decision making, being salaried, and career ladders do likely make a difference. However, the element of change itself should not be underplayed.

Putting a career ladder in place and then assuming retention will take care of itself is not likely to work satisfactorily in the long run. The organization must adopt an attitude of making changes each year to improve the lot of its nurses. It may well not be possible to improve all areas that affect nurse satisfaction in any one year. But a constant attitude of working toward improvement is needed. This may mean new major innovations each year, or it may mean modifications to past innovations. Some years changes may be financial, while other years changes may relate to nursing image. A constant approach that each year looks to see what improvements can be added is more likely to have a lasting positive impact than a dramatic, one-shot change. Nursing staff should be able to see that the organization has a commitment to the improvement of the lot of nurses each and every year.

Determining the Cost

What does it cost to retain staff? As with any decision in a health organization, the cost-benefit ratio of a retention program should be estimated in advance and also evaluated after the program has been implemented. Having accurate data on current retention patterns and knowing the organization's goal provide the first step in determining the costs of the program. Although it is often difficult to associate a particular retention program with overall retention, some estimates can be made. If a new program such as free parking is instituted, the cost of that can easily be determined. Often, however, new programs have several goals and potential benefits. A handheld computer system for nursing home visits may be intended to retain nurses who want to work in a high tech environment where charting is easier. However, the computer system is also expected to improve the quality of patient care and to decrease the time nurses spend on documentation. Other programs aimed at improving retention may have additional benefits as well. Shared governance may be instituted to improve retention, but it may improve patient care and have that benefit as well. Increasing salaries may retain staff in the short run, but as soon as the competitor across town increases its salaries, the benefits of such a program may disappear.

Determining the costs of turnover and therefore the benefits of decreasing turnover is more straightforward. What is important to remember is that the costs of turnover do not include just the costs of advertising for staff and the nurse recruiter's salary. Costs include the effect short staffing has on the remaining staff and the decreased productivity of new staff. Jones describes a detailed approach to determine the costs of turnover. She suggests that the following costs be included:

- Advertising/recruiting
- Costs of unfilled positions
- Hiring costs
- Termination costs
- Orientation/training
- Decreased new RN productivity[2]

For the hospitals studied by Jones, the mean cost per RN turnover was $10,198 (range $6,886–$15,152).

Blaufuss, Maynard, and Schollars present an alternative approach to evaluating turnover costs in response to a specific incentive.[3] They do not include general advertising and recruiting costs in their calculations. This is because they argue that hospitals must advertise regardless of turnover rates, since there will naturally be some turnover in all organizations.

They include interviewing, preparing for orientation, the orientation itself, and a learning period. They identify the individual cost of hiring each new staff member. In addition, they include estimated revenue enhancements as an offset to the recruiting cost. This is particularly important when increases in staff can lead to increasing the number of patients cared for. Essentially, if you look at the cost of attracting new staff, you must also consider the extra revenue the organization will earn if it has those new staff members.

RECRUITING STAFF

No matter how effectively an organization works to retain its existing staff, some turnover must be expected. Some staff members will retire; others will move to different parts of the country. Some replacement of staff will always be occurring. Such replacement is inherently costly. The costs of replacing staff include overtime and agency nurse costs while the position is vacant, advertising, interviewing potential employees, travel costs for recruiters, entertainment costs, moving costs, administrative processing costs, and new employee training.

Depending on the specific institution, these costs may be shared by the unit with the vacancy and the personnel department or they may all be borne by the unit with the vacancy. For example, if ads are run to replace a staff member for one unit, the cost of the ad may be charged back directly to the unit with the

---

[2]See Cheryl Bland Jones, "Staff Nurse Turnover Costs: Part II, Measurements and Results," *Journal of Nursing Administration,* Vol. 20, No. 4, May 1990, pp. 27–31, for a complete description of this approach.

[3]Judy Blaufuss, Jan Maynard, and Gail Schollars, "Methods of Evaluating Turnover Costs," *Nursing Management,* Vol. 23, No. 5, May 1992, pp. 52–61.

vacancy. If ads are run to attract candidates for a number of different units, the cost of the ad may be divided and a share of the cost may be allocated among the various units. Alternatively, the price of advertisements may be borne solely by a department responsible for recruiting, such as the personnel or nurse recruitment departments. If units share the cost of advertising, then the operating budget should contain an estimate of the number of vacancies and the cost of advertisements for the year.

Other costs related to the replacement of personnel should also be budgeted. The average length of the vacancies should be anticipated, and the extra cost of overtime and agency nurses should be included in the coming year's operating budget. Newly hired employees are often less productive than experienced staff. This may require extra hours of nursing care per patient day, often in the form of overtime. An effort should be made to anticipate turnover and the costs related to turnover. Sufficient nursing care hours should be budgeted to allow for the lower productivity of new staff. If relocation costs are charged directly to the unit, those costs should be included in the budget as well.

Marketing

One of the key elements of recruiting is an effective marketing strategy. As long as an overall shortage of talented nurses exists, there will be a winner and a loser in the effort to recruit qualified personnel. Therefore, a plan must be developed for addressing the recruiting issue.

The essence of marketing is that, based on market research, the needs and desires of a group are determined, and then an effort is made to satisfy those needs and desires. Notice that this definition does not revolve around advertising, which may or may not be part of a marketing effort. The first step is to find out what nurses want from their employment. Next, efforts must be made to ensure that the hospital meets those needs to the greatest extent possible. Finally, it is necessary to be able to convey the fact that the needs have been met.

In performing market research, a decision should first be made concerning who it is that the organization wants to recruit. Is it new nurses, right out of school? Is it experienced nurses? Nurse managers? Specialists? Local nurses? Out-of-state nurses? In trying to determine what the potential employee wants and needs, it is of critical importance to evaluate correctly the group that is to be the target of the marketing effort.

Since most health care organizations already have some staff, there must be some attractive characteristics of the organization. In relative terms, all existing organizations have some strengths. Therefore, there should not be a hopeless attitude of, "How can we compete with the rich, research-oriented medical center in town?" Perhaps many nurses would prefer to provide care in a patient-oriented rather than research-oriented setting. It is important to identify the existing strengths of the organization so that the information can be conveyed to a target group.

At the same time, weaknesses must be identified and a long-term plan designed to overcome as many of them as possible. Perhaps lack of convenient parking is the one overwhelming negative the organization has. In this case, replacing expensive advertising with a major fund-raising campaign to allow for the building of an enclosed parking garage may be an appropriate marketing strategy. This is an example of a one-shot, expensive solution to a recruiting problem.

In other cases, solutions may be less expensive but require ongoing efforts. For example, a hospital could distinguish itself through a concerted effort to develop a system of shared governance. Such efforts are not necessarily expensive. They do, however, require tremendous cooperation and commitment. The potential result is that expensive newspaper ads can be replaced with free news stories on the change at the hospital. Nursing schools can be encouraged to have the organization's staff give lectures on the shared governance approach employed by the organization. If the new system really provides something that nurses value, the word will eventually get out, even without advertising. Advertising may be employed to speed the communication process, if desired.

Note, however, that marketing does not start with advertising. It starts with the identification of the need or desire and the filling of that need or desire. These elements must precede the advertising. Only then can a specific plan be developed regarding the communication of what strengths the organization has to offer. Advertising in newspapers, television, radio, or direct mail is one approach to that communication. College visits are another. Bonuses to existing employees who bring in new employees is another.

Each of these approaches often results in inquiries by potential employees. The package of material that the organization develops to respond to those inquiries is a critical element of the overall marketing strategy. The marketing strategy should take into account all the steps in the recruiting process. Generating inquiries without a strategy to follow up effectively is one critical mistake often made by those that view marketing only in terms of advertising. If a strategy is likely to generate inquiries, the organization should not appear unorganized or uncaring when it receives those inquiries. This is the point when the organization has the chance to reaffirm the feeling that caused the nurse to inquire about the position.

Suppose a hospital runs a newspaper ad that says, "Join the nursing staff at ABC Hospital, where nurses work in an environment of shared governance and shared commitment to the highest level of patient care." Some carefully planned literature must be available for the person who asks for more information about the shared governance program. Its history, how it works, and the hospital's commitment should be included.

If the response to the inquiry leads to an interview, the interviewer should be aware that the candidate has inquired about the hospital's shared governance program. The interview should include at least some specific discussion that emphasizes or highlights the shared governance system.

Marketing is a critical element of recruiting. This does not mean that the organization has to sell people something that they don't want or need. Rather, having researched the wants and needs of a targeted nursing group, marketing should allow the organization to convey effectively to the target group the extent to which the organization has made efforts to meet those desires and needs.

Although advertising is not the first part of a marketing plan, in many instances it is an effective mechanism for speeding the word-of-mouth process. Targeted advertising can reach a potential group of employees effectively. This is particularly important in a competitive marketplace. If competing organizations are effectively communicating what they have to offer, your organization must be prepared to get its message to that group of potential employees as well.

One important element of advertising is that only a part of current advertising should be aimed at current recruitment. Another part, equally substantial, should be aimed at long-term image building. Often people associate with an organization because of its "well-known" reputation. Such reputations are built over a period of years. They are built through an effort of getting the message out year in and year out. When there is a staffing shortage, the institution advertises why it's a good place to work. It should also do so when there is no shortage of personnel. Image building is not a short-term response to shortages. By laying the groundwork over a long period of time, when the need for personnel occurs, the organization will have a head start over its competition.

In budgeting for a marketing plan, it is necessary to include the costs of advertising. However, any other costs related to the overall marketing plan should also be included in the budget. These might include consulting costs and the costs of doing market research.

Determining the Cost

Recruitment and replacement of staff is inherently costly. The costs of replacing staff include:

- Overtime and agency nurse costs while the position is vacant
- Advertising
- Interviewing potential employees
- Travel for recruiters
- Entertainment
- Moving
- Signing bonuses
- Administrative processing
- New employee training

USING ALTERNATIVE HEALTH CARE EMPLOYEES

Despite the efforts of organizations to retain nurses, nurse retention will be unable to solve all health care organizations' nursing needs. And recruitment more often results in shifting the shortage from one organization to another, rather than eliminating the shortage. Thus, despite the best efforts to retain and recruit nurses, there will probably be at least some organizations with inadequate staffing. One suggested approach to solving this shortage is the use of alternative health care employees.

There is a variety of alternative health care employees who are sometimes used. One approach is to use foreign nurses. This approach attempts to retain the concept of using RNs to the greatest extent possible. It comes to grips with a national nursing shortage by looking outside the United States. A different approach is to use non-RNs to perform activities that in the past had been performed by RNs.

Foreign Nurse Recruitment

Using foreign nurses is one possible alternative for staffing a health care institution. However, it involves a number of difficulties ranging from regulatory to language barriers. On the other hand, many foreign nurses welcome the chance to come to the United States on either a temporary or permanent basis, and this approach can be used to fill a large gap in the nursing staff.

Because of language problems, most foreign recruitment takes place in countries that are English-speaking, such as Canada, the British Isles, Australia, the Philippines, and India. Northern states may be able to recruit in Canada relatively easily, compared to other alternatives. For recruiting outside the continent, expenses of travel and relocation can become substantial. An alternative to an organization doing it all by itself is to use an agency and pay a flat fee for each nurse hired. The more nurses that will be hired, the more likely it is to be cost-effective to undertake the entire recruiting project yourself.

If a strategy of foreign recruiting is chosen, the need for careful budgeting becomes essential. The choice between using a recruiting agency versus doing it yourself can have a dramatic financial impact. By developing a budget, the costs of each alternative can be considered. For example, suppose that an agency charges one month's salary for recruiting an individual plus one month's salary for relocation expenses. It could easily cost in excess of ten thousand dollars for each nurse recruited.

There are additional recruiting costs. One cost of recruiting foreign nurses is the time between their arrival and the time when they have completed all examinations and other requirements necessary to practice as an RN. During this period they are being paid but are not fully productive. Other costs include providing convenient housing and helping the nurses settle in. Another cost is related to loss of recruits between their recruitment and their arrival. Since a fairly lengthy period is required to meet various visa and other requirements, there is a drop-out rate.

Alternative Care Givers

A drastically different approach to using foreign nurses is the alteration of the pattern of care within a health care organization to assign more activities to non-RNs. There are many types of alternate care givers. These include, but are not limited to, the traditional alternate care givers: LPNs/LVNs and unlicensed assistive personnel (UAP) such as nurses' aides. Various new positions such as hosts or hostesses are also being developed to help organizations cope. Such a person would introduce patients to the unit and respond to many of the nonclinical needs and questions of patients and their families.

In terms of clinical assistive personnel, many approaches are being tried at different health care organizations around the country. In some cases, the RN is placed in a position of greater direct supervision of other types of staff who provide more of the care. In other cases, partnerships are developed between nursing and UAP. In many cases, the ultimate impact of using alternate care givers is less bedside time for the RN and more supervisory responsibility.

At the time of the writing of this book, no single approach had emerged as the dominant path for providing nursing care in the future. The main conflict seems to be between a model that would have RNs serving as supervisors of non-RNs versus a model in which nursing activities are divided into an RN subset and a non-RN subset. In the case of the former, RNs have a decreasing bedside role but greater authority and responsibility for patient care. In the latter alternative, RNs may spend as much time in bedside care but performing only activities that require the sophistication of an RN.

There is no question that throughout the first decade of the twenty-first century we will see a great deal of experimentation in search of a model that works well. The result may be several different models, each of which works well and attracts nurses with a preference for one approach versus another. There is little question, however, that the organization of nursing services in the year 2010 will be substantially different from that observed at the start of this decade.

USING COMPUTERS

Changing the way that nursing care is provided because of a shortage of staff is a less than ideal way to evolve a profession. The changes are not the result primarily of an impetus to find better ways to give care. Rather, they are recognition of personnel availability constraints. If nursing shortages could be permanently eliminated, the approach to delivering nursing care might be substantially different. The computerization of nursing units has been put forth as a potential solution to that dilemma.

Some claims have been made that up to half of all nursing time is spent on documentation and that bedside computer terminals could save half of that time. If true, this would mean that up to one quarter of all required nursing time could be eliminated, without taking away any time from nursing care provided to patients.

Although highly touted for their timesaving potential throughout the 1990's, computer systems have yet to live up to that glowing potential. The *hardware* (equipment) capacity exists. Technological advances have reached a point where terminals by each bedside are feasible. In fact, it would be surprising to see a new building for a health care organization that did not include computer wiring to each room as part of the electrical blueprints. And gaining nurse acceptance of the use of unit or bedside computers has not turned out to be the problem that many predicted it would be. On the other hand, developing the *software* (computer programs) has been a complicated process.

Each health care institution tends to be fairly unique in its procedures. This lack of industry standardization creates difficulties in developing software. Furthermore, the process of recording the activities surrounding patient care and integrating patient care clinical and financial information with those activities is a highly complicated task.

Whether the claims of 25% savings in staff time will ever be realized is uncertain. It is likely, however, that computer software advances will be made and that computer usage by staff nurses will become commonplace in most health care organizations. In the long run, this will likely increase the quality of patient care due to more accurate and timely information, while at the same time creating at least some efficiencies in the use of nursing time. This should allow more RN time to be available for patient care. To the extent that computers reduce time spent on documentation relative to time spent in providing patient care, computerization should work to both reduce nursing shortages and increase nursing satisfaction as well.

SUMMARY AND IMPLICATIONS
FOR NURSE MANAGERS

There have periodically been nationwide shortages of nurses. Having an understanding of approaches to deal with such shortages as they occur is essential for nurse managers. These approaches include attempts to retain existing nurses, recruit additional nurses, and find ways to provide quality nursing care with fewer RN hours, whether through the use of computers, alternate care givers, or some other means.

From a budgeting perspective, the issue of retention and recruitment of staff members, whether RNs, LPNs/LVNs, aides, or other staff, is a significant one. There must be careful enumeration of all costs related to recruitment and retention. These include costs such as marketing research, consulting, advertising, travel, and relocation. They also include the costs necessary to make an organization attractive, such as training costs related to implementing a system of shared governance.

In some cases, decisions must be made regarding which budget will include the various costs related to these efforts. If alternate care providers are used, the change in staffing will clearly take place within each of the various nursing units. Computerization costs are also likely to be included in the specific capital and operating budgets of the various units. On the other hand, relocation costs for new staff are less obvious. Should they be included in the cost of the unit that will employ the staff member or in some other budget? The critical factor is that such costs must be anticipated and included in some budget, and there should be a clearly communicated understanding of whose budget that is.

One fundamental point in this process is the fact that in order for a specific organization to have an adequate staff, it must recognize a need to change over time. The environment in which health care organizations exist is in a constant state of change. Other career opportunities exist for potential staff. If a hospital job is not adequately attractive, a nurse can go into home health care or work in a physician's office. It is important to remain current in understanding what nurses desire from their employment in addition to a salary.

The successful organizations will be those that are aware of the desires of the workforce, respond to those desires, and effectively communicate to potential employees the ways in which they meet those needs and desires.

SUGGESTED READINGS

Badovinac, C.C., Wilson, S., and Woodhouse, D. (1999, July/August). The use of unlicensed assistive personnel and selected outcome indications. *Nursing Economic$.* 17(4), 194–200.

Cangelosi, J.D., Jr., Markham, F.S., and Bounds, W.T. (1998). Factors related to nurse retention and turnover: An updated study. *Health Marketing Quarterly.* 15(3):25–43.

Davidson, H., Folcarelli, P., Crawford, S., Duprat, L., and Clifford, J. (1997). The effects of health care reforms on job satisfaction and voluntary turnover among hospital-based nurses. *Medical Care.* 35(6), 634–645.

Huston, C.L. (1996). Unlicensed assistive personnel: A solution to dwindling health care resources or the precursor to the apocalypse of registered nursing. *Nursing Outlook.* 44(2), 67–73.

Irvine, D., and Evans, M. (1995). Job satisfaction and turnover among nurses: Integrating research findings across studies. *Nursing Research.* 44(4), 246–253.

Kenney, E.G. (1998, May). Creating fulfillment in today's workplace. A guide for nurses. *American Journal of Nursing.* 98(5), 44–48.

Kovner, C.T., and Schore, J. (1998). Differentiated levels of nursing workforce demand. *Journal of Professional Nursing.* 14, 242–253.

Relf, M. (1995, November). Increasing job satisfaction and motivation while reducing nursing turnover through the implementation of shared governance. *Critical Care Nursing Quarterly.* 18(3), 7–13.

Stamps, P. (1997). *Nurses and Work Satisfaction: New Perspective.* Chicago: Health Administration Press.

Winkler, J.B., Flarey, D.L., and Cameron, M.L. (1995, June). The nursing human resource budget: Design for success. *Health Care Supervisor.* 13(4), 61–69.

Yoder, L. (1995). Staff nurses' career development relationships and self-reports of professionalism, job satisfaction, and intent to stay. *Nursing Research.* 44(5), 290–297.

6

Forecasting

The goals of this chapter are to:

identify various forecasting techniques;

discuss the reasons for forecasting;

describe the types of items subject to forecast;

outline the steps in forecasting;

discuss issues related to data collection;

introduce concepts of trend and seasonality;

provide formulas for forecasting;

discuss the advantages of curvilinear forecasting;

introduce use of computers for curvilinear forecasting; and

discuss the use of Delphi and Nominal Groups for subjective forecasting.

INTRODUCTION

Preparing budgets requires a number of preliminary steps, including forecasting. Earlier, the importance of making an environmental review was discussed (Chapter 2). A budget cannot be prepared without knowing the types of patients that the organization will likely be treating. Nor can a budget be prepared without being aware of who the competition is and the actions competitors are likely to take. Similarly, a budget cannot be prepared without knowing information such as *how many* patients are likely to be treated or *how sick* they are likely to be. This is where forecasting comes in.

Forecasting techniques allow for predicting how many patients or patient days the organization or a particular unit or department will treat. Forecasting allows the manager to predict how sick the unit's patients will be. If a nurse manager were to attempt to prepare an operating budget without some prediction of these elements, there would be no way of determining how much staff is needed. Forecasting can help to estimate how many chest tubes the ICU will need or how many heparin locks a medical/surgical unit will consume. This will enable the nurse manager to plan the supplies portion of the unit's budget.

Forecasting is a tool that helps in preparing not only the operating budget but other budgets as well. If trends in the demographics of the community can be forecast, it is possible to prepare better long-range and program budgets. If it is forecast that a growing portion of the patient population will be Medicare patients, it can be determined what impact this will have on how quickly the organization gets paid. This will help in preparing the cash budget.

The range of items that can be forecast is fairly unlimited. It is possible to predict patients, patient days, various supply items, the percent of total operations performed by a specific surgeon, and so on. Generally, forecasting focuses on items that the manager must respond to rather than items that can be controlled. For example, a nursing unit may forecast how sick the patients will be. It cannot control severity of illness, but its budget must be a plan that responds to how sick the patient population is expected to be.

Forecasting should be undertaken as an early step in the budget preparation process. Virtually all managers forecast in some manner. Unsophisticated managers may forecast by simply using their best judgment or by assuming that the current year's results will occur again the next year. It has been found that more formalized analysis of historical data can yield more accurate predictions than such less sophisticated approaches. These predictions in turn form a basis for many decisions made in the planning process.

A formalized forecasting process can be divided into several steps. The first step is collecting historical data. The next step is graphing the data. The third step is analyzing the data to reveal trends or seasonal patterns. The fourth and final step is developing and using formulas to project the item being forecast into the future.

Before these steps are considered, there is one point that must be stressed. When a forecast is made, it is just an estimate of the future. Sophisticated approaches to forecasting allow the projection to be an educated estimate, but it is still an estimate. Your intuitive hunch or gut feeling should *not* be ignored. The most sophisticated methods lack the feel for the organization that a manager develops over time. Never accept forecasts on the blind faith that if it is mathematical or computerized it must be superior.

Quantitative forecasts are merely aids or supplements that managers should take into consideration along with a number of other factors, many of which often cannot be quantified and entered into formalized predictive models. The best forecasts result from neither naive guessing nor advanced mathematics but from an integration of quantitative methods with the experience and judgments of managers.

DATA COLLECTION

The first step in formalized forecasting is collecting historical data. Consider several examples. If a nurse manager wishes to make the most basic of projections—workload—she will first have to decide on a workload measure, such as patients or patient days. Then it is necessary to determine what the workload was in the past so that it can be projected into the future. This is referred to as a *time-series* approach to forecasting. Historical changes over time are used to help anticipate the likely result in a coming time period.

The methodology that will be discussed in this section is broadly applicable. If one wanted to predict diaper usage in the maternity unit, one could use historical data based on the number of diapers used. Once the number of diapers needed is predicted, it would probably be necessary to focus on the expected cost per box of diapers. If the purchasing department has a good degree of certainty about the price of diapers for next year (such as a purchase contract specifying a price), this would be a pretty accurate approach. On the other hand, if it was desired to predict the total cost for diapers directly rather than focusing first on the expected number of diapers, it would be possible to gather information on what total amount was spent on diapers in the past and use that for a direct cost estimate.

In other words, it is possible to first forecast diaper usage and then calculate the projected cost or to forecast diaper cost directly. The preferred choice would depend partly on whether information about the number of diapers to be used in the coming period is considered to be valuable information. Similarly, both the number of patient days and the patient severity of illness can be predicted; then that data can be used to project the number of nursing hours needed or historical information about the number of nursing hours consumed can be used to forecast nursing hours directly.

Appropriate Data Time Periods

There is often a tendency to try to make do with annual data. In fact, many operating budgets are annual budgets, specifying the total amounts to be spent on each line item for the coming year. However, when a manager is preparing an operating budget, it makes a lot of sense to use monthly rather than annual predictions of costs.

The easiest way to make monthly predictions is to take annual budget information and divide it by 12. In many industries it would be possible to use such a simple approach; production in one month may be much the same as in any other month. In the health care sector, such an expectation is not reasonable. The weather alone is likely to cause busy and slow periods. Winters are often busier periods of time for health care organizations than summers are. Health care organizations must be prepared to have more staff available in busier periods. It is desirable to plan more vacations in slow periods and fewer during peak periods. Thus, it is important to be concerned with month-to-month variations within each year, as well as with the predictions for the year as a whole.

Furthermore, the number of days in a month will affect monthly costs. Many health care organizations, such as clinics, labs, or radiologists' offices, might only be open weekdays. Some months have as many as 23 weekdays, while other months have as few as 20 weekdays. A 3-day difference on a 20-day base represents a 15% difference. Clearly a difference that large would have a significant impact on the resources required for the month. Similarly, for a hospital, it is quite likely that the number of weekdays will have an influence since there are some days of the week when admissions and discharges tend to be higher than other days.

Monthly budgets are also important because they can be compared to the actual results as they occur. If there is a difference (variance) between the plan and the actual results, the cause can be investigated and perhaps a problem can be corrected immediately. Such variance analysis is the topic of Chapters 13 and 14. Without monthly subdivisions of the budget, it might be necessary to wait until the end of the year to find out if things were going according to plan. By then, of course, it would be too late to do anything about it for that year.

Thus, it is important for most health care institutions to have their costs broken down on a monthly basis and to do so in some manner that is more sophisticated than dividing the year's expected cost or volume by 12. Therefore, the data collected should generally be historical *monthly* data. For each type of item to be forecast (patients, chest tubes, diapers, costs), 12 individual data points are needed per year, representing values for the item being forecast for each month.

How far back should the data go? One year seems convenient, and it provides 12 data points. However, 1 year's worth of data provides only one piece of information about January, not 12. If this January was unusual (either very costly or unusually low in cost), that would not be readily apparent. It is likely that next year would be predicted to be like this year. Therefore, more than 1 year's data is needed.

The use of 10 years of data is often suggested for forecasting, although that has weaknesses as well. It is possible that so much has changed over the last 10 years that the data are no longer relevant. For that reason, it would seem that 5 years of data (or a total of 60 months) is a reasonable rule of thumb. If a nurse manager knows that things have not changed much on the unit in a long time, using more years of data will make the estimate a better predictor. If there have been drastic changes recently, then 5 years might be too long. Judgment is needed. One of the most important things a manager does is exercise judgment. Throughout the budgeting process, as in the other managerial functions undertaken, a manager can never escape from the fact that thoughtful judgment is vital to the process of effective management.

What Data Should Be Collected?

The fact that it is necessary to collect historical data on the item to be forecast has already been discussed. Too often managers stop at that point, because this data is sufficient to make a forecast. However, these data points are not all the data that is really needed to make a *good* forecast.

Forecasting techniques mindlessly predict the future as an extension of the past, even though there are many things that change over time. Whenever forecasting is done, the manager should question whether there are factors that might have changed that will make the future different from the past. Are there in fact things that are changing? For instance, are demographics shifting? When it is predicted that next January will be like the previous five Januarys, is the fact that last July there was a large influx of refugees into the community being ignored? Is a sudden shift in population caused by the closing of the town's auto plant being ignored? The forecasting formulas to be developed will not take these recent factors into consideration. Forecasting formulas are based solely on historical information. The manager should collect additional data to use as a judgmental adjustment to forecast results.

For example, availability of personnel can have a dramatic impact. For years many health care organizations suffered from a shortage of available nurses. The result was high overtime payments to staff nurses and high agency charges for per diem nurses. If there has been a noticeable increase in the number of nurses available, then a manager should realize that the average hourly cost for nursing can now be decreased by the elimination of much overtime and agency cost. A quantitative model for forecasting will not take this into account. Information about nurse availability must be collected, and the manager should give specific consideration to this information.

Note that a unit manager does not have to be a one-person information service. The personnel department can be asked about the outlook for hiring additional staff nurses. Administrators can be asked whether changes in third-party coverage are likely to have any impact. It is unreasonable to expect a home health agency's director of nursing to budget correctly for the coming year without knowing that the number of allowable Medicare-reimbursable visits has changed. Most home health agency financial officers would quickly be aware of such a change. This information should be communicated promptly to the chief nursing officer. It is vital to open communication links with other managers throughout the organization to assure receipt of necessary information that could help in the budget process.

It will not be easy to get information about some changes. For instance, there may be no central clearing person to provide an update on changing technology that will dramatically shift the demand for nursing personnel. Nevertheless, a unit manager must try to get that information and consider its likely impact on the unit. To some extent, nurse managers may have better information on changing technology than the organization's administrators have. First, nurse managers have superior clinical knowledge to administration. Second, nurse managers are likely to know what kinds of changes physicians in their clinical area are planning to implement.

It is also important for nurse managers to be aware of the organization's long-range plan, program budgets, and capital budgets. Many hospitals tend to guard budget data closely, with an "eyes only" attitude. Only people with an immediate need are allowed to see any budget other than their own. It is important that administrators begin to understand that managers do have a need to see any budget that even indirectly may impact on their unit or department. For example, if a new service winds up consuming a significant amount of nursing time that had not been planned for, much of it will likely be at overtime rates or will result in overtime elsewhere in the hospital. Had the service been planned for, overtime premiums might have been avoided. A manager who is to be held responsible for this overtime is entitled to have the information needed to anticipate demands on the unit and to plan for adequate staffing.

GRAPHING HISTORICAL DATA

Having collected all the relevant data that might help predict the future, the next step is to lay out the historical data on a graph. In the forecasting approach to be discussed here, time is plotted on the horizontal axis. For instance, suppose that the unit manager wants to predict next year's total nursing hours starting with January. Assume that it is currently October 2001 and that historical data from the past 5 years will be used. Data for October through December of 2001 is not yet available. Therefore, the horizontal axis begins in October 1996 and goes through September 2001 (Fig. 6–1).

The vertical axis provides information on the item to be forecast. This is nursing hours in Figure 6–1. The forecasting methodologies to be discussed later in this chapter will allow a manager to predict workload estimates for the future, such as the number of patients or the number of patient days, the actual amounts of resource consumption (e.g., the number of nursing hours or the number of

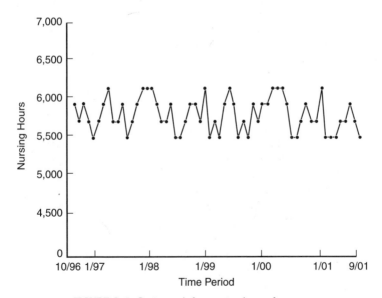

FIGURE 6–1. Basic graph for nursing hours forecast.

rolls of bandage tape), or costs. Depending on the procedures of your specific institution, some of these forecasts may be made by the accounting department rather than by nurse managers.

If costs or some other financial measure expressed in dollars are being predicted directly, the impact of inflation must be considered. If inflation is ignored as forecasting is done, the forecast becomes more complicated because it must not only predict a workload measure, such as the number of diapers for the coming year, but also the rate of inflation for the coming year. The problem of inflation and adjustments that can be made to allow for inflation are discussed in Chapter 4.

If a prediction is being made for next year's nursing hours (Fig. 6–1), the first point graphed would be the number of nursing hours worked in October 1996. The next point would be the number of nursing hours in November 1996, and so on. It is important to keep in mind that this forecasting approach is a time-series analysis—that is, the variable on the horizontal axis is always time. In time-series analysis, whether the manager is trying to predict workload, resources, or cost, the basic process is to look at how much of that item there was in the past and project that into the future. In order to make such predictions, the manager will need to be able to analyze the underlying cause of the variations in the data that has been graphed.

ANALYSIS OF GRAPHED DATA

Before any predictions can be made, it is necessary to assess the basic characteristics of the data that has been graphed. For instance, does the data exhibit *seasonality?* Is there a particular *trend?* Do variations from month to month and year to year appear to be simply random fluctuations? There may be patterns related to the passage of time that can be uncovered.

A visual inspection can usually give a good picture of the type of pattern that exists. Here it is important to focus on a reasonably long time period, at least several years, as opposed to several months. By just looking at the past few months, it is possible to get a distorted impression of what is occurring. For instance, see Figure 6–2. (Note, this is not the same data as that shown in Figure 6–1.) It appears that the number of nursing hours has a definite downward trend, but this graph covers a period of only 6 months.

Figure 6–3 shows the pattern for the full year. Now the graph gives a totally different impression. The number of nursing hours has not been steadily decreasing over time. For the first half of the year it was decreasing, and for the second half it was increasing. The pattern being observed is not likely to be indicative of a long-term decline. It is still not possible to tell, however, if some basic change has occurred that caused a downward trend to reverse or if the pattern is seasonal behavior. Next year, will the number of nursing hours continue to rise, as it appears to be doing near the end of the year, or will it turn downward,

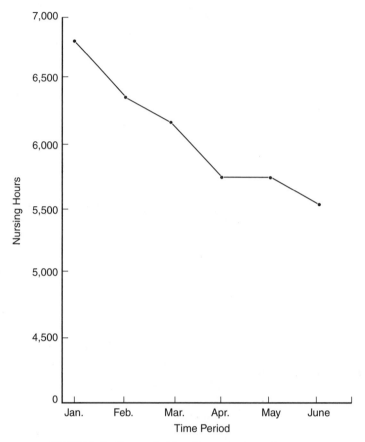

FIGURE 6–2. Six months' data for nursing hours forecast.

as it did at the beginning of the graphed year? To answer this question, it is vital that data for at least several years be graphed.

Now look at Figure 6–4, which covers a period of 5 years. A pattern of falling and then rising hours occurs each year. This is clearly a seasonal pattern rather than a trend. Each year the same pattern repeats itself.

When data for a sufficient number of years is graphed, the pattern that becomes apparent will generally fall into one of four categories. These are random fluctuations, trend, seasonality, and seasonality and trend together. Each of these patterns will be discussed.

Random Fluctuation

It would be surprising if a unit or department consumed exactly the same amount of any resource 2 months or 2 years in a row. One year the winter will be a little colder than another and more people will get pneumonia. Another year

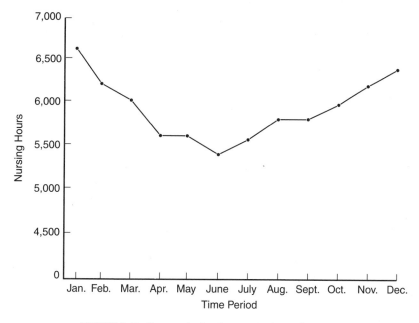

FIGURE 6–3. One year's data for nursing hours forecast.

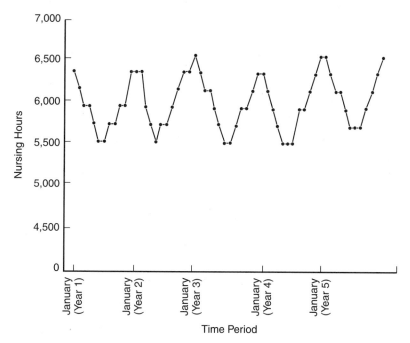

FIGURE 6–4. Five years' data for nursing hours forecast: Seasonality.

prices will rise a little faster. One year some staff members will take more sick days than another. Yet these events are not likely to be trends—it does not get colder and colder year after year. Nor are they seasonal. They are just random, unpredictable events.

When a graph exhibiting random patterns only is viewed, it should look something like Figure 6–5. As can be seen, there is no clear upward or downward trend. You will notice, for example, that each year the month of May is neither consistently higher nor consistently lower than it was the previous year. There is also no discernible seasonal pattern. May is not usually particularly busy nor particularly slow. May is a low month in the first year and a high month in the next year, relative to the values for the other months in those years.

Trend

In Figure 6–6, it should be noted that although the graph has its ups and downs, there is a clear upward trend. Because nursing hours rather than dollars are being considered here, this is not caused by inflation. Rather, it is probably caused either by an increased number of patient days or else by an increase in the amount of nursing time provided per patient day.

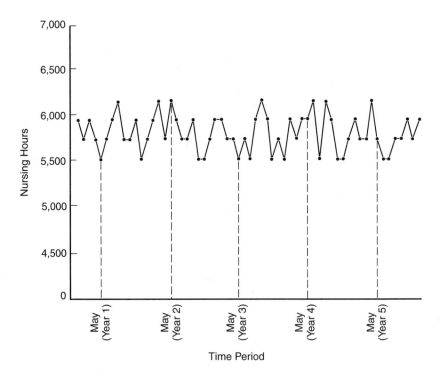

FIGURE 6–5. Five years' data for nursing hours forecast: Random fluctuations.

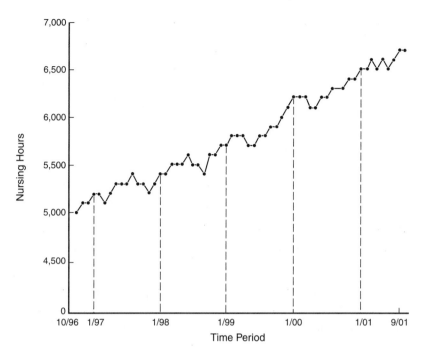

FIGURE 6–6. Five years' data for nursing hours forecast: Trend.

The underlying causes of observed patterns will not be determined in the forecasting process described here. The focus is strictly on projections of past items into the future. Whatever the cause, it appears that a definite trend exists. Unless there is information about expected patient days or a new policy regarding the relative ratio of nurses to patients, it would have to be assumed that this trend will continue. However, managers should try to understand the underlying causes of patterns such as trends. This will better enable them to forecast correctly if something does change the underlying cause of the pattern.

Note further in Figure 6–6 that although the overall trend is upward, there is no discernible seasonal pattern. For example, January does not appear to be consistently high or low each year relative to the other months of those years.

Seasonality

Seasonal patterns are sometimes visible to the eye, as was the case in Figure 6–4. In health care, one is especially likely to see seasonal patterns because of seasonal disease patterns and as a result of the weather. Winter months bring with them different ailments than those that occur in the summer. For hospitals and home health agencies, this will affect overall patient volume. On the other hand, nursing homes may be running at full occupancy all year round. Therefore, the number of patient days at a nursing home might not show any seasonality, although the specific care needs of the patients in a nursing home are likely to vary with the different seasons of the year.

Seasonality may not always be easy to spot. Therefore, it might be a worthwhile exercise to examine certain months that are known as peak or slow periods. Suppose that January is compared to June for each of the last 5 years and it is found that January almost always has higher levels of the item being forecast than June does. In this case seasonality does exist, even if it is not readily apparent when the graph is visually inspected.

Seasonality and Trend

It is common for health care organizations to experience at least some seasonality. At the same time, due to increasing patient volume or the effects of inflation, upward trends are common as well. Downward trends may also occur. It is not at all unusual, therefore, for the organization to experience both seasonal influences and trends at the same time. Figure 6–7 shows an example of a historical pattern exhibiting both seasonality and trend.

Often the trend is more obvious than the seasonality in patterns that contain both. In these cases, it becomes especially useful to make several comparisons to see if certain months are always higher or lower than other months. Valid forecasts require an awareness of seasonal patterns if they exist.

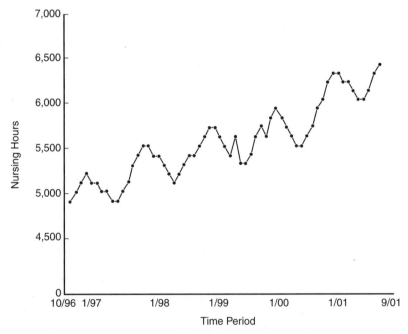

FIGURE 6–7. Five years' data for nursing hours forecast: Seasonality with trend.

FORECASTING FORMULAS

At this point, historical data has been gathered and graphed, and there has been a visual inspection of the graphs for apparent trend or seasonal patterns. It is finally time to begin using the information to make forecasts for the coming year. The approach taken for forecasting depends to a great degree on whether seasonal patterns, trends, both, or neither are present.

An approach to forecasting each of these patterns will be discussed below. First, however, it should be noted that the formulas below assume limited use of computer technology in performing the forecasting function. Much of the tedium and difficulty of the forecasting process is avoided if a sophisticated computer forecasting program is used. Although the formulas discussed below are valuable in situations in which a computer approach is unavailable, a computer solution is preferred. It takes less management time and can produce superior results. The costs of appropriate software are readily offset by the saved managerial time. A computer approach to forecasting is presented later in this chapter.

Random Fluctuations

The easiest forecasting occurs when there is no seasonal pattern or trend. For example, consider the budget for office supplies for the office of the Chief Nurse Executive. The need for these supplies may not vary much over time nor with the particular workload level faced by the clinical nurses.

The most obvious approach in this case would be simply to add up the 60 monthly data points for the past 5 years and divide by 60. This will give a monthly average. If every month is like every other month in terms of the item being forecast, this would be a reasonable approximation.

Caution must be exercised, however. Different months have different numbers of days. Even if there is no strong seasonal influence or trend, longer months may consume more of a resource. Months that have more weekdays may consume more of a resource. It may be necessary to adjust for factors such as days in a month or weekdays in a month. For example, if weekdays use much more of a resource than weekends, rather than dividing the total for the last 60 months by 60, the total could be divided by the number of weekdays in the past 60 months. The result would be a predicted value per weekday. This value would be multiplied by the specific number of weekdays in each month in the coming year to get the appropriate forecast for each month.

Seasonality

If seasonality exists in the item being forecast, it means that some months are typically low and other months are typically high. If all 60 months for the last 5 years are averaged together, the seasonality becomes lost in the broad average. An approach is needed that is more sensitive to fluctuations within each year. The most obvious approach is to add together the values for a given month for several years and divide to get an average just for that month. For example, the last five February values can be totaled and then divided by five. This provides a February average for the last 5 years that can be used as a prediction of next February.

This approach is not always acceptable. Suppose that seasonal variations do not repeat in the exact same month each year. For instance, suppose that February is usually the coldest month, causing patient days to peak because of many flu cases. Sometimes, however, January or March will be colder. Because of this variation in seasonality from year to year, a better prediction may result from adding January plus February plus March for the last 5 years. Thus, February is being based on January, February, and March. This total should be divided by 15 to get a prediction of February of next year. Then March is estimated by adding February plus March plus April for each of the last 5 years and dividing by 15.

The key to this *moving-average* approach is to add up not only the month in question for the last 5 years but also the month preceding and the month following the month being predicted. This formula will often give a good prediction. However, there are also problems with this approach. Peaks and valleys in activity will be understated. For instance, what if January were typically the busiest month of the year, with both December and February being less busy? Then, by averaging December and February with January, the slower December and February will cause the busier January to be understated in the forecast.

How can a nurse manager determine whether predictions will be improved by using calculations such as this one? Should the manager simply take an average of five Februarys or use January, February, and March information for 5 years to predict next February? One good way to make this determination is to try to use historical data (excluding data from the most recent past year) to predict the results of the past year. For instance, if 2001 has just ended, take data from 1996 through 2000 and use it to predict 2001. Since the actual results for 2001 are already known, the prediction can immediately be compared to the actual results. This is a good way to test any formula to see if it is a reasonable predictor.

Keep in mind two things, however. First, no forecast will predict the future perfectly. The future is uncertain, and all the specific events that will occur can never be fully anticipated. Therefore, the prediction should not be expected to match the actual results precisely. Second, the predictions or forecasts using formulas must be adjusted based on the manager's own knowledge about the future. The formulas just use information about the past. If a manager has some information about the future that suggests that the future will not follow the patterns of the past, this information must be used to adjust the predictions of the formulas. The role of an intelligent manager should never be relinquished to the mathematical precision of a formula.

When a formula is tested by seeing how well it can predict what actually happened last year, there should be a determination of whether the predictions based on the formula are closer to what actually happened than the predictions that would have been used in the absence of the formula. If so, then it is a useful tool. Otherwise, the formula should be either modified or discarded.

Trend

If a trend is observed, it is desirable to project that trend into the future. Trends are usually represented by a straight line. However, trends tend to have some random elements within them. If one were to draw a straight line, it would not generally go through each historical point. Some points would be above the line and some would be below the line. A manager could just eyeball the points on the graph and try to draw a line that is as close as possible to all the points and that extends into the future. However, such manual attempts are likely to be inaccurate.

If the line is drawn too high or too low, the estimates for the future will also be too high or too low. Even worse, if the slope of the line is too high or too low, the error will be magnified, as seen in Figure 6–8. In this figure, the first month is assigned a value of 1 on the horizontal axis, the second month is 2, and so on. The solid line represents the best straight line that uses the known data to forecast the future. The dashed line represents a judgmental, eyeball, estimate. Note that near the center of the graph, the two lines are relatively close. However, on the right side of the graph in the area of the forecast for the coming year, the two lines have

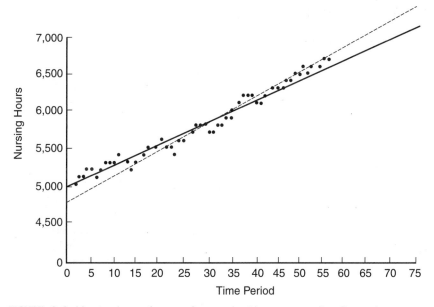

FIGURE 6–8. Nursing hours forecast for trend with no seasonality: Regression versus judgmental forecast.

diverged to the point that the number of nursing hours predicted differs a great deal depending on which line is used.

One solution to this problem is to use a statistical technique called *regression analysis*. The goal of regression analysis is to find the one unique straight line that comes closest to all the historical data points. Regression analysis can be readily performed by a nurse manager using many types of handheld calculators or on a computer using statistical software packages such as the Statistical Package for Social Sciences (SPSS), spreadsheet packages such as Excel or LOTUS 1-2-3, or forecasting packages such as SmartForecasts for Windows.

Regression analysis is a technique that applies mathematical precision to a scatter diagram. The scatter diagram used in regression analysis is a graph that plots points of information. Each data point represents a dependent variable and one or more independent variables. The independent variable is sometimes referred to as the causal variable. It is responsible for causing variations in the dependent variable.

In forecasting, time is considered to be an independent variable and a second variable is considered to be a dependent variable. For example, the dependent variable could be the number of patients treated by the organization. As time passes, the organization may have more or fewer patients. The change in the number of patients over time may reflect a random pattern, seasonal effect, trend, or seasonality and trend, as discussed in this chapter. If a trend exists, regression analysis will generate a line that is a good predictor of the future.

Regression is a tool that can help managers to manage better. The major difficulty in using regression is simply a fear of the process (and this relates not only to nurse managers but to all managers). However, when using a computer program, regression analysis does not require the user to do extensive mathematical computation. The computer carries out all the calculations.[1]

Since regression analysis requires the manager to provide numerical values, months and years cannot be used by their names for the independent variable. An independent variable cannot be referred to as January 1996. Instead, the month names can be replaced by assigning numerical values. The historical months used for the analysis can be numbered 1 through 60 instead of using October 1996, November 1996, and so forth to September 2001. Table 6–1 presents the data. After feeding the information into a calculator or computer (e.g., in month 1, there were 5,000 nursing hours; in month 2, there were 5,100 nursing hours; and so on through month 60, with 6,700 nursing hours), the calculator or computer is instructed to "run" (compute) the regression. When the computation is complete, it is possible to determine how many nursing hours would be expected in months 64 through 75, which represent the 12 months of next year. Note that months 61

---

[1]Although regression is easy to perform using a computer, the user should have some familiarity with regression to interpret the regression results and their significance. See the regression discussion in Chapter 4 or a statistics text.

TABLE 6–1. *Nursing Hours—Historical Data for Trend with No Seasonality*

Data Point	Date		Nursing Hours
1	October	1996	5,000
2	November		5,100
3	December		5,100
4	January	1997	5,200
5	February		5,200
6	March		5,100
7	April		5,200
8	May		5,300
9	June		5,300
10	July		5,300
11	August		5,400
12	September		5,300
13	October		5,300
14	November		5,200
15	December		5,300
16	January	1998	5,400
17	February		5,400
18	March		5,500
19	April		5,500
20	May		5,500
21	June		5,600
22	July		5,500
23	August		5,500
24	September		5,400
25	October		5,600
26	November		5,600
27	December		5,700
28	January	1999	5,700
29	February		5,800
30	March		5,800
31	April		5,800
32	May		5,700
33	June		5,700
34	July		5,800
35	August		5,800
36	September		5,900
37	October		5,900
38	November		6,000
39	December		6,100
40	January	2000	6,200
41	February		6,200
42	March		6,200
43	April		6,100

Continued

TABLE 6–1. *Nursing Hours—Historical Data for Trend with No Seasonality* Continued

Data Point	Date	Nursing Hours
44	May	6,100
45	June	6,200
46	July	6,200
47	August	6,300
48	September	6,300
49	October	6,300
50	November	6,400
51	December	6,400
52	January 2001	6,500
53	February	6,500
54	March	6,600
55	April	6,500
56	May	6,600
57	June	6,500
58	July	6,600
59	August	6,700
60	September	6,700

through 63 have been intentionally skipped over. There are neither historical data points nor forecast points plotted for those 3 months. This is because those months represent the remaining months of the current year, for which data is not yet available. The goal is to develop predictions for the months in the coming year.

The results are shown in the scatter diagram in Figure 6–9. The regression results are plotted as a solid line for 2002 and are extended back from 2001 to 1996 with a dashed line. The specific predictions of nursing-hour requirements for 2002, by month, are as follows:

January	6,772
February	6,800
March	6,828
April	6,856
May	6,884
June	6,911
July	6,939
August	6,967
September	6,995
October	7,023
November	7,051
December	7,079

Note in Figure 6–9 that the projections for next year all fall on the trend line, even though in the past many points are not on the extended (dashed) trend line.

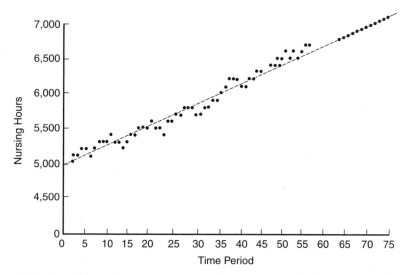

FIGURE 6–9. Nursing hours forecast for trend with no seasonality: Regression results.

Actual results for the coming year are not expected to fall right on the line; however, in the absence of any other information, the points on the trend line are the best prediction that can be made for the actual uncertain outcome. To guess higher than the trend line value would probably be too high. To guess lower than the trend line value would probably be too low.

Seasonality and Trend

Seasonality together with trend poses a more complex problem; yet it is likely to be a common occurrence, so the reader should pay special attention to the approach discussed here. This example will use the data provided in Table 6–2. The first step is to use a regression to predict a trend line for the coming year. Once a set of results for the regression is plotted for each month in the coming year (January 2002 through December 2002), it should be noted that there is no seasonal appearance to the line predicting next year. It is simply an upward trending line (see Fig. 6–10) for 2002.

The next step is to extend the trend backwards into the 5 years for which there is historical data. This is fairly straightforward, since it simply requires extending backwards a straight line that has been already located for the coming year (see the dashed line in Fig. 6–11).

Once the line has been extended backwards, the manager must calculate how much above or below the line the actual value was for each month of the last 5 years. These amounts must then be converted into a percentage. For example, in January 1997 in Figure 6–11, there were 5,200 nursing hours, but the trend

TABLE 6–2. Nursing Hours—Historical Data for Trend with Seasonality

Data Point	Date		Nursing Hours
I	October	1996	4,900
2	November		5,000
3	December		5,100
4	January	1997	5,200
5	February		5,100
6	March		5,100
7	April		5,000
8	May		5,000
9	June		4,900
10	July		4,900
II	August		5,000
12	September		5,100
13	October		5,300
14	November		5,400
15	December		5,500
16	January	1998	5,500
17	February		5,400
18	March		5,400
19	April		5,300
20	May		5,200
21	June		5,100
22	July		5,200
23	August		5,300
24	September		5,400
25	October		5,400
26	November		5,500
27	December		5,600
28	January	1999	5,700
29	February		5,700
30	March		5,600
31	April		5,500
32	May		5,400
33	June		5,600
34	July		5,300
35	August		5,300
36	September		5,400
37	October		5,600
38	November		5,700
39	December		5,600
40	January	2000	5,800
41	February		5,900
42	March		5,800
43	April		5,700
44	May		5,600

TABLE 6–2. *Nursing Hours—Historical Data for Trend with Seasonality Continued*

Data Point	Date		Nursing Hours
45	June		5,500
46	July		5,500
47	August		5,600
48	September		5,700
49	October		5,900
50	November		6,000
51	December		6,200
52	January	2001	6,300
53	February		6,300
54	March		6,200
55	April		6,200
56	May		6,100
57	June		6,000
58	July		6,000
59	August		6,100
60	September		6,300

line was at a vertical height of 5,000. The actual value was 200 hours above the trend. Because it is a trend, however, it is necessary to convert this to a percentage. In this case, it is a positive 4%, because 5,200 is 4% above the trend-line point of 5,000.

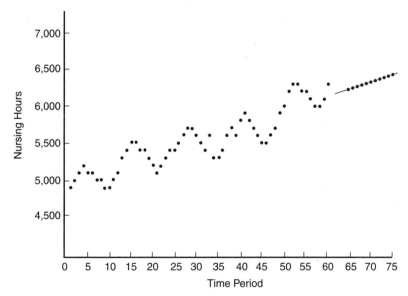

FIGURE 6–10. Nursing hours forecast for trend with seasonality: Regression results.

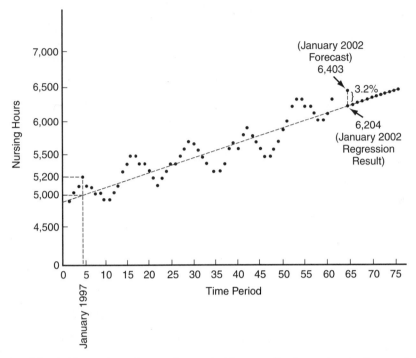

FIGURE 6–11. Nursing hours forecast for trend with seasonality: Regression results extended back into historical data.

Now simply revert to the seasonal approach. Add together the percentages that December, January, and February are over and under the trend line for the last 5 years and divide by 15. The result is a prediction of what percent above or below the trend line January will be next year. Find the point on the trend line next year for January and multiply it by the moving-average percent to find how much above or below the trend line the predicted point is. This process can be repeated for each month of the coming year.

For example, Table 6–3 shows the actual number of nursing hours incurred and the extended trend-line information for December, January, and February for 5 years.

The trend-line prediction for January 2002 from Figure 6–11 is 6,204. This is before adjustment for seasonality. In the calculation shown in Table 6–3, it was determined that for January the moving-average percentage is a positive 3.2% of 6,204. By adding 3.2% of 6,204 to the trend line value of 6,204, the resulting prediction adjusted for seasonality is 6,403. That point has been plotted for January 2002 in Figure 6–11. Similarly, to get the 2002 forecast for the entire year, this process should be repeated on a moving-average basis for each month in turn.

USING COMPUTERS FOR FORECASTING

The previous section on forecasting formulas demonstrates how complicated forecasting can become when historical data are influenced by both trend and seasonality. However, health care organizations frequently do have at least seasonality; both trend and seasonality are not uncommon. In recent years, nurse managers' ability to deal with such patterns has improved dramatically as a result of personal computers and specially designed computer software. These computer programs make the work of forecasting easier and the results more accurate.

A number of forecasting programs are available. This section discusses forecasting using one such program, SmartForecasts for Windows.[2] This program

---

[2]SmartForecasts for Windows is a trademark of Smart Software, Inc., 4 Hill Road, Belmont, MA 02178; telephone (617) 489-2743. Version 4.16 was used for Figures 6–12 and 6–13, and Tables 6–4 and 6–5 in this chapter. This chapter does not attempt to demonstrate all the capabilities of this software. The software program is used simply as an example of the use of computer forecasting. The use of the examples in this chapter does not represent a formal endorsement of the product.

TABLE 6–3. *Calculation of Moving Average Percent for January 2002*

Month		Actual	Trend Line	Difference	Difference as a Percentage of Trend Line
December	1996	5,100	4,980	120	2.4%
January	1997	5,200	5,000	200	4.0
February	1997	5,100	5,020	80	1.6
December	1997	5,500	5,221	279	5.3
January	1998	5,500	5,241	259	4.9
February	1998	5,400	5,261	139	2.6
December	1998	5,600	5,461	139	2.5
January	1999	5,700	5,482	218	4.0
February	1999	5,700	5,502	198	3.6
December	1999	5,600	5,702	(102)*	(1.8)*
January	2000	5,800	5,723	77	1.3
February	2000	5,900	5,743	157	2.7
December	2000	6,200	5,943	257	4.3
January	2001	6,300	5,963	337	5.7
February	2001	6,300	5,983	317	5.3
				Total	48.4%
				Divided by 15 =	3.2%

*Figures in parentheses indicate negative amounts.

is an example of computer forecasting software that is not limited to linear forecasting. Regression analysis produces a straight-line forecast. When there is seasonality, certain months are always above the regression line and others are always below it. Software such as SmartForecasts for Windows can generate *curvilinear* (curved line) forecasts. That means that the forecast line generated will come closer to the historical points, and therefore its projections are likely to be closer to the results that will actually occur.

SmartForecasts provides a data entry format similar to an electronic spreadsheet (e.g., LOTUS 1-2-3 or Excel), with columns and rows. Each column represents a time period, and each row represents a variable to be forecast, such as patients or nursing hours.

Reconsider the forecast for the data from Table 6–2 using SmartForecasts for Windows. After the data are entered, one of the first steps is to print a time plot graph to get a visual sense of the data. Examination of the time plot in Figure 6–12 quickly alerts the user to the upward trend; closer inspection reveals the seasonal nature of the data.

A number of different forecasting models are available within the software program. SmartForecasts allows the user to forecast nursing hours using regression analysis. However, if regression analysis is used, given the seasonality observed in the time plot, the same problem will occur as existed in Figure 6–10, requiring the same manual adjustments shown in Figure 6–11 and Table 6–3.

The key advantage of this software and other programs like it is that it allows use of a curved line for forecasting. This removes the necessity to adjust the trend line for seasonality. However, which forecasting approach should be used? Available methods include exponential smoothing, moving average, multiseries analysis, and so on.

Moving average approaches were used in the earlier section on forecasting formulas in this chapter. However, will that approach give the best result if other advanced statistical techniques are available? The best approach until one is very familiar with forecasting is to use automatic forecasting, which lets the computer choose the best approach. With the automatic approach the computer will calculate the forecast with a number of different methods to see which predicts best.

Figure 6–13 is the forecast graph generated by the software program. What does the graph consist of? The historical data points are connected by a solid line. The forecast during the historical (past) periods is dotted. Compare this dotted line with the regression line shown in Figure 6–11. During the first 5 years in Figure 6–11 the actual points are usually substantially above or below the regression line. Therefore it is reasonable to assume that as the line is used to project next year, each month's actual result is likely to be substantially above or below the forecast trend line.

Although the statistical theory is complex, effectively, the closer the forecast line comes to the actual results in the past, the more likely the forecast line is to come close to the actual results in the future. When the computer performs

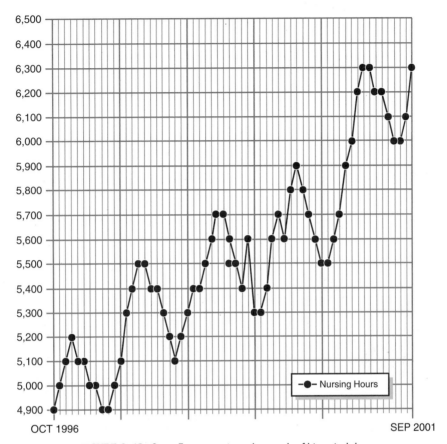

FIGURE 6–12. SmartForecasts time plot graph of historical data.

forecasting automatically, it examines how close the forecast line is to the historical actual points for each of a series of different forecasting methods. The computer can be given a command to examine the relative accuracy of the different forecasting methods examined. Table 6–4 shows the results of the competition among forecasting methods for this example. The best technique is Winters' multiplicative method. Winters' is a curvilinear approach that works extremely well for seasonal data. The data points are only 1.3% farther away from the forecast line for the next best method, another form of Winters' forecasting. However, using alternatives to the Winters' approaches generates much less accurate results.

In Figure 6–13 it is evident that the dotted forecast line for the first 5 years followed extremely closely the actual results. In some cases the solid and dotted lines are so close that they cannot be distinguished from each other. Therefore, the forecast line, when projected through 2002, is likely to give a fairly accurate estimate.

Nursing Hours

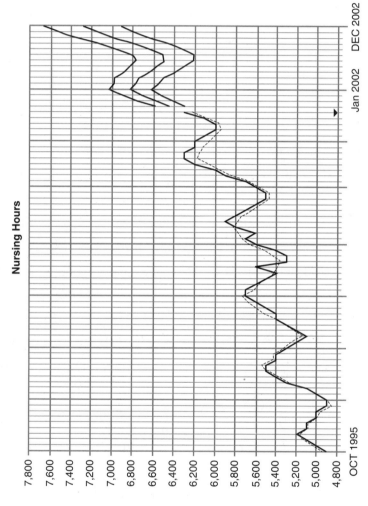

FIGURE 6–13. SmartForecasts forecast of nursing hours.

TABLE 6–4. Tournament Rankings for AUTOMATIC Forecasts of V1 Nursing Hours

Rank	Method	% Worse than Winner
1	Winters' multiplicative, weights = 22%, 22%, 22%	(winner)
2	Winters' additive, weights = 20%, 20%, 20%	1.3
3	Double exponential smoothing, weight = 8%	57.2
4	Linear moving average of 12 periods	65.0
5	Simple moving average of 1 period	118.3
6	Single exponential smoothing, weight = 59%	118.9

In the graph shown in Figure 6–13 there are solid lines above and below (bracketing) the forecast line projected into the future. These lines represent a margin-of-error interval. Forecasts can never be expected to be exactly correct. It is possible, however, to use statistics to get some idea of how large the difference might be between the forecast and the actual result. In this case, based on the statistical analysis there is a 90% likelihood that the actual result will fall somewhere between these solid lines. But graphs, while visually informative, are hard to read when it is time to write the actual forecast. Another computer command provides a numerical table of the forecast results. See Table 6–5 for the forecast results.

This table shows not only the forecast but also the margin of error or

TABLE 6–5. Forecasts of V1 NURSING HOURS Using Multiplicative WINTERS' METHOD

| Time Period | Approximate 90% Forecast Interval | | |
	Lower Limit	FORECAST	Upper Limit
OCT 2001	6,284	6,434	6,584
NOV 2001	6,405	6,572	6,740
DEC 2001	6,520	6,704	6,888
JAN 2002	6,622	6,821	7,020
FEB 2002	6,549	6,766	6,983
MAR 2002	6,502	6,737	6,973
APR 2002	6,391	6,641	6,891
MAY 2002	6,306	6,570	6,834
JUN 2002	6,210	6,493	6,775
JUL 2002	6,205	6,507	6,809
AUG 2002	6,311	6,633	6,956
SEP 2002	6,449	6,788	7,126
OCT 2002	6,634	6,996	7,358
NOV 2002	6,769	7,143	7,516
DEC 2002	6,897	7,282	7,666

confidence interval above and below the forecast. If desired, that interval can easily be changed so that there is 95% or 99% confidence that the actual result will fall within the range of values between the lower limit and upper limit estimates. If the percentage is raised to a higher confidence level, the interval around the forecast line becomes wider. For example, for January 2002 the prediction is 6,821 nursing hours, and there is 90% confidence that the actual nursing hours will not be less than 6,622 nor more than 7,020. If a manager wants to be 99% confident that the actual results will not exceed the boundaries of the projection, the lower limit value becomes lower and the upper limit higher.

In practice it is rarely necessary to be so precise. While 95% or 99% confidence may be important for academic research studies, in practice, managers tend to have a greater degree of latitude. In fact, the SmartForecasts software program is preset by the manufacturer to give a 90% confidence. While it is simple for the user to change that confidence level, given the way the software is set up, one must question whether it is desirable. Essentially, a 90% confidence interval implies that nine times out of ten the actual result will fall within the bounds of the interval. That is an extremely good result for most managers' forecasts.

Compare the result from Winters' multiplicative method (Table 6–5, Fig. 6–13) with the earlier result obtained by the combined regression analysis-moving-average approach (see January 2002 in Fig. 6–11). As can be seen, the results differ. This is because the approach used earlier is less accurate than the Winters' method. Earlier the January 2002 number of nursing hours was projected to be 6,403, while the Winters' method predicts it to be approximately 6,821. In fact the earlier estimate is below the lower limit value of the 90% confidence interval. It is clear that using more sophisticated techniques can generate results that differ markedly from the manual approaches used before computer software was readily available. It is probable that the manual moving-average calculation will be more accurate than simply a judgmental guess. However, the computer-based Winters' solution is likely to be even more accurate.

It is also possible to refine Winters' method even further. The computer makes some general assumptions when it performs forecasts under the automatic approach. If Winters' method was immediately selected as the forecasting method instead of selecting automatic, some additional options would be provided to improve the forecast further. Specifically, the SmartForecasts software can be informed of the relative importance of the most recent level, trend, and seasonal factors. If the user knows that the trend is changing due to shifts in the underlying demographics of the community population, it is possible to give more weight to the most recent trend, as compared with the trend in the earlier years.

Not only can information be supplied to enable the computer to be more accurate, such as the relative importance of the recent trend, but it is also possible to modify the results of the computer analysis. Results can be adjusted directly on the forecast graph, or historical data points can be modified on the basis of some judgment or knowledge the user has that is not reflected in the historical information. This is especially helpful when there is an outlier data point. For example, suppose that a rare event caused data for 1 month to be atypical. That data point can cause the forecast to be thrown off substantially. A better forecast may be obtained by judgmentally adjusting that data point's value. Judgmental adjustments are also needed because computer-generated forecasts assume that factors that affected nursing hours remain the same in the future as they were in the past. That may not be the case.

Most managers initially use a forecasting program only to forecast one item at a time. However, as one becomes more adept at using computer-based forecasting, the program would probably be used to generate forecasts on a number of different variables. The user will also want to be able to save the data file to avoid having to reenter data each time an analysis is to be performed. The SmartForecasts program has its own data files, and the data can also be stored in a wide variety of formats for future use, including LOTUS 1-2-3 worksheet files, ASCII (generic) files, or DIF files. By the same token, data in another format such as LOTUS, ASCII, or DIF can be read into SmartForecasts.

SmartForecasts is one of a number of forecasting programs that can be used on a personal computer. The most significant aspect of using sophisticated software programs is that they can generate a substantially improved result. The ability of the forecast line to curve in synchronization with the actual historical seasonal pattern decreases the required effort by the manager substantially, while enhancing the result.

DELPHI AND NOMINAL GROUP FORECASTING

The discussion of this chapter has assumed that reasonably reliable historical data is available. However, there will be many instances, especially in the case of new ventures, where a forecast will be needed for a budget, even though there is no reliable historical data. Subjective estimates will be required. In such cases, regression analysis or even computerized curvilinear forecasting will be inadequate to provide a solution. Two approaches commonly used to aid in making reasonable subjective forecasts are the Delphi and Nominal Group techniques.

In both approaches, a team or panel must be selected who are likely to have reasoned insights with respect to the item being forecast. Although no one may have direct knowledge or experience, an attempt should be made to select a qualified group. Industrial experience has shown that by arriving at a consensus among a team of experts, subjective forecasts can be reasonably accurate.

The Nominal Group technique is one in which the group of individuals are brought together in a structured meeting. Each member would write down their forecast. Then all the written forecasts are presented to the group by a group leader without discussion. Once all of the forecasts have been revealed, the reasoning behind each one is discussed. After the discussions, each member again makes a forecast in writing. Through a repetitive process, eventually a group decision is made.

Obviously, there are weaknesses to the Nominal Group technique. One problem concerns lack of information. If different forecasts are made based on different assumptions, it may be impossible to reach consensus. Another problem concerns politics and personalities. As members of the group defend their forecasts, extraneous issues having to do with whose idea it is may bias the group decision.

With the Delphi technique, the group never meets. All forecasts are presented in writing to a group leader, who provides summaries to all group members. For those forecasts that differ substantially from the majority—either high or low—a request is made for the reasoning behind the forecast. This information is also shared with all group members. Then a new round of forecasts are made. This process is repeated several times, and then a decision is made based on the collective responses.

Delphi has several particular advantages. By avoiding a face-to-face meeting, confrontation is avoided. Decisions are based more on logic than personality or position. The dissemination of the respondent's underlying reasoning allows erroneous facts or assumptions to be eliminated.

These two methods both make use of the fact that individual managers cannot be expected to think of everything. Different individuals, bringing different expertise and different points of view to bear on the same problem, can create an outcome that is superior to what any one of them could do individually. It is a cliche to say that two minds are better than one. Nevertheless, it is true that in many forecasting instances, the Delphi and Nominal Group approaches can substantially improve results.

SUMMARY AND IMPLICATIONS FOR NURSE MANAGERS

Forecasting is an essential part of the budgeting process. There are a number of items, such as patients, length of stay, and acuity, that are essential ingredients of an operating budget. Preparing an operating budget cannot begin without some prediction of the values for these variables. The same holds true for other types of budgets.

Managers have great flexibility in selecting the variables that they choose to forecast. They can forecast the number of patients, patient days, the quantity of a resource that will be consumed (e.g., the number of chest tubes needed or the number of nursing care hours), the amount that will be spent on supplies or personnel, or the acuity level of patients. Any variable for which historical data is available can be forecast using the methods of this chapter.

The forecasting process consists of collecting data, graphing the data, analyzing the graphed data, and preparing prediction formulas. Care must be exercised regarding consideration of things that are changing and that will prevent the future from being like the past. For example, a change in federal regulations concerning types of treatments covered by Medicare might have a dramatic impact on volume. While managers are aware of such changes, computerized formulas are unlikely to take discrete, recent changes into account. The human role in the forecasting process is critical to generating accurate forecasts.

Analysis of the graphed data will help a manager determine whether the item to be forecast has been exhibiting seasonal or trend behavior, both, or neither. Formulas can then be used to make predictions of the future.

It is important for managers to not only use common techniques of management but also to be prepared to be leaders in developing new uses. The first decade of the twenty-first century will likely see a rapid increase in the use of computers by health care managers. The first wave of microcomputer use saw widespread introduction of personal computers in positions where the same rote function was performed over and over. Computers clearly increase productivity by being faster at performing a calculation currently done many times. The next wave of computer use often represented a novelty. Computers were widely introduced but in many cases were used only as sophisticated typewriters (word processors).

Now, however, the average manager will start to use personal computers to manage better—not just to do an existing calculation faster or to type nice-looking letters. Forecasting is one area where the results of a manager's efforts will be superior because the use of a computer can allow a greater degree of sophistication to be merged with the already existing judgment and experience of the manager.

At the same time, one must always bear in mind that the sophisticated techniques of forecasting lack the judgment and experience of managers. Therefore, whether one is using a subjective Delphi technique or an objective computer program, the role of the manager in making the final forecast should never be understated.

SUGGESTED READINGS

Bauer, J.C. (1995). *Statistical Analysis for Decision Makers in Healthcare: Understanding and Evaluating Critical Information in a Competitive Market.* Chicago: Irwin.

Corley, M.C., and Satterwhite, B.E. (1993, March–April). Forecasting ambulatory clinic workload to facilitate budgeting. *Nursing Economic$.* 11(2), 77–81, 114.

Fass, S. (1997, June). Forecasting techniques improve hospital budgeting. *Hospital Cost Management & Accounting.* 9(3), 1–8.

Finkler, S.A., and Kovner, C.T. (2000). *Financial Management for Nurse Managers and Executives,* Second edition. Philadelphia: W.B. Saunders.

Finkler, S.A., and Ward, D.R. (1999). *Cost Accounting for Health Care Organizations: Concepts and Applications,* Second edition. Gaithersburg, MD: Aspen Publishers.

Horngren, C.T., Foster, G., and Datar, S.M. (1999). *Cost Accounting: A Managerial Emphasis,* Tenth edition. Englewood Cliffs, NJ: Prentice-Hall.

Zimmerman S. (1996, March). Forecasting and its importance to health managers in the ever-changing health care industry. *Hospital Cost Management & Accounting.* 7(12), 1–8.

7

Strategic Planning and Business Plans

The goals of this chapter are to:

define strategic management, its importance to health care organizations, and the benefits of the strategic planning process;

describe the evolution of strategic management from long-range planning to strategic planning to strategic management;

distinguish between broad, long-term goals and time-oriented, specific, measurable objectives;

introduce the concept of process improvement;

discuss each element of a strategic plan;

stress the importance of strategic thought by all managers in carrying out the operating budget;

explain the role of the long-range budget and strategic plan in the planning process;

define program budgeting and discuss the zero-base budgeting technique, stressing the importance of examining alternatives; and

outline the uses and elements of a business plan.

INTRODUCTION

Strategic management is the process of setting the goals and objectives of the organization, determining the resources to be allocated to achieving those goals and objectives, and establishing policies concerning getting and using those resources.[1] This process includes an environmental assessment and depends heavily on data concerning the organization's external environment. The strategic management process is critical to the organization's success. Managers and their

---

[1]John C. Camillus, *Strategic Planning and Management Control,* Lexington Books, Lexington, MA, 1986, p. 18.

staffs must not only do the things they do well but also carefully decide what must be done.

One planning text quotes Henry Thoreau: "It is not enough to be busy—the question is, what are we busy about?"[2] This simple question should cause nurse managers to pause and consider their role in the budget process. Day-to-day routine activities often cause nurse managers to become overloaded. Managers become so busy that they have little time to plan for the future or to introduce innovations. It is important for all managers to structure their jobs so that planning does not become pushed aside by the pressing day-in and day-out issues.

Strategy applied in managing organizations is still a developing field. In the middle of the twentieth century, businesses began to place a growing reliance on *long-range planning*. Long-range plans focus on general objectives to be achieved by the organization over a period of typically 3 to 5 years. By the 1960s the term *strategy* became commonplace, and long-range planning started being referred to as *strategic planning*. It was contrasted with operational planning—the development of a detailed plan for the coming year.

When strategic planning was introduced, the concept of strategy was that operational planning is tactical, whereas long-range planning is strategic. Under strategic or long-range planning an organization prepares a set of goals, then a strategy is developed for accomplishing them. That strategy is formalized into a plan of action generally covering a horizon of 3 to 5 years.

In the late 1980s and the 1990s experts in the area started to use the more generic term *strategic management* to define better the role of strategic thought in organizations.[3] Such experts argue for a broad view of strategic planning. The primary focus remains the identification of broad, long-term goals and the creation of plans to achieve them. However, the current view of strategic management or strategic planning relies on the use of strategic thought in guiding all plans and actions in an organization. This relates to short-term operational plans as well as long-range plans. Thus the operating budget discussed in the next chapter must always be viewed in its context within the long-term strategic plan of the organization.

Strategic planning is no longer simply long-range planning with a new name, as it was in the 1970s, 1980s, and 1990s. Strategic management "stresses three points: that the strategic planner is clearly the advisor and facilitator to line management decision-makers; that the program executive, not the strategic planner, is the key strategist; and that strategic planning is always integrated with other functions of the program management process—program design, organiz-

---

[2]Darryl J. Ellis and Peter P. Pekar, Jr., *Planning for Nonplanners*, Amacom, New York, 1980, p. 24.

[3]Jack Koteen, *Strategic Management in Public and Nonprofit Organizations*, Praeger, New York, 1989, pp. 19–21.

ing, budgeting, staffing, controlling, and evaluating."[4] Long-range planning is still a part of strategic planning, but it is no longer the only feature.

The current philosophy is that thinking strategically should not be the sole domain of the strategic planners of the organization. Planning by planners is important but insufficient. Strategic thought should be an element of the job description of all managers throughout the organization. Nurse managers have a central role in strategic planning in this new philosophical approach. The way a nursing unit is organized to provide care, the way it establishes patterns of staff to provide care, and the financial budgets it develops to gain authorization of needed resources to provide care should all be outcomes of a strategic process managed at the unit level. The principal change from earlier views of strategic planning is the emphasis on bringing all managers into the direct process of working to achieve the organization's primary goals instead of focusing narrowly on specific short-term objectives.

This chapter first discusses the definition, aims, and benefits of strategic planning and strategic thought. It then focuses on several specific aspects of strategic management, namely, long-range plans, program budgets, and business plans.

PROCESS IMPROVEMENT

A theme for the provision of health services in the twenty-first century is improved quality of care at a decreased cost. During the 1980s and 1990s, process improvement focused on reengineering, total quality management (TQM), and continuous quality improvement (CQI). These represent philosophies concerning the production of an organization's goods and services. Arikian notes that "TQM emphasizes a preventive approach to management, one that addresses problems before they arise, and handles concerns with a studied, long-term commitment to continuous improvement in product and service."[5] From a strategic management perspective, production in America has been dominated by an attitude of getting it done and then fixing it if it is wrong. Observations of the Japanese production process, however, have taught us that if more time is spent on planning, less will be done wrong and less will have to be fixed.

Many American corporations learned this lesson as they lost some of their competitive edge. To regain that edge corporations have adopted procedures that focus on avoiding the costs associated with poor quality. Examples of the change in attitude are apparent in the slogans adopted by corporations. For example, Ethicon, a manufacturer of sutures, adopted the policy, "Get it right the first time, every time."

Quality costs money. However, so does lack of quality. TQM focuses on the issue of being responsive to the needs of customers, while at the same time

---

[4]*Ibid.*, p. 21.

[5]Veronica Arikian, "Total Quality Management: Applications to Nursing Service," *Journal of Nursing Administration*, Vol. 21, No. 6, June 1991, p. 46.

reducing waste. Kirk notes in examinations of Japanese firms: "The most significant discovery related to their determination to *build quality into the product (or service)* rather than to inspect for errors and assume that error removal would lead to quality. Many Japanese managers bought into the concept of planning and followed through on it—unlike many American managers who use the ready-fire-aim approach. 'We don't have time to plan,' some American managers say. Contrarily, many Japanese businessmen say 'We don't have time *not* to plan.' "[6]

Various authors have identified different elements of TQM and CQI. Deming, the pathbreaker in the field, established fourteen points related to TQM.[7] These include such factors as a focus on education and training of employees, viewing employees not only as providers but also as customers, quality insurance, and a constant focus on finding ways to improve quality.

TQM and CQI are not financial management tools per se. We will not go into a detailed analysis of the methods here.[8] However, TQM and CQI have tremendous financial implications. Historically, health care organizations have minimized planning and maximized control over day-to-day operations. The lesson of TQM and CQI is that managers will be more likely to achieve their objectives if they can redesign their work to allow much more time for planning and innovating. Such activities are not occasional but rather should be viewed as a major element of the management function. We must learn to focus on improving the service we provide rather than simply making sure we get it provided.

As we enter the twenty-first century, the focus is shifting from TQM and CQI to value-added analysis. We must only spend money on activities that add value. All non-value-added functions represent wasted resources. The key, however, is not reengineering, TQM, CQI, or value-added. It is process improvement. Managers must focus on how they can change the way things are done to achieve higher quality at lower cost. In the long run increased focus on improvement of quality will lead to more satisfied staff and patients, higher quality of care, and lower costs.

STRATEGIC PLANNING

As noted earlier, strategic management calls for setting objectives, allocating resources, and establishing policies concerning those resources. Under this strategic planning approach, all managers become involved in this process.

---

[6]Roey Kirk, "The Big Picture: Total Quality Management and Continuous Quality Improvement," *Journal of Nursing Administration,* Vol. 22, No. 4, April 1992, p. 24.

[7]T. Gillem, "Deming's 14 Points and Hospital Quality: Responding to the Consumer's Demand for the Best Value in Health Care," *Nursing Quality Assurance,* Vol. 2, No. 3, 1988, p. 70.

[8]The interested reader is referred to the readings on the topic listed at the end of this chapter.

To establish and achieve goals, strategic planners have found it useful for the managers of an organization to focus on a series of key questions. The following questions are the most essential an organization must consider:

- Why does the organization exist?
- What is the organization currently?
- What would it like to be?
- How can we make the transformation to what it wants to be?
- How will it know when it is done?

These questions in turn lead to a large number of other questions. What are the organization's strengths? Its weaknesses? Its opportunities? Its threats? Who are the organization's primary customers? Are they being well served? Does the organization learn from its mistakes? Does the organization have a vision for the future? These questions are related to the organization as a whole, but they also relate to each department and unit within the organization.

Managers need to step aside from the current day-to-day activities and assess the nature of the existing organization. Has the organization over the years lost track of its reason for existence? Is the current status of the organization the desired one? If not, then the organization needs to address formally the issue of how it can change things to become the type of organization it believes it should be. Again, this is true for departments and units as well as for entire organizations.

Strategic planning asserts that the way to become the type of organization you want to be is to establish a set of clear goals and objectives and then a plan for achieving them. Goals are defined as the broad aims of the organization, while objectives are specific targets to be achieved to attain those goals.[9]

Once goals and objectives are identified, then specific tactics can be designed to move the organization toward those goals. Tactical plans require resources. When managers prepare operating budgets they often fail to include the resources necessary to achieve the goals of the strategic plan. That is one reason that strategic management now takes a more global perspective.

In developing a short-term operating budget for the coming year, the unit manager must decide whether to place more emphasis on short-run profits or long-term growth. Spending extra money on quality improvements now will generate expenses not offset by revenues. But the reputation for quality will generate more revenues in the future. If strategic plans and operating budgets are treated as being separate, it forces managers with responsibility for operating expenses to focus on reducing short-run expenses. That tends to be exactly the opposite of the long-run strategic goals of the organization as designed by preparers of the strategic plan. Therefore managers must balance the short-term objectives of their units or departments with a long-range vision for the

---

[9]The planning literature is inconsistent in the definition of goals and objectives. In some instances the definition used here for goals is assigned to objectives, and vice versa.

organization. Developing and carrying out the operating budget should not be done without knowledge of the organization's strategic plan.

It is not clear if any organization will ever get where it wants to be. The target goals tend to be modified over time in reaction to changes both inside and outside the organization. However, to make progress toward the goals, the organization should constantly be attempting to answer the various questions stated earlier and to take necessary actions based on the answers to the questions.

The Elements of a Strategic Plan

Strategic plans must be adapted to specific situations. The elements of a plan for one organization may not be perfectly suited to another. Flexibility is a positive attribute in the strategic planning process. For most organizations, however, the basic elements of a strategic plan would include:

- Mission statement or philosophy
- Statement of long-term goals
- Statement of competitive strategy
- Statement of organizational policies
- Statement of needed resources
- Statement of key assumptions

The Mission Statement or Philosophy

The first step in strategic management is the development of a *mission statement* for the organization, department, or unit. What is the purpose of the organization or unit? An organization cannot begin to plan goals effectively and allocate resources sensibly until it first clearly determines its reason for existence. Strategic planners refer to an organization-wide statement of purpose or focus as the mission statement. In the department of nursing this is often referred to as the philosophical statement.

A great deal of care should be taken in developing a mission statement. The mission statement of the organization should focus the organization by defining what it does. Some health care organizations set their mission statement either too broadly or too narrowly. At one extreme they wind up running restaurants or other nonhealth facilities that sap time and energy and often fail because the organization lacks expertise in that area. At the other extreme, growth and change are not encouraged by the statement, and the organization stagnates.

Some degree of limitation in the mission statement is beneficial, forcing the organization to concentrate on what it knows how to do. At the same time, the mission statement should allow growth and diversification. The mission statement should be defined in such a way as to prevent the organization from exceeding its manageable boundaries but encouraging exploration within those boundaries. Camillus notes that a

health care organization engaged in providing eye-care services can describe itself as fulfilling the mission of examining eyes and writing prescriptions for corrective lenses or the mission of protecting and improving human vision. The first statement is essentially a description of activities in which the organization is engaged. The second statement, in contrast, identifies consequences rather than activities and thus leads to the identification of such possibilities as opening clinics where eye surgery is carried out, engaging in the development and possibly the manufacture of devices for rectifying faulty vision, and running programs for educating the public about the proper care of eyes.[10]

The key to designing the mission statement is to focus not on what the organization does right now as much as think about the range of possible types of activities one would see as a logical extension for the organization over time.

Statement of Long-term Goals

Goal setting is the organization's attempt to set the direction for itself as it tries to meet its mission. Often an organization will have both quantitative and qualitative goals. Quantitative goals may relate to financial outcomes, such as rates of growth in the number of patients served and in revenues. Qualitative goals may relate to patient satisfaction and general reputation.

In developing the long-term goals of the organization, their timeless nature should be kept in mind. Objectives are intended to be attained within a specific time frame. Goals tend to stay in force over long periods. Providing the needs of an increasing percentage of the community's citizens is a long-term goal. Increasing the number of patients by 8% in the coming year is a specific measurable objective.

While statements of objectives are necessary, the statement of goals is of greater concern in strategic management. As managers attempt to respond in their operations to specific, time-oriented objectives, they should bear in mind the overriding goals that the organization wants to achieve. Innovations that allow the organization to make major steps forward toward achieving its long-run goals should constantly be sought by all managers.

Statement of Competitive Strategy

The organization's competitive strategy is its plan for achieving its goals, specifically, what services will be provided and to whom. The development of this strategy relies to a great extent on a thorough internal and external review. What are the organization's strengths and weaknesses, its opportunities and threats?

Competitive strategy is the planning of what care will be provided and to whom. To develop such a plan the organization must consider what competitors are or are not doing and what expertise the organization does or does not possess. Based on that information the organization can decide where it should expand and perhaps where it should contract.

---

[10]John Camillus, *op. cit.,* p. 47.

Essentially the organization must evaluate its mission and goals in light of its particular strengths and weaknesses and in light of the demand for services and competition in the external environment. Based on that evaluation it can make a plan that will take advantage of opportunities that present themselves and plan a reaction to the threats that exist.

Statement of Organizational Policies

The role of policies is to specify what are and are not acceptable practices by the organization. The establishment of a mission and objectives incorporates a set of values. It integrates the values of the organization's founders, the values of its management and staff, and the values of the community. Those values should be incorporated in the decisions made by the organization.

In most organizations no single person can review each and every decision and decide if it is appropriate. A set of policies that clearly indicates what actions are appropriate and what actions are not removes an unreasonable burden from managers throughout the organization. It removes the necessity for guesswork by individual managers in many specific situations.

Policy statements are substantially different from mission statements, statements of goals, and statements of competitive strategy. In each of those earlier statements there is a need to encourage creativity. Each one leaves room for the organization to innovate or grow. In contrast, policy statements are generally limiting. They provide the constraints that the organization wants to place on managerial discretion.

Surprisingly, such constraints can ultimately enhance organizational growth. Without specific policies, managers may find that they are chastised for specific actions without any rhyme or reason. They become uncertain as to when it is okay to take initiative and make changes and when higher levels of management want things done just the way they always have been done. This high degree of uncertainty will lead managers over time to become reluctant to innovate in any respect. The availability of specific procedures clearly delineates where innovation is not allowed. However, that also provides the manager a sense of where innovation is allowed and welcomed.

Statement of Needed Resources

Strategic planning cannot be held apart from the reality of the resources needed to carry out the plan. These include resources in terms of personnel, the facilities for the personnel to work in and with, and the other requirements for accomplishing the goals of the organization. Without linkage between the plan and the resources to carry it out, there can be little hope of achieving the organization's goals.

Statement of Key Assumptions

Part of the planning process is development of a statement of key assumptions. Since strategic management calls for a decentralization of the planning process, there must be a set of guidelines that all managers use in common. If management expects to have additional contracts with managed care organizations, that will affect the entire organization. The same assumption about such contracts should be used consistently by all managers. This will make plans consistent and will also improve coordination of plans throughout the organization. It will also help in determining whether variations from the plan are due to carrying out the plan or the accuracy of the underlying assumptions.

Benefits of the Strategic Planning Process

One can think of a number of benefits that result from having a strategic planning system. One of the most predominant benefits is that it forces the organization to determine its long-run goals and come up with an approach to accomplish them. Establishing long-run goals forces managers to decide what the organization's purpose is and to formalize that purpose. Many health care organizations were established long before any of the current employees worked for the organization. The original goals of the organization can easily become lost among the personal needs and desires of the current management and staff. The process of establishing a formalized mission and goals gives a sense of direction to the organization.

A strategic planning system also promotes efficiency. Managers working toward clear goals are less likely to be inefficient. When everyone clearly knows what the organization is trying to achieve, there is a likelihood that less effort will be spent on unnecessary activities.

The strategic planning process provides a means of communication among the various hierarchical levels of the organization. In large organizations (and sometimes even in relatively small ones) communication between organizational levels becomes difficult. The managers on the lower rungs may know that things are not being done efficiently. The managers at the upper rungs may believe that the systems they have in place do generate efficiency. Inadequate channels exist for moving information up or down through the ranks. Innovation in such cases is expected to be dictated from the higher levels of the organization. In fact, often the need for and opportunities for improvements are most visible at the lower levels. A strategic management process should allow new ideas to flow smoothly down or up.

Lower-level managers will learn more about why changes are taking place if they share the strategic plan and can see how changes relate to achieving the plan's goals. Higher-level managers will receive better information if lower-level managers focus some of their attention on factors that affect the organization's long-run goals.

The strategic planning process provides managers with an improved sense of the needs of the organization and of its environmental constraints. It has often been found that a partnership approach to management works better than a dictatorial approach. Managers who are told that they must live within constraints resist them. Managers who are asked to become part of the team to solve the problem of constraints learn to understand the difficulty in the constraints and are more willing to work cooperatively instead of adversarially.

The strategic planning process increases the level of organizational creativity in addressing problems. Successful organizations encourage rather than resist change. Things are done very differently now than they were twenty years ago. Change, however, doesn't occur at some arbitrary point every twenty years. It occurs gradually in an evolutionary process. The fact that most organizations do things a certain way now that they didn't do twenty years ago indicates that someone tried a new approach and found it superior. Who is that someone? Is it the lucky one who accidentally fell upon an improved approach?

Generally, this is one area where organizations make their own luck. Creativity cannot be forced upon people. One cannot tell employees to be creative and to develop innovative improvements. However, creativity can be either fostered or stifled. A strong commitment to strategic management throughout the organization will convey the organization's view of creativity as a positive rather than a negative element.

Implementing a Strategic Management Process

This chapter has alternatively referred to the strategic plan and to the strategic planning or management process.

The specific development of a strategic plan will be discussed in the next section of this chapter. However, strategic management relies not just on a plan but on a broad planning process. That process is one of making managers aware of the need to think strategically as they carry out all their management activities. In developing the long-range plan, managers must relate the plan to the mission. In designing specific program budgets or business plans, the manager must consider how the program will help the organization achieve its goals. In developing the specific details of the operating budget, again the manager should be trying to link the details with how they help the organization reach its long-term aims.

The remainder of this chapter focuses on several of the long-range elements of strategic planning. Specifically, long-range planning, program budgets and business plans are addressed. As the reader proceeds to Chapters 8 through 12 on operating, revenue, capital, performance, and cash budgets, the notion of trying to link operational activities with strategic thought should be kept in mind.

LONG-RANGE PLANNING

In developing the long-range budget the organization begins the process of translating its general goals and objectives into a specific action plan. Long-range budgets or long-range plans are often referred to as the organization's strategic plan. Such plans generally cover a period of 3 to 5 years.

Given a strategic management process that calls upon managers to focus on the organization's goals, is a strategic plan essential? The answer is clearly yes. Long-range planning is critical to the vitality of an organization. For organizations to thrive, they must move forward rather than being stagnant. The staff of an organization should be able to look back and see the progress that has been made over an extended period. Budgeting for one year at a time does not allow for the major types of changes that would take years to plan and implement. Yet that lengthy process is needed for the efforts that will substantially move the organization forward.

For example, suppose that one goal of the organization is to move from being a primary care community hospital to a regional tertiary care center. This cannot be accomplished by having each department attempt to modify its operating budget. An overall organizational plan is needed. Which of the new tertiary services can or should be added in the next 5 years? Which programs already exist but need to be expanded in the next 5 years to accommodate the changing role of the organization? These questions are specifically addressed in the strategic plan or long-range budget.

Nursing should be involved in this planning process. The success of the plan will depend on how well it is carried out. If the plan does not have adequate nursing input when it is prepared, it is unlikely that the nursing staff will support it fully. Nurses must push their organizations to incorporate nursing leadership into the planning process not only for the good of nurses and nursing but also for the ultimate success of the organization.

The strategic plan may lay the groundwork for a fund-raising campaign to precede and parallel expansion of services. Or the plan may indicate that each year for 5 years growth in specified existing profitable areas must be undertaken to offset the start-up losses on the introduction of major new programs. Specific dollar amounts of additional revenue and new program cost may be projected only in terms of an extremely rough estimate. Although quite general, such a plan does give the organization enough specific information about the implications and requirements for the expansion into a tertiary care center to allow for the development of specific programs to move the organization toward that ultimate goal.

The strategic plan may be somewhat more detailed, showing projections of the dollar amounts expected to be available (and their sources) as well as which specific programs will be adopted and what their approximate costs will be. Since a strategic or long-range plan projects at least 3, and up to 10, years into the future, it is unlikely that revenue and cost estimates will be highly accurate. Therefore while rough estimates are often included in such plans, they are generally not overly detailed or refined.

The plan should not focus only on major program additions. The services and programs that already exist are equally important to an organization. Expanding a service, contracting one, or even deleting a program or service requires the same consideration and planning as the addition of a program or service. A part of the planning process should be to address explicitly whether those services and programs that make up the majority of operations of the organization are being retained at a steady-state level or whether they are to be contracted or expanded in scope.

One serious potential problem arises if this issue is ignored in preparing strategic plans. If existing programs are implicitly assumed to continue unchanged, a plan that includes a number of new programs may appear feasible. However, it may not be feasible when technological and other changing factors are explicitly considered for the ongoing operations of the organization. Therefore, expectations regarding existing programs should be reviewed explicitly and included as part of the plan.

Once the plan has been finalized and formalized, it serves as a guide for a number of years. Long-range plans are typically prepared only once every 3 or 5 years. Creating a new plan each year would only lead to constant changes in the organization's direction. This would lead to wasted efforts and frustrated managers. However, such plans should be reviewed each year. Assumptions may turn out to be wrong. A cure for cancer could change patient volume. The external environment can change dramatically. An influx of refugees could change the demand for services. Annual reviews allow the organization to adjust the strategic plan to react to current events.

Each year elements of the plan are brought into the current activities of the organization. The operating budget should be prepared based on an understanding of the strategic plan. It should be designed to assist the organization to achieve the goals and objectives of that strategic plan. To make the transition from the plan into operations, many proposed additions or changes require a thorough evaluation. This may be accomplished through the development of a program budget.

PROGRAM BUDGETING AND ZERO-BASE BUDGETING

Program budgeting is the part of the overall strategic planning process that focuses on all the costs and benefits associated with a specific program. The program may be an existing one that the organization is considering expanding, contracting, or eliminating, or it may be a new program that the organization is thinking of adding. Program budgeting examines alternative programs to meet the organization's objectives and examines feasible alternative ways to accomplish each given program.

Some program budgeting is done within a nursing unit or department. Often, however, the program changes generated by a strategic plan have interdepartmental impacts. Such program changes are much more complicated because of the need for coordination between departments. It is vital that nursing participate fully in such interdepartmental planning. Working on key committees is essential not only to protect the interests of nursing but also, as noted earlier, to ensure that any plans developed make sense from a nursing perspective and can be supported by the nursing staff.

In most cases program budgets relate directly to the strategic planning of the organization. The projects being evaluated are under consideration because they relate directly to moving the organization toward the achievement of its long-term goals.

Program budgets are substantially different from other types of budgets. Long-range budgets or strategic plans look in general terms at the entire organization over a period of years. Their information is based on rough approximations rather than being highly detailed. Operating and cash budgets look in great detail but only at the coming year. A program budget combines a great amount of detailed information for a long period for one specific program. Further, while most budgets focus on a given department's revenues and costs, program budgets compare revenues and expenses for an entire program, cutting across departments or cost centers.

A program budget compares all its costs and benefits to evaluate the entire program's effect on the organization over its lifetime. In doing this the program budgeting methods identify costs and benefits of different programs aimed at the same purpose or of different approaches to one program. Because resources are limited, program budgeting often focuses on trade-offs. That is, program budgeting considers the extra benefit to be gained by spending additional money on a program. Alternatively, program budgeting considers how much of the benefit of a program would be lost if less money were spent on the program.

Zero-Base Budgeting

Zero-base budgeting (ZBB) is a popular program budgeting technique that gained fame for its strong push toward analysis of all costs. All costs from a base of zero must be justified. Until the introduction of ZBB, it was common for budget negotiations to revolve around the appropriate amount of the increase in a budget. How much more should be spent next year than was spent in the current year? Implicitly, such an approach assumes that all current-year spending continues to be reasonable and justified for the next year. Only the amount of the increment is subject to examination and discussion.

In reality, as technology and diseases change, some departments have growing financial needs, while other departments could get by with decreasing resources. The concept of requiring a zero-base evaluation is attractive because it means that budgets would not be allowed to become "fat" over time. Many organizations use ZBB analysis to see exactly how money is being spent within a unit or department. Such an approach requires existing programs to justify their continued existence. Rather than basing the future budget on the past budget, all expenditures in the proposed budget must demonstrate why they are needed.

Additionally, the ZBB approach pays great attention to the alternative ways that any one given program can be offered. ZBB collects information regarding a program into a *decision package*. A decision package contains documentation in support of the program and summaries of the analyses performed. In that sense, the decision package is just a mechanism to ensure a formal, systematic review of each budget.

Each package contains a statement of the purpose of the program, the consequences of not performing the program, and the ways that the costs and benefits of the program can be measured. More interestingly, the package also includes statements of alternatives. These statements are the heart of ZBB.

ZBB provides a great degree of sophistication in the analysis of alternatives. Not only may different programs with separate decision packages be compared, but ZBB also compares three major types of alternatives within the decision package for each individual program. The first alternative involves ways to produce the treatment, service, or other output. The second set of alternatives relates to the quantity of treatments, service, or output to be provided. The third set of alternatives considers varying levels of quality.

For many nurses, considering trade-offs such as these is counter to their traditional education. Nurses, as health care professionals, are trained to provide the best possible care to each patient. At the larger level of organizational planning, however, it must be acknowledged that no health care provider can provide everything to everyone. There simply are limited resources. ZBB forces recognition of the need to determine the greatest overall good that can be provided to the entire population served by an organization, in contrast to the view of providing care to a specific individual.

Perhaps the best way to understand how these alternatives are examined is to work through a potential program budget problem.

ZBB Case Study–Hemodialysis

Suppose that the hypothetical Wagner Hospital has decided on the basis of its environmental review that there is a pressing need for additional hemodialysis services in the community. In Wagner's long-range plan the introduction of a hemodialysis program has been included, although the plan does not include much in the way of specifics other than to note that within the next 5 years some form of hemodialysis program should be instituted. This program was highly placed when priorities were established, although it would have to vie for funds with several other important new programs that were also included in the long-range plan, such as a new primary care center.

Wagner has compiled a decision package for the hemodialysis program. The formal documentation in the package first notes the name of the program (hemodialysis) and the sponsoring department within the hospital (internal medicine). The stated purpose of the program is to reduce levels of mortality and morbidity currently experienced in the community due to insufficient hemodialysis facilities. The resources needed for the program are stated in general terms.

They include dialysis machines, physicians, nurses, technicians, supplies, and overhead items such as electrical power and physical space.

If Wagner were not a user of ZBB, it is likely that the renal specialists in the hospital would have designed a first-class hemodialysis center, perhaps as a new hospital wing, with five machines to satisfy all community needs. The proposal would have been a take-it-or-leave-it package, with strong political emphasis on its acceptance.

There is nothing wrong with wanting everything to be first class. It is not wasteful to provide top-quality care. However, that does not mean that an organization can afford to provide that care. Having a first-class hemodialysis center may mean that there will not be enough resources left for adequate cancer treatment.

Because Wagner Hospital uses ZBB, the hemodialysis plan cannot be approved until an analysis is performed that examines a number of alternatives. The first issue concerns the level of output. How much treatment will be provided? Suppose that five machines would take care of the entire community demand now and for the foreseeable future. Suppose that the estimated annual cost of this alternative were $2 million including depreciation, supplies, personnel, overhead, maintenance, and so on. A second alternative may be to purchase only four machines. Suppose that at this level it would still be possible to eliminate all mortality and morbidity, but some of the machines might have to operate two or three shifts per day, causing some inconvenience for nurses and physicians.

Four machines might cost a total of $1,700,000. Note that while the number of machines would fall 20%, from five to four, the costs would fall only 15%. That would be possible because some costs associated with the program are likely to be fixed. As discussed in Chapter 4, fixed costs do not change in total as the output level increases. Does this mean that five machines would be better than four, since the hospital would get 20% more machines for only 15% more cost? Not necessarily. That is the wrong comparison. The goal is to provide cost-effective, high-quality health care to the community. The goal is not to buy unnecessary equipment to minimize the cost per machine.

The alternative of four machines instead of five would save $300,000. Although there would be some inconvenience, the reduced cost would not result in any extra mortality or morbidity. The extra convenience gained by having five machines must be compared to the benefits available by spending $300,000 for some other program. Also, one must determine if the extra machine generates any additional revenue or solely affects scheduling.

Other alternative levels of output might be the use of three machines, which would eliminate all mortality and 50% of the morbidity for a cost of $1,400,000; two machines, which would eliminate only 80% of the mortality at a cost of $1,100,000; and one machine, which would eliminate only 40% of the mortality at a cost of $800,000.

Itemizing the costs and benefits of the alternative output levels is informative.

Unlike the usual all-or-nothing presentation for a new program, either five machines or no program at all ("We don't practice second-class medicine here!"), the choice is not that dramatic. In fact, in a constrained environment it may well be that upon seeing all the alternatives, the choice will focus between either three machines or four machines. Less than three may be considered inadequate to accomplish the long-run objectives; more than four may raise questions of priorities.

It is not only the amount of output that is a question here. The ZBB system requires that alternative ways to produce the output also be considered. Is there a choice? Isn't it hemodialysis machines or nothing? Perhaps the answer is yes, but one of the major roles of ZBB is to ask questions such as these. The next question might be, Does hemodialysis have to be performed in the hospital? The answer is no. While one alternative would be to perform all dialysis in the hospital, another alternative would be to perform all dialysis in one clinic location. Another alternative would be to have a series of external locations spread throughout the community, one location for each machine. It is also possible to use one mobile van for each machine, allowing dialysis to be performed at many locations. Each of these alternatives would be matched with one, two, three, four, and five machines.

Other alternative options must also be considered. Can the patient be on the machine for a shorter period, thus increasing the number of people who have access to it? Can money be saved by buying machines with fewer accessories? Such questions almost certainly hit upon issues of quality. However, the trade-offs between quality and cost must be examined.

Trade-offs are always made, and they sometimes impact on the quality of care. If one person dies of heart disease, it may be because not enough resources were devoted to having the latest open heart surgery equipment. That person suffered from a lack of high-quality care. More resources devoted to heart surgery equipment might have saved that individual. Perhaps the hospital should cut back in another area and pursue the very best heart surgery. In the vast majority of cases, that would simply result in other people dying in the other area. The budgeting system must attempt to select a set of projects that are carried out in a way that minimizes the overall negative impact on quality. That may mean undertaking two new services, each at less than the optimal level of care, rather than totally sacrificing the existence of either service so the remaining one could be run on an optimal basis. Table 7–1 provides a summary of the hemodialysis decision package and its focus on trade-offs in this hypothetical example.

The difficult part of the analysis is to explicitly and creatively seek and examine trade-offs from alternatives. Specifically, it is necessary to ask whether more lives could be saved by the organization if it spent $300,000 less on hemodialysis and got four machines instead of five. Could even more lives be saved in some other program if dialysis was cut to three machines and $600,000 less was spent on this? Three machines might mean less care and lower quality care—less time on the machine for each noncritical patient. What could $600,000 do elsewhere in the

TABLE 7–1. ZBB Decision Package—Hemodialysis

1. Name of program: Hemodialysis
2. Department: Internal Medicine
3. Purpose: Reduce mortality and morbidity due to lack of hemodialysis facilities
4. Resources required; Dialysis machines, physicians, nurses, technicians, supplies, overhead
5. Quantity or level of output alternatives

Level	Medical Implications	Cost
Five machines	Eliminates all mortality and morbidity; no inconvenience to staff	$2,000,000
Four machines	Eliminates all mortality and morbidity; some inconvenience to staff	1,700,000
Three machines	Eliminates all mortality and 50% of all morbidity	1,400,000
Two machines	Eliminates 80% of mortality	1,100,000
One machine	Eliminates 40% of mortality	800,000

6. Alternative ways to produce the output: This section should consider the various approaches to providing the product and the cost of each. For instance, it should consider providing the care in the hospital, in clinics, or in mobile vans. For each way of providing the output, each output level (i.e., one machine, two machines, etc.) should be considered.
7. Alternative levels of quality of care: This should consider the cost of using different types of machines and/or changing the amount of time each patient is on the machine for each way of producing the output and for each level of output in terms of numbers of machines.

organization? Would $600,000 spent elsewhere provide enough benefit to justify less care and lower-quality care in this area?

Suppose that in addition to hemodialysis, a primary care center has also been proposed. A first-class primary care center might cost $1 million per year (the numbers here are hypothetical). This primary care center would provide access to care for 50,000 visits per year (or about 12,000 people). However, a ZBB review of primary care indicates that for $600,000 a total of 35,000 visits could be handled. All children in the community could get immunizations, but some older patients would have to travel to an existing clinic.

Because of the large capital investment, the Wagner Hospital does not have sufficient cash to establish both a primary care center and a hemodialysis service at the ideal first-class levels. It is highly likely that without a zero-base review, the hospital might well select either hemodialysis or primary care—and the choice would likely depend largely on politics. The well-being of the community can get lost in the struggle between vested interest groups within the organization.

There might, however, be enough resources to provide both hemodialysis and primary care at slightly reduced levels of care. The hospital could add three dialysis machines and a primary care unit.

The zero-base review forces the examination of alternatives. It forces recognition of the fact that more lives would be saved by scaling back the size of hemodialysis and primary care and then providing both services. Given the explicit information contained in the ZBB reviews, both vested interest groups are likely to be more willing to accept the resulting compromise.

The ZBB Cost Matrix

Looking at the descriptions of alternatives in Table 7–1, it becomes apparent that presenting various possible alternatives can become complex. To help with this logistical problem, the ZBB decision package for each program can be summarized in the form of a matrix (Table 7–2). Each cell in the matrix provides the cost of providing a certain level of care, produced in a particular way and with a particular approach to quality. This makes all trade-offs explicit. In picking a particular cell from the matrix, the organization knows exactly what it is getting and at what cost. All cells meeting minimum requirements should be calculated.

In Table 7–2, the rows represent the cost of various numbers of machines placed in a variety of types of locations, such as all machines in the hospital or all machines in one clinic. All possible locations and all quantities of machines are included. The columns present the various possible types of machines. They are referred to as the best, moderate, and minimum. Alternatively, specific types of machines could be listed in the various columns. Similarly, assuming that the length of time a patient is on a dialysis machine is variable, one could think of the best, moderate, or minimal amounts of time.

Notice that the columns in Table 7–2 combine all quality of care possibilities. It is possible to have the best machine and the best amount of time on the machine. Or the hospital might have the best machine with a minimal amount of time, or the minimum acceptable machine with the best amount of time, and so on.

For any given cell in the matrix, the cost of a particular type of machine and length of treatment time for each patient, as well as the number of machines and location, is calculated. It is possible that some cells will not be feasible and will not have a value. For instance, if only two machines are purchased, it might not be possible for patients to have the longest (and best) amount of time on the machine.

If the hospital were to decide to spend $600,000 on primary care and $1,400,000 on hemodialysis, all cells on this hemodialysis matrix that have a cost over $1,400,000 could be eliminated. Then the organization could focus on the different combinations of quantity of care, quality of care, and ways to produce hemodialysis care that cost $1,400,000 or less. The most preferred alternative from among those that are feasible for $1,400,000 or less could then be selected.

Ranking Decision Packages

Since the resources of the organization are always limited, it is rare that all proposed packages can be accepted. Therefore ZBB requires each manager to rank the alternative decision packages. The best alternative would be ranked number 1.

TABLE 7–2. ZBB Cost Matrix—Hemodialysis

Alternative Ways to Produce and Alternative Quantities	Alternative Quality Levels								
	Quality of Machine/Patient Time on Machines								
	Best/Best	Best/Moderate	Best/Minimum	Moderate/Best	Moderate/Moderate	Moderate/Minimum	Minimum/Best	Minimum/Moderate	Minimum/Minimum
In Hospital									
5 machines	$2,000,000	$1,750,000	$1,500,000	$1,750,000	$1,500,000	$1,250,000	$1,625,000	$1,375,000	$1,125,000
4 machines	1,700,000	1,500,000	1,300,000	1,500,000	1,300,000	1,100,000	1,400,000	1,200,000	1,000,000
3 machines	1,400,000	1,250,000	1,100,000	1,250,000	1,100,000	950,000	1,175,000	1,025,000	875,000
2 machines	1,100,000	1,000,000	900,000	1,000,000	900,000	800,000	950,000	850,000	750,000
1 machine	800,000	750,000	700,000	750,000	700,000	650,000	725,000	675,000	625,000
In One Clinic									
5 machines	1,800,000	1,550,000	1,300,000	1,550,000	1,300,000	1,050,000	1,425,000	1,175,000	925,000
4 machines	1,500,000	1,300,000	1,100,000	1,300,000	1,100,000	900,000	1,200,000	1,000,000	800,000
3 machines	1,200,000	1,050,000	900,000	1,050,000	900,000	750,000	975,000	825,000	675,000
2 machines	900,000	800,000	700,000	800,000	700,000	600,000	750,000	650,000	550,000
1 machine	700,000	650,000	600,000	650,000	600,000	550,000	625,000	575,000	525,000

Multiple Clinics									
5 machines	1,075,000	1,325,000	1,575,000	1,200,000	1,450,000	1,700,000	1,450,000	1,700,000	1,950,000
4 machines	950,000	1,150,000	1,350,000	1,050,000	1,250,000	1,450,000	1,250,000	1,450,000	1,650,000
3 machines	825,000	975,000	1,125,000	900,000	1,050,000	1,200,000	1,050,000	1,200,000	1,350,000
2 machines	700,000	800,000	900,000	750,000	850,000	950,000	850,000	950,000	1,050,000
1 machine	575,000	625,000	675,000	600,000	650,000	700,000	650,000	700,000	750,000
Mobile Van									
5 machines	775,000	1,025,000	1,275,000	900,000	1,150,000	1,400,000	1,150,000	1,400,000	1,650,000
4 machines	700,000	900,000	1,100,000	800,000	1,000,000	1,200,000	1,000,000	1,200,000	1,400,000
3 machines	625,000	775,000	925,000	700,000	850,000	1,000,000	850,000	1,000,000	1,150,000
2 machines	550,000	650,000	750,000	600,000	700,000	800,000	700,000	800,000	900,000
1 machine	475,000	525,000	575,000	500,000	550,000	600,000	550,000	600,000	650,000

During the process of budget review and negotiation, managers at higher levels of the organization will receive ranked decision packages from a number of subordinate managers. For example, a nurse manager with responsibility for a number of units might receive packages from each unit nurse manager. The packages from all these different units must be ranked in order of importance by the manager responsible for the group of units. Then the packages will continue up through the organization. The CNE and her administrative staff will rank all the packages received from all the different nursing areas.

In large organizations the ranking process can become quite tedious. However, it is a necessary evil if the goal of the program budgeting process is to compare all the alternatives available to the organization and ultimately to allocate the organization's resources to those projects that best lead to attainment of the organization's goals.

BUSINESS PLANS

One approach to program budgeting that first became widely used in the latter part of the twentieth century is the business plan. This technique, long used in industry, became popular in health care as it became clear that health care organizations would have to take a more businesslike approach to providing their services in an ever more difficult financial environment. It is a method that is still gaining support in all types of health care organizations.

What Is a Business Plan?

A *business plan* is a detailed plan for a proposed program, project, or service including information to be used to assess the venture's financial feasibility. Business plans are used by nurse managers to assess the likelihood of success for a wide variety of ventures. Nurse entrepreneurs should certainly prepare a business plan before starting a new venture. In addition, nurse managers working for an organization should prepare business plans for new programs or services to be offered by the organization. Often the plan is used as a sales document that makes the case for undertaking a new project. However, despite its advocacy role, the plan should provide an honest appraisal of the project. If in fact the proposed project is not good for the organization, that should be determined at the planning stage rather than after a large financial investment has been made to implement it.

The first step in planning a new program should be to understand which goals of the organization the program promotes. Does the proposed project fit with the organization's mission statement? In developing the plan, sufficient information must be gathered to indicate whether the proposed program will move the organization closer to its goals. In evaluating the plan, it is important not to lose sight of the original organizational goal to which the project relates.

For example, one business plan might relate to the development of a community education program for diabetics, while another plan focuses on providing home health care. Both of these new programs might fit nicely within a mission of providing health care services to the community. It is possible, however, that the former program on community education would not be expected to be financially self-sufficient. It fits into the element of mission that concerns providing important services on a charitable basis. On the other hand, the home care plan may be based on the notion of earning profits to be used to subsidize the charitable elements of the organization's mission. The organization cannot provide some services at a loss unless it provides some at a profit or receives donations to offset the loss.

Even the program aimed at the charitable mission would require a business plan. The fact that it is not expected to earn a profit does not remove the need to understand just how much of a subsidy it might require. At the same time, if home care is being proposed to earn profits to subsidize the other operations of the organization, we should not lose sight of that fact during the planning process.

The plan should define the tactics that are being taken to accomplish the organization's goal. It should clearly state the objectives of the proposed project and provide a linkage that shows how the plan's objectives will lead to accomplishment of the organization's goal.

The plan must clearly communicate the concept of the project. It must also communicate the organization's ability to carry out the project. One can think of a business plan as a document that answers the questions one should ask before investing money in a project:

- What exactly is the proposed project?
- To what extent does the organization have the capabilities to undertake the project?
- Where will the organization acquire the capabilities that it lacks?
- Will the project make or lose money?
- How much?
- Does the organization have the financial resources to undertake the project?
- If not, where can those resources be obtained?
- How will the new product or service be marketed?
- What alternative approaches have been considered?
- Why is the proposed approach considered better than the alternatives?

The Steps in Developing a Business Plan
Project Proposal

The first step in developing a business plan is the proposal of a new product or service or an expansion of an old one. Nursing is often involved in new products and services, either in a support role or as the principal proponent. For example, the addition of a new type of laser surgery would clearly have implications for nursing. Changes would likely occur in the operating room as well as the med/surg units. The project might be proposed by the surgeons, with the nursing department providing valuable assistance in developing the business plan. On the other hand, the decision to add an outpatient surgery unit might be suggested by the nursing director of the operating room. As such, it would be primarily a nursing business plan. Nurses can become involved in developing a variety of different programs and innovative services. Nurse entrepreneurs developing a new home care agency or additional home care services for an existing agency, developing a nursing agency, and developing an educational or counseling clinic are just a few examples of projects that should have business plans.

Business plans can be developed for new ventures or ongoing organizations. When planning a new venture, it is important to consider market opportunity, resource needs, resource sources, and risks. Market opportunity refers to identifying the unfilled existing need. The entire venture rests on this issue. What do people need that no one is providing to them? If that need does not exist, the venture is not likely to succeed. If the need does exist, what resources would be required to meet that need? Where might you get the resources from? Finally, what could go wrong? No one should ever enter a new venture without careful thought to the possible risks involved.

Existing organizations should consider strengths and weaknesses, opportunities and threats. New initiatives or programs can be developed to enhance an area in which the organization is already strong or to offset some weakness. At times the primary goal is to enhance a strength to make it even more difficult for competitors to challenge that strength. At other times the goal is to shore up a weakness. Existing organizations should also be on the lookout for opportunities or threats. At times a new program may be developed to ward off potential competition. At other times, competition falters and a temporary opportunity exists. Successful organizations try to anticipate or at least identify opportunities and threats and to respond to them on a timely basis.

Product Definition

Once a program has been proposed, the product or service must be carefully defined. What is the specific product; what are the ways it can be provided; what are the resources needed to provide it? Are the patients homogeneous or mixed in terms of diagnoses; in terms of acuity? Are the required resources limited to labor and other operating items, or are capital investments needed as well? How long will it take to get the program up and running? Are there economic or technological trends that could impact on patient demand in the future?

Market Analysis

Having defined the product, the next step is a market analysis. Are there people who want that product and are willing to pay for it? How many potential buyers are there, and how many other organizations offer the product or service? What *market share* can this organization get? Market share refers to a percentage of the total demand or volume for the product or service. For example, if there are 10,000 patients in your community who will be treated and your organization gains a 10% market share, it will expect to treat 1,000 patients. The organization must be convinced that there will be sufficient demand to justify the investment in this project as opposed to some other project.

As part of the market study, it is necessary to consider change. Is the market likely to grow? That is, will there be a growing number of patients? Will competition grow? Will there be more and more providers competing for the patients? If so, will this organization's market share fall?

The issue of competition is critical. Is there competition? Is there the potential for competition? What will competition do when they see this organization's new program or project? What are the strengths and weaknesses of the competition?

The market analysis must consider who the patients will be and who the payers will be. Is the population largely insured; largely indigent? Having enough patients is the first step. Equally important, however, is knowing the mix of patients.

Mix of patients refers to different types of ailments and different types of payers. The types of ailments must be known so that the expected costs can be calculated. The mix of payers is also important. What percentage are Medicare patients, Medicaid, HMO, other insurance? The program's revenue can vary dramatically based on who will ultimately be responsible for paying the organization's charges. The charges represent gross revenues. Generally, however, only a portion of total charges is collected because of government-mandated rates or special discount arrangements or because the patients are uninsured and unable to pay. The ultimate cash receipts must be known in addition to the volume of patients.

If the market analysis shows little demand or excessive competition, the planning process for this specific program may be discontinued. If it appears that there is demand for the product or service and a reasonable potential market share for the organization, the planning can continue.

Rough Financial Plan

After the market analysis is completed indicating a demand exists for the product, a rough financial plan can be developed. The purpose of this rough plan is to determine whether the project warrants further attention. The rough financial plan revolves around an operating budget.

The operating budget includes rough estimates of both revenues and expenses. The revenues can be calculated based on the demand projections from the market analysis. The expenses can be based on rough approximations of the types and amounts of various resources needed.

The results of a rough financial plan are imprecise. The purpose of the plan is to arrive at one of three findings. The first possible finding is that the cost of the program will far exceed the revenues under any reasonable set of assumptions. In that case, managers should save their time by discontinuing the planning process if the project is being evaluated solely on financial merit. A second finding is that the program looks as if it will definitely be profitable. In that case the manager can proceed with the substantial time investment required to develop a fully detailed plan. A third finding is that it is unclear whether the project will be profitable.

The third result creates some difficulty for managers. A major potential danger in program planning is that the manager working on the data collection will begin to push harder and harder for the project, the more time the manager has invested in the analysis. The more time managers invest, the greater their psychological need to justify that investment by having the plan indicate that the project is favorable. This could result in a bias in the collection and interpretation of data concerning project feasibility.

Given the unknowns that one encounters in putting any new program into place, there should be a healthy degree of skepticism about any new project. "If it's such a good project, why isn't someone else already doing it" is a reasonable thought. Therefore, one should always continue with analysis cautiously. There may be a good answer to the question of why someone isn't already doing it. But the issue should be considered. Generally, if the rough analysis indicates just borderline profitability, then plans should be discontinued unless factors lead the manager to believe that a more detailed analysis may in fact produce information in the project's favor. More often than not there are unanticipated problems that reduce profitability as a project progresses. If the project was borderline in the beginning, losses may well result. It is better to discontinue work on such projecs sooner rather than later.

Detailed Operations Plan

Assuming that planning for the project is still continuing after the rough financial plan, the next step would be to develop a detailed operations plan. The essence of this plan is to consider the entire impact that the new project will have on the existing operations of the organization.

The first element of the plan is to consider the physical location and structure required by the program or project. Next one must consider the specific human resources required. Equipment and supplies must also be taken into account. These are all direct costs of the project. It is possible, however, that the project will also cause indirect costs to vary. For instance, the admitting department may need more personnel. The marketing department may have to make a substantial effort to get the new service off the ground. The engineering department may have to devote many personnel hours to the project. It is necessary to account for the impact of the program on all the organizational overhead components.

Detailed Financial Plan

Once a thorough analysis has been made concerning the various impacts of the proposed plan on the operations of the organization, a detailed and thorough financial plan can be developed. This financial plan incorporates all the information from the operations plan, considering the financial impact of the resources to be used. This information will ultimately be used to determine whether it is possible to go ahead with the new program.

The financial plan has three critical elements: a break-even analysis, preparation of budgets, and the development of a set of pro forma financial statements. Pro forma financial statements present a prediction of what the financial statements for the project or program will look like in the future.

The break-even analysis provides information on the minimum volume of patients that must be achieved for the new program not to lose money. Many new programs or projects start with low volume and gradually attract more patients. The pattern of growth in the volume of patients is predicted as part of the market analysis. Break-even analysis is valuable because combined with the volume projection it can help give the organization a sense of how long it will take before the new program stops losing money. The techniques of break-even analysis were discussed in Chapter 4.

Budget preparation includes the development of an operating budget, a cash budget, and a capital budget. These budgets are prepared for 3 to 5 years into the future, from the start of the venture. The cash and operating budgets are often prepared on a monthly basis over that time. Many new ventures take several years to become operational. If we were to prepare budgets for just 1 year into the future, we would not get a full sense of the mature entity. Often there are few patients when a venture first starts. Minimal staffing levels may cause losses in the first quarter or half year for even the most successful initiatives. Longer range detailed budgets can provide a better picture of what is likely to happen once the organization is fully operational and has a stable (although hopefully growing) patient population.

Although many nurse managers in large organizations are only responsible for expenses of their units, that is rarely the case in new ventures. The developers of the business plan must critically consider the revenue flow. The revenue budget must include estimates of patient demand, broken down by type of care or services to be consumed. The payer mix must be estimated as well. In other words, the developers must determine what percent of the patients will receive each type of treatment offered and what percent of patients will be Medicare, Medicaid, and so on. The amount to be charged for each service must be decided, and the expected amount to be collected by payer for each service must be forecast. All this information is used to estimate the amount of revenue to be earned. See the Chapter 9 discussion of revenue budgets.

Various expenses also have to be planned based on the same patient demand estimates used for revenue. Preparation of the expense budget requires that decisions be made concerning how large a facility is needed to house the service at the start and later as it grows. Will the venture start with a small amount of space and add additional space as required or start out from the beginning with enough space to handle expected patient volume for at least several years into the future? Will all the equipment be purchased at the start, or will it be acquired in phases?

How much staff is needed when the venture opens for business, and at what volume levels will additional staff be hired? Clearly, business plan budgets must address many questions about the timing and amount of expenses that do not come up in running an ongoing department of an existing organization.

The capital budget considers the acquisitions the organization will have to make for buildings and equipment with multiyear lives. Unlike ongoing departments that focus capital budgets on additions or replacements, new ventures are faced with evaluating many capital acquisitions all at once. However, it is important to give each acquisition the same careful consideration one would if only a few capital assets were being acquired. Capital acquisition errors made by a start-up venture can be costly. If it turns out that a $500,000 piece of equipment is really not adequate and has to be replaced with a $600,000 alternative that was considered but rejected as being too expensive, the attempt to "save" $100,000 on the initial purchase can be devastating to the financial success of the start-up venture.

The cash-flow budget provides information on how much cash the program or project will spend each year and how much cash will be received. This information is not available from the operating budget for the program. That budget will focus on revenues and expenses. However, revenues are generally received some time after the patients are treated. In many cases it takes payers (including Medicare, Medicaid, HMOs, and others) weeks or months to pay for the services provided. On the other hand, cash outlays at the beginning of the project may be substantial. In addition to paying salaries on a current basis, the organization will need to acquire supplies, equipment, and, in some cases, buildings.

In the case of salaries and supplies, the time between cash payment and ultimate cash receipt may be a matter of months. In the case of buildings and equipment, substantial amounts of money may be needed to start the program, while the receipt of cash from the use of the buildings and equipment may stretch out over a period of years. Therefore it is important for the organization to know the amount of cash required. That information will allow the organization to decide if it has sufficient cash available to undertake the project. Cash budgeting is discussed further in Chapter 12.

Pro forma financial statements present a more comprehensive summary of the financial implications of the plan than is provided by the budgets developed as part of the rough financial plan.

Pro Forma Financial Statements

Every organization has a set of financial statements that are financial summaries used to indicate the financial position of the organization at a point in time, as well as the financial results of its activities for a period of time. Often financial statements are used to indicate the organization's financial position at the end of its fiscal year and its revenues and expenses and cash receipts and payments for an entire fiscal year. The most typically used financial statements are the balance sheet (also called the statement of financial position), the statement of operations (also called the activity statement or the income statement), and the statement of cash flows (or the cash flow statement).

The balance sheet provides a listing of all the resources and obligations of the organization. The resources owned by the organization are called assets. The obligations of the organization are called liabilities. If the assets exceed the liabilities, the difference is called *net assets* or *owners' equity.* The assets will always equal the total of the liabilities plus the net assets or owner's equity. Therefore the balance sheet will always be "in balance."

The operating statement is a listing of all the revenues, less all the expenses. The difference is sometimes referred to as the net income. Many health care organizations refer to the difference as the excess of revenues over expenses or the change in unrestricted net assets. This is the primary measure of an organization's profitability.

The statement of cash flows is a categorized listing of all the organization's cash receipts and cash payments.

Using the budgets and the various projections and assumptions about the proposed program or project, the key financial statements are projected for each year into the future, usually for a period of 3 to 5 years. Any predictions beyond 5 years are generally considered unreliable. Any predictions fewer than 3 years fail to give a picture of what the financial impact of the program is likely to be once it is fully up and running.

Pro forma statements allow the user to determine some basic financial information about the proposed program or project. The pro forma balance sheet will indicate for each future year what the year-end obligations are likely to be relative to the resources. One would want to always have sufficient resources to be able to pay obligations as they become due. The pro forma operating statement will tell the project's expected profitability for each future year. The pro forma cash flow statement provides a summary of the information from the cash-flow analysis discussed above.

Forecasting

The detailed financial plan, as noted above, includes a break-even analysis, budgets, and a set of pro forma financial statements. To get the information needed for these elements, the business plan relies heavily on forecasts.

To prepare a cash-flow analysis and to generate pro forma financial statements, a great number of items must be forecast. These include, but are not limited to, inflation, regulation, revenues, wage rates, availability of personnel, detailed expenses, cash flows, and patient volumes. To make these forecasts, the techniques discussed in Chapter 6 are employed.

Sensitivity Analysis

In developing the detailed financial plan, a helpful technique is sensitivity analysis. Sensitivity analysis is concerned with the fact that often a number of assumptions and predictions are made in calculating the financial aspects of a business plan. The number of expected patients used to develop pro forma financial statements is the result of a forecast, which may not be exactly correct. The revenues are based on a stated average charge, which is an assumption. The actual rates charged may be higher or lower. Sensitivity analysis is a process whereby the financial results are recalculated under a series of varying assumptions and predictions. This is often referred to as "what-if" analysis.

Suppose that the pro forma financial statements lead one to believe that the proposed project will be a reasonable financial success. Using sensitivity analysis, one could then say, "What if there are 5% fewer patients than expected? 10% fewer? What if there are 5% more patients than expected? 10% more? What if the average amount charged is raised by 10%? What if the number of staff nurses needed is three FTEs greater than anticipated? What if the construction costs are $30,000 more than expected?

Essentially, sensitivity analysis provides recognition of uncertainty. Uncertainty creates risk. Before a final business plan is put together and accepted, one needs to have some idea of the magnitude of risk involved. By going through the what-if analysis, one can get a sense of how unfavorable the financial results would be if some things do not occur just as hoped for or expected. If a project can show an expected favorable financial result over a range of what-if questions, it can provide an extra degree of assurance. If that is not the case, then one must carefully question whether the potential benefits are worth the risk that must be undertaken.

Examination of Alternatives

A final consideration in the development of a detailed financial plan is the examination of alternatives. There is often more than one way to do a new program. The alternatives relate to factors such as the capacity of the program, the approach to providing the service, and the quality of the program. The business plan should be based on having selected one specific approach after having considered a wide variety of potential alternatives. Calculations regarding the costs and benefits of the various alternatives that have been considered become part of the final business plan package.

The Elements of a Business Plan Package

With business plans, as with great cooking, presentation of the finished product is an essential component of the process. Business plan development requires a significant amount of time and effort. The finished result is often a long document. Unless carefully presented in a final package, the benefits of much of the work may be lost.

The first and most critical element is a concise executive summary. The executive summary should be brief. Ideally it is no more than one paragraph or one page. It may be two or three pages if absolutely necessary. The summary should convey what the project is, why it is being proposed, and what the projected most likely results are. This should be able to be done in just a few brief sentences. If the information in the summary indicates that the project is worth pursuing, the reader will read further.

The next part of a business plan should be a detailed abstract. Such an abstract is generally about 20 or 30 pages long. This should provide a much greater amount of detail than the executive summary. However, it still is a summary or abstract. It does not include all the specific documentation for the calculations that underlie the plan.

The abstract should describe the mission of the organization and the way that the proposed program fits in with the mission. It should provide a description of both the product or service and its potential consumer. The abstract should explain how the new product fits in with the organization's existing services. It should explain why there is a belief that the organization has a competitive edge for this product or service that will allow it to gain and maintain a certain level of market share. The profitability of the program should be discussed in greater detail than that provided in the executive summary. The pro forma financial statements should be included.

It is essential that the abstract discuss potential risks. Regulation and other elements that would impede the project should be discussed as well. Finally, the abstract should include some estimate of the requirement for management time needed to implement the program and a statement of commitment by the manager who will bear primary responsibility for the implementation of the program.

The final part of the business plan package is the detailed analysis of each element. At this point all remaining data are included: detailed descriptions of the product and service, a detailed market research plan indicating market potential and competition, a detailed time line for implementation of the plan, a detailed marketing plan for attracting patients, and a detailed financial plan including the analyses used to develop the pro forma statements. Some of the data may be organized into appendixes to the detailed analysis.

By grouping the business plan into these three sections—executive summary, detailed abstract, and full detailed analysis—the manager allows other managers less familiar with the project to understand it. This will allow the project to get a fair examination and should lead to a reasoned final decision on whether to implement the proposed program.

Readers who plan to prepare a business plan should read one of several books on the topic listed in the Suggested Readings at the end of this chapter.

SUMMARY AND IMPLICATIONS FOR NURSE MANAGERS

Often nurse managers at all levels of the organization have insights that can result in significant operational changes that will move the organization closer to its strategic goals. That is why strategic management takes the view that strategic planning is not limited to the development of the long-range plan and program budgets. Strategic management must exhibit itself through strategic thought by managers throughout the organization. All nurse managers should make themselves aware of their organization's mission and goals as well as its specific objectives and policies. Knowing only the philosophical statement of the nursing department alone is too narrow a view.

The organization-wide goals developed in the strategic management process are used as a point of reference in assessing where the organization has been, where it is going, and what it hopes to accomplish in the coming years.

Strategic management requires a significant effort from managers at all levels. However, that effort is rewarded. Careful planning reduces the extent to which managers move from crisis to crisis. It promotes the efficient use of resources and the financial health of the organization. It results in goal setting and the establishment of a vision for the organization. Strategic planning helps ensure that managers will identify opportunities and take reasonable risks to take advantage of those opportunities. Strategic management promotes organizational change within a stable framework of constant mission and goals.

The strategic plan or long-range budget indicates which programs are to remain at a steady state, which are to be reduced in size or eliminated entirely, which are to be expanded, and which are to be added. This gives impetus to specific program budgets in which a unit, department, or program undergoes a complete assessment.

Using a method such as ZBB, the organization's managers can systematically examine all the implications of a program over its lifetime. The program can be compared to others that would achieve the same end. The program can also be assessed in terms of alternative ways to produce the output, alternative levels of quality, and alternative levels of quantity of output.

Program budget analyses can uncover unneeded costs in existing programs. There is waste in health care organizations as in virtually all organizations. Further, program budgeting can help the organization to make effective choices of how to best use limited resources. Trade-offs among various alternatives can be more clearly assessed with the increased information program budgets provide about the impact of different available options.

The organization can settle for a less-than-first-class bedside computer system but can also have new unit-based video cassette recorders (VCRs) for patient education. Alternatively, it can have a new first-rate bedside computer system and forgo having unit-based VCRs. This book cannot say which of the choices would be best. However, there should be an awareness that the alternatives do exist. The organization should not blindly get a first-rate bedside computer system because of internal political pressure and then simply accede to the fact that there is no money for VCRs. The alternatives should be considered and an explicit choice made.

Program budgeting techniques are equally effective for reviewing the operations of an ongoing unit as they are for evaluating a new program. The way a nursing unit performs its tasks may go unchanged from year to year. A ZBB review, however, can force the manager to consider whether there are alternative ways or levels of effort that could be used to accomplish the unit's goals.

Performing a zero-base review for a nursing unit, department, or organization is expensive. It takes a substantial amount of time to evaluate all the cost elements of a budget. It is much simpler to just indicate the next year's operating budget will be 2% more than the current year's. However, the chances of making a significant positive gain for the organization are much higher when a thorough justification of each and every expenditure is undertaken. Managers tend to accept the status quo. Instead, managers should spend less time on day-in and day-out routine activities and more time on being innovative. Examining all aspects of a unit's operations can result in significant and lasting benefits for the unit and the entire organization.

Business plans are documents that are becoming essential for the introduction of new programs. Such plans help managers to complete a comprehensive examination of a proposed program. By making such a thorough review, the manager and the organization gain an in-depth understanding of the program as well as its financial implications for the organization.

Strategic management has broader implications than just for use in specific areas such as zero-base reviews or business plans. Managers should be creative in their applications. For example, there are many models for the delivery of nursing services. Each one has financial, quality, and other implications. A nurse manager who understands strategic management can apply its principles when the organization makes choices among alternative delivery care models. In this way the choice made will reflect consideration of the wide range of factors that relate to that decision.

SUGGESTED READINGS

Arkebauer, J.B. (1995). *Guide to Writing a High-Impact Business Plan.* New York: McGraw-Hill.

Ballein, K.M. (1997, Winter). Entrepreneurial leadership characteristics of SNEs emerge as their role develops. *Nursing Administration Quarterly.* 22(2), 60–69.

Campbell, S. (1997, March). The newest gatekeepers: Nurses take on the duties of primary care physicians. *Health Care Strategic Management.* 15(3), 14–15.

Cortes, T.A. (1996, May). Zero-based budgeting for a radiology service: A case study in outsourcing. *Hospital Cost Management & Accounting.* 8(2), 1–6.

Crow, G.L. (1996, Summer). The business of planning your practice: Success is no accident. *Advanced Practice Nursing Quarterly.* 2(1), pp. 55–61.

Etinger, W.H., Jr. (1998, January). Consumer-perceived value: The key to a successful business strategy in the healthcare marketplace. *Journal of American Geriatric Society.* 46(1), 111–113.

Finkler, S.A., and Ward, D.R. (1999). *Cost Accounting for Health Care Organizations: Concepts and Applications,* Second edition. Gaithersburg, MD: Aspen Publishers.

Haag, A.B. (1997, January). Writing a successful business plan. *Journal of American Association of Occupational Health Nursing.* 45(1), 25–32, 33–34.

Holman, E.J., and Branstetter, E. (1997, September–October). An academic nursing clinic's financial survival. *Nursing Economic$.* 15(5), 248–252.

Hough, D.E., and Bolinger, J.E. (1998). *Developing a Managed Care Business Plan*. Chicago: American Medical Association.

Lambert, V.A., and Lambert, C.E., Jr. (1996, January–March). Advanced practice nurses: Starting an independent practice. *Nursing Forum*. 31(1), 11–21.

McLaughlin, C.P., Kaluzny, P., and Arnold, D. (1997, Fall). Total quality management issues in managed care. *Journal of Health Care Finance*. 24(1), 10–16.

McNiel, N.O., and Mackey, T.A. (1995, July–August). The consistency of change in the development of nursing faculty practice plans. *Journal of Professional Nursing*. 11(4), 220–226.

Nagaike K. (1997, Winter). Understanding and managing change in health care organizations. *Nursing Administration Quarterly*. 21(2), 65–73.

Newland, J.A., and Rich, E. (1996, September). Nurse-managed primary care center. *Nursing Clinics of North America*. 31(3), 471–486.

Olsen, S., and McFarlin, J. (1998, November). The Tapestry model: An innovative strategy for futuristic strategic planning. *Aspen's Advisor for Nurse Executives*. 14(2), 1, 3–5.

Parker, M. (1997, Winter). The new entrepreneurial foundation for the nurse executive. *Nursing Administration Quarterly*. 22(2), 13–21.

Porter-O'Grady, T. (1997, Fall). The private practice of nursing: The gift of entrepreneurialism. *Nursing Administration Quarterly*. 22(1), 23–29.

Shames, K. (1997, May). Holistic nurse entrepreneur—growing a business. *Beginnings*. 17(5), 7, 13.

Simpson, R.L. (1997, March). Take advantage of managed care opportunities. *Nursing Management*. 28(3), 24–25.

Simpson, R.L. (1997, Winter). From nurse to nursing informatics consultant: A lesson in entrepreneurship. *Nursing Administration Quarterly*. 22:2, 87–90.

White, K.R., and Begun, J.W. (1997, Winter). Nursing entrepreneurship in an era of chaos and complexity. *Nursing Administration Quarterly*. 22, 2, 40–47.

Wilson, C.K. (1997, Winter). Mentoring the entrepreneur. *Nursing Administration Quarterly*. 22(2), 1–12.

8

The Operating Budget

by Christina M. Graf, RN, MS

The goals of this chapter are to:

explain the various factors in preparing an operating budget;

describe the financial structure of health care organizations;

review the planning elements of an operating budget;

discuss the elements of an activity budget;

explain the types of patient classification systems and the related issues of reliability and validity;

provide a detailed approach to developing an operating budget, including determining unit workload, other units of service, the revenue budget, staffing requirements, the personnel budget, the positions/hours budget, the salary budget, and the nonsalary budget;

define FTEs and variations in definitions of FTEs;

discuss the impact of alternative coverage patterns on the preparation of the operating budget;

describe the role of productive and nonproductive time;

explain calculations of differentials, premiums, and overtime;

create an awareness of the need to account for float, on-call, callback, and agency nurse time;

describe the rationale for and approach to budget negotiation;

discuss the elements of budget finalization; and

discuss budget implementation.

The operating budget is a plan that projects the health care organization's anticipated activity, required resources, and associated revenue and expense for a specified period of time—generally 1 year. The framework for the operating budget is reflected in the financial structure and reporting system of the organization.

FINANCIAL STRUCTURE

Most health care organizations follow the same general format in financial structures and systems, with some variation in specifics. The format for the financial structure is the organization's *chart of accounts*. The chart of accounts gives structure to the recording and reporting of a firm's transactions. It organizes this data to make it useful and meaningful for management of the enterprise. The chart of accounts identifies both areas of responsibility that constitute the work of the organization and the categorization of transactions occurring within these areas. It is specific to an organization and reflects that organization's unique reporting needs.

The financial structure is based on the *responsibility center,* a program or area of activity within the organization. This term emphasizes the concept of the manager's control of and accountability for a defined area of activity. These centers may be either *revenue-producing,* such as pharmacy and laboratory, or *non-revenue-producing,* such as housekeeping and administration. On this basis, the chart of accounts may term these areas *revenue centers* or *cost centers.* Individual departments may be single cost centers or may be composed of several cost centers.

Typically, nursing departments are made up of multiple cost centers that describe discrete physical locations or operational areas: individual patient care units, operating room, postanesthesia recovery, ambulatory clinics, emergency department, administration, and so on. In many settings, particularly inpatient settings, nursing is not directly reimbursed for its services in the same way that, for example, pharmacy is reimbursed according to the type and amount of drugs provided. Nursing services are included in overall routine charges for room and board, procedures, or visits, as are services such as housekeeping and dietary. If these routine charges appear on nursing cost center reports, the cost centers may be designated as revenue-producing for accounting purposes. Operationally, however, nursing in these organizations is not seen as revenue-producing. In some hospitals, nursing costs have been accurately described, separated from the routine charges and used as the basis for determining nursing charges. In these circumstances, nursing's contribution to revenue generation for the organization is defined explicitly. In other settings, the revenue generated by nursing is clearly delineated. Visits by nurse clinicians in the home care setting or by nurse practitioners in the ambulatory setting, for example, directly generate revenue for the organization. (See Chapters 9 and 16 for further discussion.)

The financial reporting system for the responsibility center and the department identifies the revenue generated and expenses incurred for each accounting cycle (generally one calendar month or one 28-day period). Cumulative totals for the fiscal year-to-date (YTD) are also reported, as are totals (both for the month and year-to-date) for departments and the total organization. The organization's revenue is based initially on *charges,* or the prices that it sets for specific services. The sum of these charges is described as gross *patient revenue.* However, not everyone pays the full charge for their services. Under the federal Diagnosis Related Group (DRG) system, for example, Medicare pays a fixed amount per inpatient admission based on the patient's discharge diagnosis, which may or may not cover the charges generated during that admission. Medicaid systems vary from state to state, but they usually pay an amount less than charges. Other third-party payers such as Blue Cross and managed care organizations frequently negotiate a discounted payment rate that is less than charges. The difference between the charge and the discounted rate is referred to as a *contractual allowance.* Typically, health care organizations also provide some level of *free care or charity care,* which also reduces the amount the organization expects to be paid. These allowances are identified as *deductions from revenue,* and the gross revenue less deductions from revenue is called *net revenue.* (Note that *bad debt,* bills that patients are able but unwilling to pay, are considered a business expense and not a deduction from revenue.) Revenue reported in the individual responsibility center, however, generally reflects only the gross charges for specific services provided for that area of activity.

Expenses reported in the responsibility centers are generally limited to *direct expenses,* those expenses that can be specifically and exclusively related to the activity within that area. Note that direct expenses can be further subdivided into direct and indirect patient care costs. This subdivision differentiates those unit costs that can be specifically related to providing care for individual patients (direct) from those that support the overall operation of the unit (indirect). In this differentiation, salaries paid to staff nurses for hours spent providing care to patients would be considered direct care costs, while the salaries paid for hours devoted to orientation or continuing education would be considered indirect care costs. Similarly, dressing supplies or IV fluids would be identified as direct care costs, while notepads and similar office supplies would be identified as indirect. Both direct and indirect patient care costs, however, would be classified as direct *unit* expenses. *Indirect expenses,* such as administrative and personnel costs or heating and lighting expenses, are shared by all departments. These expenses are usually not allocated to individual cost centers in the revenue and expense report or are allocated according to standard costing methodologies and are referred to as *overhead.*

Within the monthly financial report, individual revenue and expense items are sorted into like groupings and reported by account. For example, expenses incurred within a given time period are separated into two major categories: employment costs and nonsalary expenses. Within these two categories, expenses may be further subdivided. Employment costs can be reported according to types of employees (RN, non-RN), types of hours (straight time, overtime, vacation, sick), types of differentials (evening, night, on call), and categories of fringe benefits (FICA, health insurance). Nonsalary categories could include subgroupings such as patient care supplies, instruments, office supplies, equipment, and subscriptions. Supply expenses identified as *interdepartmentals* refer to those expenses initially incurred by one department and later charged to the end-user department. For example, pharmacy may purchase bulk supplies of stock drugs, then charge them to the individual patient care units as unit stock supplies are replaced. Telephone bills may initially be charged to a central communications office, then allocated to individual areas based on actual utilization of services. Although these expenses are not purchased directly from the vendor by the end-users, they are real expenses to the responsibility center and require the same level of management as other supply expenses. The chart of accounts provides the identifying numbers and descriptions of these accounts.

RESPONSIBILITY CENTER: 611 GENERAL SURGERY				REPORT FOR: JANUARY, 2001		
THIS MONTH			**ACCOUNT**	**YEAR TO DATE**		
Actual	Budget	Variance	NUMBER/DESCRIPTION	Actual	Budget	Variance
			311. Revenue			
($371,026)	($365,800)	$5,226	010 Routine	($3,244,410)	($3,221,400)	$23,010
(2,987)	(3,153)	(166)	020 Other	(27,590)	(27,768)	(178)
($374,013)	($368,953)	$5,060	Total Operating Revenue	(3,272,000)	(3,249,168)	$22,832
			411. Salary Expense			
$ 85,115	$ 85,127	$ 12	010 Salaries—Regular	$ 730,881	$ 749,665	$18,784
2,758	0	(2,758)	020 Salaries—Per Diem	2,758	0	(2,758)
3,209	4,101	892	030 Salaries—Overtime	40,128	36,115	(4,013)
10,885	11,220	335	040 Salaries—Differential	97,995	98,810	815
7,168	7,066	(103)	050 FICA	61,285	62,222	937
7,235	7,363	129	060 Health Insurance	62,125	64,846	2,721
2,212	2,358	146	070 Pension	19,855	20,766	911
1,896	1,915	19	090 Other	17,228	16,868	(360)
$120,478	$119,150	($1,328)	Total Salary Expense	$1,032,255	$1,049,292	$17,037
			611. Supply Expense			
$4,976	$4,084	($892)	010 Patient Care Supplies	$41,692	$35,961	($5,731)
118	202	84	020 Office Supplies	1,097	1,780	683
371	366	(5)	030 Forms	3,111	3,224	113
0	127	127	040 Supplies Purchased	1,210	1,122	(88)
250	191	(59)	050 Equipment	1,553	1,683	130
125	149	24	060 Seminars/Meetings	1,163	1,309	146
25	17	(8)	070 Books	145	150	5
0	112	112	080 Equipment Rental	385	987	602
31	64	33	090 Miscellaneous	388	561	173
$5,896	$5,312	($584)	Total Supply Expense	$50,744	$46,777	($3,967)
			911. Interdepartment Expense			
$ 934	$ 921	($ 13)	010 Central Supply	$ 7,828	$ 8,114	$ 286
1,137	1,121	(16)	020 Pharmacy	9,527	9,868	341
1,915	1,888	(27)	030 Linen/Laundry	16,046	16,628	582
105	297	192	040 Maintenance	977	2,618	1,641
211	212	1	060 Telephone	1,962	1,870	(92)
0	21	21	070 Photocopy	124	187	63
0	13	13	090 Miscellaneous	165	112	(53)
$4,302	$4,473	$171	Total Interdepartment Expense	$36,629	$39,397	$2,768
$130,676	$128,935	($1,741)	Total Operating Expense	$1,119,628	$1,135,466	$15,838

FIGURE 8–1. Sample revenue and expense report.

Figure 8–1 is a sample revenue and expense report for one cost center. This report lists both actual and budgeted revenues and expenses for the month and year-to-date, as well as a variance (budget minus actual). The expenses in this example are listed as positive numbers, and the revenues are listed as negative numbers. Some organizations would show revenue as positive and expense as negative. In the variance column the mathematical sign indicates actual performance against budget. In our example, negative variance (parentheses) for either revenue or expenses means that the unit did not do so well as projected; positive variance (no parentheses) means that the unit did better than projected. Some organizations may reverse this, using a positive variance as unfavorable. Other organizations eliminate variance signs altogether and designate variances as favorable to budget or unfavorable to budget. As long as the reporting is consistent within the organization, it does not matter which approach is used.

COMPUTERIZING THE BUDGET PROCESS

It is appropriate at this point to discuss the value of computerizing the budget process. The most important aspects of preparing the budget for the nurse manager are those that involve creativity and critical thinking—analyzing data, setting goals, projecting resource needs, determining effective mix shift allocations of staff, and the like. Throughout the budget process, the manager will identify or be asked to consider variations in the budget assumptions, operational goals, or unit plan. These variations will require recalculation of the impact of potential changes on the proposed budget. Unless technologic support is available throughout this process, the manager is likely to spend time doing endless mathematical calculations rather than analyzing the effect of the variations on the operations of the patient care area.

Ideally, with an integrated computerized management information system, the manager accesses the existing workload and personnel databases and describes options for the unit's workload and resource requirements. The system calculates the impact of various options, including revenue, personnel costs, and supply expense, according to the methodologies and formulas established for the organization and the individual responsibility center. The manager then reviews and evaluates the operational impact of the various options and uses this information during the budget process. When the final budget is approved, the system is programmed to produce the budget seasonalized according to defined parameters, relevant targets, and comparisons of actual experience to both fixed and variable budget.

Most health care organizations provide some level of computer support for the budget process, for example, determining annual salary and differential costs, calculating fringe benefit expenses, producing a seasonalized budget, and comparing actual experience to fixed budget. This level of support is helpful in eliminating the repetitive, tedious work of calculation. When this support is available, it is extremely important that the manager understands the methodology for producing budgetary data in order to insure that it is being analyzed and utilized appropriately.

However, the level of sophistication that provides integrated computerized support for unit- and discipline-specific analysis of workload data and projection of required resources is frequently unavailable. In the absence of that level of technological support, it is still possible for the manager to simplify budget calculations using software available for microcomputers. Spreadsheets can be developed for calculations related to all the budget components and can be customized to reflect the specific approaches of the institution and the requirements of the individual unit. The advantages in simplifying the process and promoting accuracy in calculation more than justify the time taken to create budget spreadsheets. To the extent that these spreadsheets are consistent across units, summarization by department and division is also facilitated.

There are several key elements in developing a spreadsheet:

1. Describe the mathematical processes. What are the variables involved? How are they related? What are the calculations or formulas used to express those relationships?
2. Limit data entry and maximize computer calculation. Set up the spreadsheet to enter data only once. Reference the initial entry cell for additional uses of the same data element. Create calculations using cell references, even if a number in a formula is unlikely to change.
3. Test the spreadsheet against a known entity to ensure accuracy of calculations.

Relatively simple and useful spreadsheets can be developed with some basic computer skills. For the more experienced computer user, the ability to link spreadsheets, create macros, and utilize database programs can be valuable assets in developing the operating budget. All the examples in this chapter and the sample budget forms in the appendix can be converted to spreadsheets.

PLANNING FOR THE OPERATING BUDGET

Executive management is charged with the overall responsibility for the operating budget of the organization, and the fiscal staff provides support and direction throughout the budgeting process. However, effective administration of the operating budget requires the active primary involvement of the responsibility center manager in planning, preparing, and implementing the budget.

Planning for the individual responsibility center takes place within the context of the total organization and department. The nurse manager must identify and consider those factors that affect the activity of the area and therefore affect the operating budget. Obviously, the overall goals and objectives of the organization, as defined in the programming process, are an essential element. Definitions of the philosophy and objectives of nursing consistent with those of the larger organization are also necessary. The organizational structure and nursing care delivery system must be clearly defined, as these will affect the level and mix of nursing personnel required. In addition, analysis and planning, occurring on all levels, will generate specific budget assumptions and operational goals.

The *budget assumptions* incorporate those more global projections that are not the responsibility of any single department but that affect all—or most—areas of the organization. Much of the data needed is obtained from forecasting, as described in Chapter 6. Assumptions may include (a) significant activity projections, such as total admissions, length of stay, patient distribution by DRG, and patient day distribution or occupancy by unit, visits or procedures; (b) revenue projections, such as rate changes or payor mix changes; (c) wage and salary decisions, such as general and merit increase rates or changes in fringe benefit levels; and (d) factors to be used for projecting supply expense, such as inflation rates. The budget assumptions may also describe overall parameters or targets for total revenue, expense, or profit margin.

Operational goals include organization, department, and unit plans, and may be related to patients, staff, or systems. Patient-related goals may involve a change in service, such as developing a general surgery unit into an orthopedic specialty unit; expanding an existing service, such as increasing the number of telemetry monitors on a medical unit; or adding to available services, such as implementing a pediatric play therapy program. Staff-related goals may include planned changes in staffing mix, implementing a clinical ladder program, or defining expanded continuing education requirements. System-related goals address such things as implementing computerized documentation or expanding the quality assessment program. Once these goals are established and defined, they must be prioritized.

In addition to the goals for the organization and nursing department and unit, the nurse manager must also be aware of projections or changes within other departments that will affect nursing. If the pharmacy department plans to implement a computerized medication administration system or the communications department changes its method of allocating telephone charges, the operating budget for the nursing department could be affected significantly.

The nurse manager's *unit plan* addresses both unit goals and the context, as described above, in which these goals will be implemented. The format for presenting the plan is determined both by the manager's need for clarity and in consideration of the environment in which the budget will be reviewed. That the budget is a logical representation of the unit plan may not be apparent to others. If the plan is described in clear and concise language, with accurate and pertinent documentation, the manager can effectively explain and defend specific components of the budget.

ACTIVITY BUDGET

The *unit of service* is a measurement that describes the activity of the organization or a part of the organization. It is the basis for both determining revenue generation and describing resource requirements.

At its most basic level, an activity report will simply total the number of times a particular activity occurred within a given time period. It may identify patient days, discharges, procedures, or visits, as the units of service for this purpose. In the inpatient setting, the *census* is the most frequently reported activity measurement. Within this report, several consistent definitions are used:

Beds = number of beds available for occupancy.

Census = number of patients occupying a bed at a specific time of day (usually midnight).

Percent occupancy = census ÷ beds available × 100.

Patient day = one patient occupying one bed for one day.

Average daily census (ADC) = patient days in a given time period ÷ number of days in the time period.

Average length of stay (ALOS) = patient days in a given time period ÷ number of discharges or admissions in the time period.

The activity measures most frequently used in health care are often inadequate in measuring nursing activity and workload. In the operating room, for example, activity can be described as the number of operative procedures performed. But a dilatation and curettage (D&C) that takes 30 minutes and an exploratory laparotomy that takes 2 hours will generate different personnel requirements, supply needs, and charges. Measuring operating room activity in terms of time will give a clearer picture of the workload. If the unit of measurement—the unit of service—is 30 minutes of operating time, then the D&C and the exploratory laparotomy together total five "time" units of service instead of two "procedure" units. This system still does not completely describe the workload, however. Depending on the nature of the surgery and the condition of the patient, the exploratory laparotomy may require only two nurses present, or it may require three or four. The D&C requiring two nurses will utilize two "resource units" (30 minutes of nursing time), whereas the exploratory laparotomy requiring three nurses will utilize 12 "resource units." An activity total of "two procedures" does not reflect the actual level of nursing resources required.

The ability to describe workload accurately in terms of required resources, particularly personnel resources, becomes even more difficult on the inpatient care units. As a measure of activity, the census assumes that all patients are equal and have the same nursing care needs. In fact, patients' needs vary significantly not only as a result of their medical condition but also of their age, economic condition, psychological status, family situation, and other factors. It is because of this diversity of patients' needs for nursing care that many organizations have now implemented some form of patient classification system (PCS).

Patient Classification System (PCS)

Patient classification is a process of grouping patients into homogeneous, mutually exclusive groups. The DRG system, for example, is one method of patient classification. For nursing, patient classification groups patients according to their requirements for nursing care.

The two approaches to PCS most frequently used are prototype and factor evaluation. The *prototype* instruments describe the characteristics of patients in each category. Individual patients are then assigned to the category that most closely reflects their nursing care requirements. The *factor evaluation* instruments identify selected elements of care—critical indicators—that are the most likely predictors of nursing care needs. Individual patients are then assessed for the presence or absence of these critical indicators and, based on this, assigned to a category. Other approaches to patient classification, using frameworks based on nursing diagnosis or measures of nursing intensity, have also been developed. Particular systems may classify patients *retrospectively,* identifying what nursing care needs were met, or *prospectively,* anticipating what the nursing care requirements will be.

In addition to grouping patients into similar categories based on nursing care needs, the PCS also quantifies the workload within the categories by assigning a *relative value* to each category. The system describes the resources required for each category as either ranges or averages of nursing care time and, based on these times, assigns relative weights to each of the categories. Thus, a classification system with four categories might identify relative values as:

Patient Type	Care Hours in 24 Hours		Relative Value
	Range	*Average*	
1	0.5– 2.9	2.0	0.4
2	3.0– 6.9	5.0	1.0
3	7.0–15.4	10.0	2.0
4	15.5–24.0	22.0	4.4

Note that the numbers under Patient Type have no real value but are simply descriptors. They could as easily be labeled A,B,C,D. The indication of nursing resources required is in the Care Hours in 24 Hours column. To determine Relative Values, one category is assigned arbitrarily the value of 1.0, and all other categories are assigned values in relation to it. In this example, the type 2 patient, with average care hours of 5.0 has been assigned the 1.0 value. Because the type 3 patient requires 10 average hours of care, or twice as much as the type 2 patient, the relative value for this category is 2.0. Similarly, the type 1 patient requires an average of only 2 care hours, or 40% of the hours required by the type 2 patient, and therefore has a relative value of 0.4.

The relative value scale can then be used to describe workload for a given unit or organization. Within each category or type, the number of patients is multiplied by the relative value for that type, and the resultant category workloads are added for a total workload. The actual census is thus weighted to reflect the acuity of the patients.

Patient Type	Number of Patients	Relative Value	Workload
1	4	0.4	1.6
2	8	1.0	8.0
3	5	2.0	10.0
4	1	4.4	4.4
Total	18		24.0

In this example, the unit census of 18 generated a workload of 24.0. The average relative value or *average acuity* for this patient group is:

$$\text{Workload} \div \text{Census} = \text{Acuity}$$
$$24.0 \div 18 = 1.33$$

Using this workload, it is possible to describe the difference between units with the same census but with dissimilar patient populations or to identify trends in patient populations.

In some organizations the average Care Hours in 24 Hours, also referred to as hours per patient day (HPPD), is used instead of the relative value scale. In order to be meaningful, the appropriate HPPD must be identified for each category, as it is with the RVU methodology. The calculation of workload then applies the average HPPD identified for each patient category to the number of patients in that category.

Patient Type	Care Hours in 24 Hours *Range*	Care Hours in 24 Hours *Average*	Number of Patients	Workload
1	0.5– 2.9	2.0	4	8.0
2	3.0– 6.9	5.0	8	40.0
3	7.0–15.4	10.0	5	50.0
4	15.5–24.0	22.0	1	22.0
Total			18	120.0

In this approach, the average hours becomes the expression of the relative values for each of the categories. The description of average acuity for this population could be expressed as:

$$\text{Workload} \div \text{Census} = \text{Acuity}$$
$$120.0 \div 18 = 6.67$$

It is important to understand that this process of patient classification only identifies workload or units of service, a measurement of the activity that generates the need for resources. The advantage of the relative value scale over the average required hours scale is that the former clearly describes the patient population while the latter may be confused with a calculation of resources to be allocated. The determination of the actual resources required for a particular unit or organization is a separate process that will be discussed later in this chapter.

In order to be useful, the PCS must be credible both to the nursing staff and to those outside nursing—administrators, financial officers, and others—who will be exposed to the PCS data. Both the validity and reliability of the system must therefore be clearly established.

A PCS is developed using a specific framework that defines the elements of workload to be measured. The *validity* of the tool is the degree to which it actually measures what it intends to measure. Validity testing should occur as the tool is being developed and results of that testing be made available to users and prospective users. The validity of a tool may be compromised, however, if significant definitions are changed or if the tool is otherwise adapted to reflect the idiosyncrasies of a particular organization. Also at issue may be the currency of the framework and the definition of the elements of workload. This is of particular concern if a PCS tool is not updated and revalidated periodically. Tools that were developed in the eighties may still measure what they were originally intended to measure. However, these tools may not be valid in the nineties if they have not been updated to reflect the significant changes that have occurred in health care, nursing practice, and patient requirements for care.

The *reliability* of the PCS tool addresses the consistency of rating. Different observers assessing the same patient at the same time should generate the same rating. The prototype tools are more subjective, making this degree of reliability more difficult to achieve. The factor evaluation tools are more objective, but their reliability depends on clear definition and consistent interpretation of the critical indicators. Although initial reliability testing is part of the development of the system, continuous measurement of reliability must be the responsibility of the users. Ongoing reliability testing generally involves two or more raters independently assessing a defined percentage of classified patients at specified intervals. Reliability scores of 100% (no discrepancies in ratings) are always the target. With the prototype tools, reliability only addresses agreement of type. With the factor evaluation tools, reliability will ideally be demonstrated by agreement on both patient type and individual critical indicators.

Skepticism about PCS on the part of the nursing staff frequently relates to questions of validity—does this tool really measure our workload? Extensive discussion of the framework and methodology of the system may be needed in order to generate the acceptance and support of the staff. Skepticism about PCS on the part of those outside of nursing may relate to questions of validity but more frequently focus on issues of reliability. The PCS is usually administered by the nursing department and involves the unit staff who will be affected by the outcome. This may lead to questions about the possibility of manipulating the data to the advantage of nursing, particularly if the data demonstrates increased workload and increased need for resources. These are pertinent and legitimate questions, and nursing must be prepared to respond by demonstrating system reliability.

Alternate Workload Measurement Systems

Most patient classification systems focus on the patient in the acute care inpatient setting. Less numerous but equally needed are systems that describe nursing workload in other clinical settings. In the operating room, for example, workload is driven by the number and types of cases and case lengths. In postanesthesia recovery the number of patients, length of recovery, and variable intensity of care needed over the course of the recovery period determines workload. Workload in home care and ambulatory settings reflects number of visits, visit length, and care rendered during the visit. The primary indicator of workload in nursing homes may be the level of independence of residents related to activities of daily living. This may also be an indicator in rehabilitation facilities. With the decreasing length of stay in acute care facilities, however, rehabilitation hospitals are seeing more acutely ill patients whose rehabilitation needs are complicated by medical needs formerly not seen. These organizations may find that a PCS similar to that used in an acute care setting is appropriate for describing workload.

Workload measurement systems for these various settings may be available via either commercially produced programs or established organizational systems. In the absence of adequate workload measurement systems, it is possible for a manager to develop a measurement system that provides more complete information on nursing workload. One approach that has been used successfully in a variety of situations is to differentiate the existing, less precise measures according to resource requirements generated, aggregate those with similar resource requirements, and weight them in relationship to one another. This approach, using a *relative value unit (RVU),* creates a representative and consistent measure of workload that can be valuable in projecting, measuring, and evaluating performance. Although the RVU methodology does not provide an absolutely precise level of measurement of inputs, its advantage is that it adjusts for variations among patients and their needs without excessively complicating the data collection process.

Construction of a relative value scale is conceptually simple. Different activities (outputs) are described according to the standard, expected, or target resources (inputs) they require. The required resources are measured in a consistent unit, such as dollars or staff hours or minutes. The activities are then aggregated into categories based on similarity of required resources. One of the categories is selected as the benchmark, with a value of 1, and all other categories are given relative values based on the relationship of their required resources to those of the benchmark category. For example, if the benchmark category requires resources amounting to $500, then a category with required resources of $750 will have a relative value of 1.5, and a category with required resources of $400 will have a relative value of 0.8.

The methodology for developing a relative value scale is as follows:

1. *Identify resource drivers:* What are the significant activities that generate resource utilization?
2. *Specify significant elements of these resource drivers:* Among these drivers, what accounts for variations in resource utilization (e.g., length of procedure or visit, number of staff required)?
3. *Determine which activities or elements are being measured and reported and can be accessed easily:* These may include only volume statistics or another descriptor of complexity such as visit or case length. The relative value scale will be developed for the elements already being reported.
4. *Measure or quantify resource utilization for unreported elements related to reported elements, using the desired unit of measurement such as minutes or hours or dollars:* The unreported elements can be quantified using focused audit, that is, measuring the real time or dollars for a representative number of each of the drivers and calculating the average. Existing standards or targets can also be used to quantify the elements.
5. *Calculate total resource requirement for the reported activities:* For each reported driver, sum the total resource requirement using the actual average, standard, or target measurements.
6. *Determine the benchmark that will constitute a relative value of 1:* This can be a unit of measurement (for example, 1 RVU = 1 hour of staff time or 1 RVU = $100 of expense), or it can be the average resource utilization for one driver (e.g., the most frequently occurring procedure). Selection of the benchmark is at the discretion of the developer of the RVU scale, and is whatever works best in the situation.
7. *Calculate relative values for all reported drivers:* Calculation divides the resource requirement for each driver by the resource requirement for the measure identified as having a relative value of 1.

For example, a home visit program may identify visits as the primary resource driver. Variations in resource utilization result from the length of the visit (typically 15, 30, or 45 minutes) and the time required for the associated documentation (usually 5 minutes, except for initial visits, which are generally 30 minutes in length but require 15 minutes for documentation). This results in four visit categories. Category I is selected as the benchmark, and 1 RVU = 20 minutes of staff time.

Type	Visit Time	Documentation	Total Time	RVU
I	15	5	20	1.00
II	30	5	35	1.75
III	45	5	50	2.50
IV	30	15	45	2.25

If the developer selected category III as the benchmark instead, then 1 RVU = 50 minutes of staff time, and a category I visit has an RVU of 0.40.

Type	Visit Time	Documentation	Total Time	RVU
I	15	5	20	0.40
II	30	5	35	0.70
III	45	5	50	1.00
IV	30	15	45	0.90

The value of the benchmark changes in each of these examples, but the relative value of each procedure to the other remains the same. Category III has 2.5 times the resource requirement of category I in each situation.

For subsequent workload measurement the reported procedures can be weighted using the relative value unit to identify changes in total resource requirements and compare and contrast them over time. For example, Figure 8–2 contrasts the number of procedures and the RVU-based workload for two time periods. Although the volume in period 2 has decreased by 3% over period 1, from 131 units of service to 127 units, the workload has increased by almost 7% from 241.5 relative value units to 258.3 RVU.

With the conversion of 1 RVU = 20 minutes of staff time, it is easy to quantify the difference in staff time required in period 2 compared to period 1:

Period 1: 241.5 RVU × 20 minutes = 4,830 minutes/60 minutes = 80.5 hours
Period 2: 258.3 RVU × 20 minutes = 5,166 minutes/60 minutes = 86.1 hours

Instead of requiring fewer staff hours in period 2, as the number of procedures suggests, the RVU-based workload calculation demonstrates that, because of the change in mix of procedures, more staff hours were required.

In the process of budgeting or performance measurement, the relative value–based workload volume measure is the basis for determining resource requirements. It quantifies the need for direct nursing care, to which will be added the calculation of other resource needs such as coverage for indirect time, benefit time, and "down time."

Developing a relative value scale can be a time-consuming process. It is certainly not needed if existing reported volume measures accurately reflect variations in nursing care requirements. However, if reported volume statistics do not differentiate between activities requiring more or less nursing care time, then the time and energy expended in developing an RVU scale may be justified as it

PERIOD 1				PERIOD 2			
PROCEDURE	N	RVU	WORKLOAD	PROCEDURE	N	RVU	WORKLOAD
I	28	1.00	28.0	I	10	1.00	10.0
II	55	1.75	96.3	II	53	1.75	92.8
III	37	2.50	92.5	III	46	2.50	115.0
IV	11	2.25	24.8	IV	18	2.25	40.5
Total	131		241.5	Total	127		258.3

FIGURE 8–2. Calculating workload for home visits.

will provide a more accurate and realistic quantification of care requirements. As new procedures are added, relative value units can be incorporated using the same methodology. It is also useful periodically to review and update the calculation of the relative value units. This can be done by repeating the focus audits and reevaluating the standards and targets, an activity that is a logical companion to the annual budget planning process.

DETERMINING UNIT WORKLOAD

The individual inpatient nurse manager is generally not involved in projecting patient admissions, mix, and length of stay, and only infrequently in allocating patient days to individual patient care units. Once this determination is made, however, the manager will identify the projected workload for the unit. Using current and historical data available from the patient classification system, average acuity is determined. Current actual acuity may be the most reasonable predictor for budgeting purposes unless the patient population is expected to change significantly.

Assume, for example, that a 35-bed general surgical unit has a year-to-date average census of 28.7 and an average workload of 34.7. The unit is budgeted for 11,133 patient days in the coming fiscal year, and the proportionate distribution among patient type, and therefore the average acuity, are expected to remain the same. Calculating the projected average workload becomes relatively simple, as demonstrated in Figure 8–3. The projected workload is increased solely because of the increase in projected census from an ADC of 28.7 to an ADC of 30.5.

If, however, there is a projected change in the patient population, then the calculation becomes more complex. Given the same current PCS data for this unit, assume that the projections for the coming fiscal year predict the following:

- 1,533 days (4.2 ADC) of current type 1 patient days will be lost to expanded outpatient services.
- 2,190 days (6.0 ADC) will be added, based on the relocation of subspecialty patients from another unit.
- The relocated patients currently generate two thirds of the days as type 2 and one third of the days as type 3.

The projected workload in this example (Fig. 8–4) has increased not only because of the increase in projected census but also because of the change in the mix of patients and their average acuity. Obviously, the workload can be very different for the same number of patients when identifiable changes in patient population are factored into the calculations.

DETERMINING OTHER UNITS OF SERVICE

Often nurse managers may need to project units of service other than patient days and related workload: clinic visits, surgical procedures, deliveries, hemodialysis procedures, and the like. To do this, the manager will identify the most

FY _02_

RESPONSIBILITY CENTER: _611 - GENERAL SURGERY_

CURRENT PCS ACTIVITY:

PATIENT TYPE	AVERAGE DAILY CENSUS	RELATIVE VALUE	AVERAGE WORKLOAD
1	6.3	0.4	2.5
2	15.0	1.0	15.0
3	6.4	2.0	12.8
4	1.0	4.4	4.4
Total	28.7		34.7

Workload _34.7_ ÷ ADC _28.7_ = Average Acuity _1.21_

Projected Workload:

Patient Days _11,133_ ÷ 365 = Average Daily Census _30.5_

ADC _30.5_ × Average Acuity _1.21_ = Workload _36.9_

FIGURE 8-3. Workload/units of service budget.

FY _02_

RESPONSIBILITY CENTER: _611 - GENERAL SURGERY_

PATIENT TYPE	CURRENT ADC	PROJECTED CHANGE	REVISED ADC	RELATIVE VALUE	PROJECTED WORKLOAD
1	6.3	-4.2	2.1	0.4	0.8
2	15.0	+4.0	19.0	1.0	19.0
3	6.4	↑2.0	8.4	2.0	16.8
4	1.0	—	1.0	4.4	4.4
Total	28.7	+1.8	30.5		41.0

Workload _41.0_ ÷ ADC _30.5_ = Average Acuity _1.34_

FIGURE 8-4. Workload/units of service budget.

representative and discrete units of service for which data is available. Since these will be used for determining revenue as well as for describing resources required, the units of service should also reflect the charging structure. For example, if clinic visits are categorized by time (e.g., 15 minutes, 30 minutes, 45 minutes) or by type (e.g., screening, limited, intermediate, extended, comprehensive), then the units of service should be projected in each of the categories. The forecasting methods described in Chapter 6 can be used in predicting these units of service. With a workload measurement system and historical data about volume of units of service and distribution across workload categories, the manager can then calculate the workload in the same manner as that described for the inpatient care units.

REVENUE BUDGET

The actual calculation of revenue for specific units of service is a straight-forward one: units of service multiplied by the price per unit. Obviously, if similar activities or procedures are priced differently, then each price type must be projected and calculated individually. For example, if the room charges vary for private and semiprivate rooms, then the revenue projections must be based on the number of patient days projected for each type of room.

However, with the advent of the DRG-based prospective payment system for Medicare patients and the proliferation of alternative reimbursement systems and managed care programs in the private sector, calculating revenue has become increasingly complex. Distribution of patients by DRG, special discounts or allowances, and projections for free care must all be factored when determining revenue. In addition, individual state regulations may affect the revenue that an organization will be able to generate. These calculations are generally done by the finance department for the total hospital.

At the same time, individual responsibility centers may still calculate revenue based on charges and units of service, although this does not represent the actual revenue to the organization. It does, however, provide useful data to the organization in projecting total revenue and determining changes in pricing structures and reimbursement formulas.

More importantly, it serves to quantify the relationship of particular services to total revenue generation. For this reason, it is vital that nursing, which has traditionally been considered to be non-revenue-producing, design methodologies to cost nursing services and to identify nursing's contribution to revenue generation. Where nursing has been able to separate itself from umbrella service charges, this contribution is readily apparent. (Revenue budgeting is discussed more extensively in Chapter 9, and costing nursing services in Chapter 16.)

PERSONNEL BUDGET

The personnel budget generally represents the greatest expenditure for the nursing cost center and is also the part of the budget over which the nurse manager has the most control. It is therefore the most time-consuming portion of budget preparation. Within the personnel budget, the nurse manager must identify FTEs, positions, and employment costs.

FTEs and Positions

To prepare and manage the personnel budget, it is important to understand the concept of *full time equivalent* (FTE) and to differentiate between that and *position.*

A position is one job for one person, regardless of the number of hours that person works. Personnel reports generally describe positions by job category and regularly worked hours (full time, part time, or per diem), and identify the number of people by cost center and department. Position control, vacancy, and turnover reports are also generated using positions.

A full time equivalent is a conversion of hours to a standard base of one employee working 8 hours a day, 5 days a week, 52 weeks a year, as follows:

	Total Hours	**8 Hour Shifts**
Per year	2,080	260
Per month	173.3333 ...	21.6666 ...
Per 4-week payroll period	160	20
Per 2-week payroll period	80	10
Per week	40	5

Per month is rarely used in FTE calculations because the conversion is not in whole numbers.

The value of FTE conversion becomes readily apparent in reviewing payroll reports, which describe the employee population in terms of hours paid. In analyzing these reports, it is useful to identify trends and to compare current levels of utilization with previous levels. Paid time reported in total hours is cumbersome and inefficient for management purposes. If, for example, a manager has paid 15,892 hours in the first quarter (13 weeks) of the fiscal year and 4,992 hours in the next 4 weeks, are the paid hours increasing or decreasing? And if this week's paid hours total 1,185, how does this relate to previous experience? The application of the FTE standard will enable the manager to compare and analyze these hours. Simply take the number of paid hours in each time period and divide by the number of hours that the standard full-time employee would be paid during the same time period. A full-time employee would be paid 520 hours in 13 weeks (13 weeks × 40 hours per week), 160 hours in 4 weeks, and 40 hours in 1 week. Figure 8–5 demonstrates the results of the FTE calculations.

The most recent week's experience thus demonstrates a decrease from previous reporting. The manager may then question whether this represents a decrease in available care hours. It will be helpful, therefore, to determine whether

NUMBER OF WEEKS REPORTED (A)	TOTAL HOURS PAID (B)	TOTAL HOURS PER FTE (C)	TOTAL FTEs PAID (D) = (B) ÷ (C)
13	15,892	520	30.56
4	4,992	160	31.20
1	1,185	40	29.63

FIGURE 8–5. Calculating FTEs from total paid hours.

the variation is related to productive or nonproductive time. *Productive* (worked) time includes straight time and overtime. *Nonproductive* (benefit) time includes paid sick, vacation, holiday, and other paid nonworked time. These can be calculated using the same methodology (Fig. 8–6).

This demonstrates for the manager that, although there is a slight change in productive time, the most significant factor influencing paid FTEs is the fluctuation in nonproductive time. The same methodology can be used to determine whether the variations are related to changes in use of full-time versus part-time staff or of professional versus nonprofessional staff. These conclusions are not readily apparent by simply looking at the total hours.

Variations on FTE Definitions

In some institutions, the standard work week has been determined to be something other than 40 hours or the equivalent of five 8-hour days. For example, in a number of hospitals the standard work week is 37½ hours, or five 7½ hour days. If in fact a full-time employee is considered to be based on this standard work week, then the calculations for FTE are as follows:

	Total Hours	7½ Hour Shifts
Per year	1,950	260
Per month	162.5	21.6666 . . .
Per 4-week payroll period	150	20
Per 2-week payroll period	75	10
Per week	37.5	5

Note that the difference from the previous description of FTE is a result of the decrease in the number of hours per shift. Therefore, the total hours are fewer, although the total number of shifts remains the same.

Another scheduling variation that may affect the definition of FTE is the employee who works and is paid for seven 10-hour days in a 2-week period. This would total 70 hours in 2-weeks, or an average of 35 hours per week. If this is

NUMBER OF WEEKS REPORTED (A)	TOTAL HOURS PAID		TOTAL HOURS PER FTE (D)	TOTAL FTEs PAID	
	PROD (B)	NONPROD (C)		PROD (E) = (B) ÷ (D)	NONPROD (F) = (C) ÷ (D)
13	13,244	2,648	520	25.47	5.09
4	4,082	910	160	25.51	5.69
1	1,030	155	40	25.75	3.88

FIGURE 8–6. Calculating productive and nonproductive FTEs.

considered the standard for a full-time employee, then the calculations for FTE would be:

	Total Hours	10 Hour Shifts
Per year	1,820	182
Per month	151.6666 ...	15.6666 ...
Per 4-week payroll period	140	14
Per 2-week payroll period	70	7
Per week	35	3.5

In this example, both the number of shifts and the total hours are affected by the variation in the definition of the standard.

In identifying the appropriate calculation for FTE in a given organization, it is important to describe the full-time employee in terms of *total hours paid*. In the example given above, for instance, the full-time employee who works 70 hours in a 2-week period may in fact be paid for 80 hours in that same 2-week period, with the additional 10 hours considered to be paid nonproductive time. In this case, the FTE equivalent in paid hours would be 2,080—the same total hours as the FTE in the original example. The definition of an FTE will be determined by the personnel and payroll policies of the organization. If the manager clearly understands the definition appropriate to that organization, then the formulas and calculations described throughout this chapter can be easily adapted to the particular situation.

Statistical Relationships

Analysis of historical and current paid FTE and hours data relates paid hours to activity and workload, using a variety of statistical ratios. Hospitals frequently use the following statistical relationships:

EPOB (employee per occupied bed) = paid FTEs ÷ ADC
HPPD (hours per patient day) = paid hours ÷ patient days

Obviously, the elements of the equations (FTEs, ADC, hours, days) must cover the same time period. Also, the formulas may use either *total* paid FTEs or hours, or *productive* (worked) FTEs or hours. This must be clarified in the description of the data. Similar formulas can be developed for other areas (paid hours per OR case hour, for example, or total paid FTEs per 100 clinic visits), provided that the formulas express logical relationships.

For individual managers, the most useful staffing reports relate workload to the hours available to manage that workload. Thus, nonproductive (benefit) time is not included in this reporting, and productive time is reported as hours per unit of service. In some systems, this productive time can be further subdivided so that the *direct* hours, which vary based on workload, are separated from *indirect* hours, which may be fixed (such as nurse manager's hours) or vary by number of staff (such as educational or meeting hours).

Determining Staffing Requirements

The most critical step in preparing the personnel budget is to determine the staffing required for the projected activity. Where a PCS is being used to calculate workload, this requirement can be described as hours per workload unit (HPW).

It is important to remember that the determination of care hours in the PCS framework is used primarily as a means to establish relative values for the various classification categories. In the system example described earlier in this chapter, the requirement of 5 hours of care in 24 hours for a type 2 patient may or may not fit a specific institution or unit situation. Staffing requirements are influenced not only by patients' needs for nursing care but also by the nursing care delivery system in place, nursing and physician practice patterns, physical environment, staffing mix, level of support services, and degree of computerization, among other factors. These are rarely consistent from one organization to another and can even vary among units within one organization. Each organization, therefore, must determine its own target hours per workload unit. This can be done in several ways.

One approach is to employ the techniques of management engineering, such as time and motion or work sampling studies. These studies quantify actual time spent in caring for patients of different types and can yield valid projections of hours requirements. However, this approach assumes that what is currently being done is what should be done, and this underlying assumption may not be accurate. In addition, the studies can be time-consuming and expensive, and should be repeated periodically to determine the impact of changes in practice or other factors.

Probably the simplest but also the least appropriate approach is to adopt some local, regional, or national standard of required hours. Frequently, this is the basis for comparison among nursing departments using the HPPD measurement. It assumes that organizations can be—and should be—similar in their requirements for nursing hours. As we have seen, however, requirements can vary widely from one setting to another as a result of multiple factors other than patient type. Targets for nursing care hours, therefore, cannot be transferred from one organization to another, nor can one standard be applied equally to all institutions.

Arriving at target nursing care hours by a process of analysis and negotiation may be a less formally structured approach but can ultimately be more appropriate and effective. This approach assumes that the manager, using professional management judgment, can describe nursing staffing requirements based on analysis of staffing and outcome data specific to that unit, on an understanding of the environment in which care is given and on a realistic assessment of what is possible within that environment. In some organizations, a single target may be determined for all units with exceptions identified for individual unit situations. In others, each unit may develop a target, with the overall organizational target derived from the cumulative unit totals.

Target Hours per Workload Unit (HPW)

The HPW target reflects the nursing care hours required in 24 hours for each unit of work. It is important to clarify what is and is not included in that target. The HPW target includes only productive or worked time. Within this time, however, the manager must account for:

- Direct patient care—time actually spent with patients.
- Indirect patient care—activities related to individual patients' care but performed away from the patient, such as preparing medications.
- Unit activity—activities not related to a specific patient, such as report, rounds, or stocking supplies.
- Other support activities—meetings, educational programs, and orientation, for example.
- Personal time—paid only; excludes unpaid meal breaks.

The manager must understand which of these activities is included in the ongoing reporting of the HPW. The calculation of the projected HPW will be assumed to contain the same elements. Any elements not reflected in the HPW must be budgeted separately.

The HPW target reflects *variable* staff (i.e., those that tend to fluctuate based on workload). The requirements for *fixed* staff, such as the nurse manager or secretary, are not driven by workload and are budgeted in addition to the variable staff.

The HPW target only identifies total hours required for the workload described. It does not describe either the type of hours (i.e., mix of staff) or the distribution of hours by time of day or day of week. These elements are generally expressed as percentages that are applied after the total required hours per 24 hours is calculated. Together with the total required hours, they will be used to determine the daily staffing pattern.

Calculating Total Hours Required

For the general surgical patient care unit described earlier, using the work-load calculated in Figure 8–4, let us assume that the target set for the budgeting process is:

$$HPW = 3.5$$

This target will include all the worked hours categories described above, with the exception of orientation time. The average workload times the target hours for each unit of workload will give the total hours of nursing care required in 24 hours for the unit. We see in Figure 8–4 that a total of 41.0 workload units are expected, so we can calculate the hours of care required:

$$\text{Workload} \times \text{HPW} = \text{Hours/24 hours}$$
$$41.0 \times 3.5 = 144$$

Using a basic 8-hour shift, we can then determine the number of staff needed during the 24-hour day.

$$\text{Hours/24 hours} \div 8 = \text{Shifts/24 hours}$$
$$144 \div 8 = 18.0$$

Thus, we will need 18 nurses each working an 8-hour shift to cover the 144 hours of work.

Impact of Required Minimum Staffing

In many inpatient settings, the minimum staffing for a patient care area, if there are any patients on the unit, is two. In other areas, the definition of required minimum staffing may be driven by a commitment to availability of services. In the operating room, for example, the requirement may be that a specified number of rooms be available for a specified period of time. In the ambulatory setting, this may translate to having the capability of some set number of visits per day. Minimum staffing requirements lead to productivity inefficiencies whenever the level of required nursing care is less than the hours provided by the minimum staffing. However, the benefits from the minimum staffing requirements may outweigh the costs of productivity inefficiency. For example, the requirement of two staff on an inpatient unit provides a safety factor in the event of medical or environmental emergencies. In other areas, the ability to schedule procedures or visits without extensive delays may have significant implications for patient care or patient and physician satisfaction or may have marketing effects that will lead to increased volume and thus increased productivity.

Whatever the rationale, minimum required staffing must be factored into the calculation of FTEs. On inpatient units the total number of staff in 24 hours calculated using workload may be greater than the minimum required. However, when the shifts are distributed throughout the day based on the distribution of care needs, it may be evident that the night shift will have fewer than two staff routinely assigned. In this situation, the manager will adjust the staffing pattern for nights to match the minimum (without altering the day and evening allocations, since these are necessary to meet patient care needs). This adjusted staffing pattern will be used as the basis for determining other worked time, benefit time, and total FTEs. Generally in areas like the operating room, the required staffing levels for the number of rooms available at different times of the day and on different days of the week is the basis for determining staffing. Analyzing activity and calculating workload is done in conjunction with this, not only to address productivity but also to identify times when the usual activity surpasses these minimums and requires additional staffing. Whatever the situation, it is important in the budgeting process to look at minimum staffing issues together with staffing required by workload in order to present a true picture of resource requirements.

Distribution by Mix and Shift

The next step in the process is to design a daily staffing pattern that distributes the staff according to mix and shift. Distribution by skill mix varies significantly from one organization to another, as well as within one organization. It is driven not only by patient acuity but also by organizational and departmental goals and by availability of particular categories of personnel. Distribution by shift exhibits more similarities than dissimilarities for patient populations with similar levels of acuity. In general, the more acute the patient population, the closer the distribution comes to equal numbers of staff on all shifts.

Distribution by mix and shift is initially calculated according to identified percentages and then adjusted based on the reasonableness of the projections and the unique needs of the unit. If the nurse manager initially projects a 70% staff nurse mix and anticipates needing a shift distribution of 40% on days, 35% on evenings, and 25% on nights, then the calculation for the number of staff nurses on days is:

$$\text{Total staff} \times \%\,\text{RN} \times \%\,\text{days} = \text{Staff nurse shifts on days}$$
$$18.0 \times 70\% \times 40\% = 5.04$$

The same distribution can be used for all other shifts and categories (Variable Staff [Preliminary] in Fig. 8–7). The numbers are then adjusted to reflect the actual number of staff who will be scheduled each day. Based on the needs of the unit, the nurse manager may determine that four staff are sufficient on the night shift and redistribute the balance of the night shift coverage to days and evenings. In addition, the unit needs may support only one nursing assistant on each shift. The balance of the nursing assistant hours would then be redistributed to other categories. Fractions of shifts, if they occur at all, are generally rounded to one decimal place. This indicates that on a given percentage of days an additional staff person may be scheduled.

FY _O2_

RESPONSIBILITY CENTER: _611- GENERAL SURGERY_

Bed Complement ___35___ Total Patient Days _11, 133_ % Occupancy _87.1%_

ADC _30.5_ × Average Acuity _1.34_ = Average Workload _41.0_

Average Workload _41.0_ × Target HPW _3.5_ = Hours/24 Hours _144_

Hours/24 Hours _144_ ÷ 8 = Shifts/24 Hours _18.0_

DAILY STAFFING PATTERN
Variable Staff (Preliminary):

SHIFT DISTRIBUTION		_40_ %	_35_ %	_25_ %	
Mix	Position	7–3	3–11	11–7	Total
_70_ %	Staff Nurse	5.04	4.41	3.15	12.6
_10_ %	LPN/LVN	0.72	0.63	0.45	1.8
_20_ %	Nursing Asst	1.44	1.26	0.90	3.6
	Total	7.20	6.30	4.50	18.0

Variable Staff (Adjusted):

SHIFT DISTRIBUTION		_42_ %	_36_ %	_22_ %	
Mix	Position	7–3	3–11	11–7	Total
_72_ %	Staff Nurse	5.5	4.5	3	13
_11_ %	LPN/LVN	1	1	0	2
_17_ %	Nursing Asst	1	1	1	3
	Total	7.5	6.5	4	18

Support Staff:

Position	7–3	3–11	11–7	Total
Secretary	1	1	1	3
Unit Aide (M–F)	1	1	—	2
Total	2	2	1	5

Fixed Staff: Nurse Manager _1.0_ Clinical Specialist _1.0_

FIGURE 8–7. Personnel budget worksheet.

The final staffing pattern (Variable Staff [Adjusted] in Fig. 8–7) reflects these adjustments and will form the basis not only for calculating the total required FTEs but also for generating the unit work schedule. Mix and shift percentages can be recalculated based on the adjusted staffing pattern and used as targets against which performance will be measured.

Because both the workload and the required hours have been expressed as daily averages, the staffing pattern reflects this average and does not address variations based on day of the week. If a particular unit experiences significant, consistent changes in workload based on the day of the week or on weekday and weekend variations, the total weekly workload can be calculated (average daily workload × 7) and redistributed using unit specific trend data. The staffing patterns for each day of the week, or for weekdays versus weekends, can then be calculated individually. Where variations are less dramatic, the average daily staffing pattern is usually sufficient for budgeting purposes, and the variations are managed in day-to-day scheduling and staffing.

CALCULATING COVERAGE FOR DAYS OFF AND NONPRODUCTIVE TIME

The average daily staffing pattern for this unit must be maintained 7 days a week. But the 18 staff identified in our variable staffing pattern will only work 5 days a week. In addition, they will sometimes be ill, on vacation, or on holiday—time for which they will be paid but during which they are not available for patient care. Therefore, these 18 FTEs must be supplemented by enough additional FTEs to maintain the daily staffing pattern.

Since five shifts per week is equivalent to 1 FTE, then one 8-hour shift equals 0.2 FTE and the coverage for days off for 1 FTE equals 0.4 FTE, or 2 days off out of each 7-day week. For every shift required in 24 hours in the daily staffing pattern, 1.40 FTEs must be budgeted to account for weekday and weekend coverage.

$$\text{Shifts/24 hours} \times 1.4 = \text{FTE for 7-day week}$$
$$18 \times 1.4 = 25.2$$

Each of these 25.2 FTEs, however, will take paid nonproductive time, for which coverage must also be provided if the staffing pattern is to be maintained. To calculate the coverage required for paid nonproductive time, use existing payroll data to identify the nonproductive time as a percent of the productive time. In the example shown in Figure 8–8, nonproductive time is subtracted from total paid hours to identify productive hours. Nonproductive hours are then divided by productive hours to identify the nonproductive time as a percent of the productive time. This unit is therefore paying productive time plus an additional 17.4% of productive time in nonproductive hours. (It is important to recognize that this is not equivalent to 17.4% of total paid time. The total paid time will include the productive time plus the nonproductive time. In this example, the nonproductive time represents 14.8% of the total paid time, or 6,368

FY _O2_

CALCULATION OF NONPRODUCTIVE TIME

Factor for days of nonproductive time:

YTD as of _Payroll period #20 ending 2/18/01_

(a) Total paid hours _43,008_

(b) Total paid nonproductive hours _6,368_ (sick + vacation + holiday + other paid nonworked)

(c) Total paid productive hours (a) – (b) _36,640_

(d) % paid nonproductive (b) ÷ (c) _0.174_ (convert % to decimal)

(e) Factor = $1 \times 1.4 \times 1(d) = 1 \times 1.4 \times$ _1.174_ = _1.64_

CALCULATION OF TOTAL REQUIRED FTEs

CATEGORY	SHIFT/24 HOUR	FACTOR (e)	TOTAL FTEs REQUIRED	BUDGET FTE	
				ST	OT
Nurse Manager	1.0	—	1.0	1.0	—
Clinical Specialist	1.0	—	1.0	1.0	—
Staff Nurse	13.0	1.64	21.3	21.0	0.3
LPN/LVN	2.0	1.64	3.3	3.2	0.1
Nursing Assistant	3.0	1.64	4.9	4.6	0.3
Secretary	3.0	1.64	4.9	4.8	0.1
Unit Aide (M–F)	2.0	1.174	2.4	2.4	—
Total	25.0		38.8	38.0	0.8

FIGURE 8–8. Personnel budget worksheet.

nonproductive hours ÷ 43,008 total paid hours. However, at this point in the budget process, we have only identified productive time requirements, and using 14.8% as the nonproductive coverage requirement would understate the unit needs.) By combining the above, we can determine a single factor:

Shifts/24 hours × Coverage for days off ×
Coverage for nonproductive time = Total FTEs required

$$1 \times 1.4 \times 1.174 = 1.64$$

Therefore, for every person required in 24 hours, 1.64 FTEs must be budgeted to maintain the daily staffing pattern for a 7-day week and to cover for nonproductive time. Using this factor, the required FTEs can be identified by position and also by shift within position, if needed, by simply applying the factor to each category of the daily staffing pattern. Note that in the example in Figure 8–8, the factor is not applied to the nurse manager or clinical specialist, since their particular responsibilities are not assumed by someone else in their absence. Also, although a single nonproductive percent was calculated for the entire staff, it is possible with detailed personnel data, to calculated nonproductive percents for each role group separately. This may be advantageous if there is significant variation in the actual among those groups. Finally, in this example, coverage for the unit aide, scheduled only for Monday through Friday, is calculated only for nonproductive time. Coverage for days off is not included, since the unit aide is not replaced on the weekend days off.

CALCULATION OF OTHER WORKED HOURS

In our example, the target HPW included all activities related to the variable staff with the exception of orientation. Suppose, however, that the reported actual HPW does not reflect off-unit activities for the variable staff, such as meetings, educational programs, and the like. The target HPW will reflect only those elements that are reflected in the reported HPW, and the manager will need to project other worked hours. Using the same approach as described in the calculations for nonproductive time, the other worked hours can be calculated as a percent of the direct/indirect worked hours. If in 13 weeks the average HPW is 3.4 for an average workload of 34.7, then the total direct/indirect hours would be:

Workload	×	HPW	×	7 days	×	13 weeks	=	Total direct/indirect hours
34.7	×	3.4	×	7	×	13	=	10,763 hours

If in that same 13 weeks, the manager paid 11,052 productive hours, then:

Paid productive hours	−	Direct/indirect hours	=	Other worked hours
11,052	−	10,736	=	316 hours

Other worked hours	÷	Direct/indirect hours	=	% Other worked hours
316	÷	10,736	=	2.9%

Thus, for every FTE budgeted for direct/indirect care, an additional 0.029 FTEs must be budgeted for other worked hours. A combined factor can then be derived:

Shifts/24 hours × Coverage for other worked hours × Coverage for days off × Coverage for nonproductive time = Total FTEs

$$1 \times 1.029 \times 1.4 \times 1.174 = 1.69$$

In this circumstance, for every shift required in 24 hours, 1.69 FTEs must be budgeted to provide complete coverage. Obviously, it is important that the nurse manager clearly understands what is included in the reported and target HPW in order to calculate accurately the FTEs that must be projected.

ALTERNATE COVERAGE PATTERNS

For those settings that do not require relatively consistent 7 day a week coverage, the approach to identifying both productive and nonproductive coverage requirements must be adapted. In ambulatory settings, for example, coverage is generally not required for weekends or scheduled holidays. In perioperative areas, staffing requirements are generally reduced significantly on the weekends. In these circumstances, it is more appropriate to identify the varying levels of coverage required and calculate annual requirements for productive time.

An ambulatory clinic, for example, might be covered from 8 AM to 6 PM on weekdays, except for nine scheduled weekday holidays. Coverage requirement is for four staff nurses each day. Total productive hours required, therefore, will be:

$$52 \text{ weeks} \times 5 \text{ days} = 260 \text{ days} - 9 \text{ holidays} = 251 \text{ days}$$
$$251 \text{ days} \times 10 \text{ hours} \times 4 \text{ staff nurses} = 10,040 \text{ hours}$$

If the experience of this setting is that nonproductive time historically has accounted for 14.8% of total paid time, then on the average each full-time staff nurse's productive time is 85.2% (100% − 14.8%) of total paid time. This can be converted to hours:

$$2,080 \text{ hours (1 FTE)} \times 85.2\% = 1,772 \text{ productive hours}$$

If one FTE works a total of 1,772 productive hours in the year and the ambulatory clinic requires 10,040 productive hours per year, then the total FTE requirement will be:

$$10,040 \text{ hours required} \div 1,772 \text{ worked hours per FTE} = 5.7 \text{ FTEs}$$

The same approach can be used for perioperative areas that function 7 days a week but are staffed differently on different days. Staffing patterns can be developed separately for weekdays and weekends or even for each day of the week, if that more accurately reflects the needs of the unit. Total annual hours can then be calculated, and the total required FTEs identified using the same method as described for the ambulatory setting. For example, assume that the surgery suite is generally staffed with a total of 40 eight-hour shifts on Mondays through Fridays. On Saturday, however, only 12 shifts are required, and on Sundays and scheduled holidays, only 6 shifts. Total annual productive hours required, therefore, are:

$$251 \text{ weekdays} \times 40 \text{ staff} \times 8 \text{ hours} = 80,320 \text{ hours}$$
$$52 \text{ Saturdays} \times 12 \text{ staff} \times 8 \text{ hours} = 4,992 \text{ hours}$$
$$61 \text{ Sundays/holidays} \times 6 \text{ staff} \times 8 \text{ hours} = 2,928 \text{ hours}$$
$$\text{Total required} = 88,240 \text{ hours}$$

Again using the experience of 14.8% nonproductive time as a percent of total paid time, the average productive hours for 1 FTE = 1,772. Therefore:

88,240 hours ÷ 1,772 hours/FTE = 49.8 FTEs required

IMPACT OF FLEXIBLE STAFFING PATTERNS

In an effort to respond to the needs of their staff as well as those of their patients, many hospitals have instituted various forms of flexible scheduling, including shifts of varying lengths (4-, 6-, 8-, 10-, and 12-hour shifts are not uncommon) or varying weekly schedules (such as 7 days on and 7 days off or two 12-hour and two 8-hour shifts per week). In general, these different flexible staffing patterns have a greater impact on managing the budget, and particularly on the scheduling process, than they do on preparing the budget.

Provided that the flexible patterns result in the same average number of hours available for the workload of the unit, the approaches to budgeting already described are sufficient. For the general surgical unit described above, instead of having 18 staff scheduled for 8 hours each, the flexible schedule might result in 4 staff working 12 hours each and only 12 staff working 8-hour shifts.

4 staff	×	12 hours	=	48	hours
12 staff	×	8 hours	=	96	hours
16 staff				144	hours

This means that there are only 16 staff working that day, but the available hours remains the same (144 hours). The budget calculations therefore remain the same.

However, if the schedule variation leads to a change in the available hours, then the budget can be affected. One example of this is the implementation of a 10-hour 4-day work week. Suppose that 4 of the 18 staff required for the unit's staffing pattern work a 10-hour day. In fact, they are providing 40 hours of care during the 24-hour period, the equivalent of 5 staff working 8-hour shifts. In this situation, only 13 additional staff should be needed to meet the 144 hour total staffing requirement.

4 staff	×	10 hours	=	40	hours
13 staff	×	8 hours	=	104	hours
17 staff				144	hours

However, if the additional 2 hours of each of the 10-hour shifts are overlapping hours occurring at times when the workload does not support the additional hours, then problems can arise. Either the unit has fewer hours than needed at some other time during the 24 hours or the schedule provides for the original total of 18 staff, resulting in the scheduling of 8 hours more than workload supports.

$$
\begin{array}{lcrcl}
4 \text{ staff} & \times & 10 \text{ hours} & = & 40 \text{ hours} \\
14 \text{ staff} & \times & 8 \text{ hours} & = & 112 \text{ hours} \\
\hline
18 \text{ staff} & & & & 152 \text{ hours} \\
\end{array}
$$

Some flexible scheduling patterns will have a greater effect on nonproductive time. For example, if staff nurses working 32 hours per week on nights are paid for 40 hours for the week, then the additional hours may in some organizations be considered paid nonproductive time. This will significantly affect the calculation of nonproductive time and may require a separate determination of nonproductive factor for that category of staff. Other variations in scheduling may affect the total paid hours per FTE, as discussed earlier in this chapter. The formulas presented here for determining required FTEs will be applicable in those situations, provided the FTE hours represent the particular variation.

Impact of Alternate Sources of Coverage

In calculating the total FTEs required for the unit, the initial assumption is that all FTEs will reflect regular positions on the unit and that the unit staff will provide coverage for days off and nonproductive time. In most organizations, however, at least a part of this coverage is provided by overtime. This is particularly likely to occur when absences are unplanned. In other situations, a centralized float staff, per diem staff or agency staff may be used regularly to provide this coverage. All the hours provided by these alternate sources of coverage must be covered by the total hours allocated to the unit. Therefore, the nurse manager must identify those FTEs or portions of FTEs that will be needed to support this supplemental staff.

Using the current and historical unit data, the nurse manager can estimate the overtime, float, per diem, or agency hours that will be needed or are most likely to be used. These hours are converted to FTEs and deducted from the total FTE complement for the unit. (Allocation of overtime hours is shown in Figure 8–8.) The remaining hours and FTEs will be identified as specific positions into which the nurse manager is authorized to hire. If float, per diem, or agency staff are used only rarely to cover temporarily vacant positions, then the dollars allocated to the vacant positions can be assumed to cover the alternate staff and the nurse manager can be authorized to hire into all positions. Overtime, on the other hand, should always be budgeted, unless unit history indicates that it is not used, because it is generally paid at a much higher rate.

Impact of Vacancies

In some organizations, the nurse manager is asked to project a vacancy factor. This approach is based on the assumption that, particularly in larger departments such as nursing, there is always a certain amount of turnover and therefore always some vacancies and that the budget can be reduced on the strength of those vacant positions that do not generate salary costs. The flaw in this thinking is that, if the budget does in fact accurately reflect workload and the resources required for that workload, alternate sources of coverage for the vacant positions will be required and the monies in fact will be used. To the extent that it is possible, however, the nurse manager should attempt to estimate turnover and vacancy for the unit, in order to plan both for sources of coverage for vacancies and orientation of replacement staff.

Callback Time

In some specialty areas (such as the operating room), the staff may be subject to being called back in urgent situations to cover workload that is unanticipated and not projected in the baseline budget. Generally, these hours are overtime hours for the regular staff; however, they are productive hours in addition to those already calculated (unless the workload-generated staffing patterns clearly incorporate callback time) and must be added to the budget. The projection of callback hours is usually based on analysis of historical data, and the hours are converted to FTEs.

Orientation

The Department of Nursing will normally experience some turnover during the year and may also identify necessary staffing increases. This will lead to the recruitment of new staff members, who will require some period of orientation. During the orientation period, new staff are not considered to be contributing to meeting the workload requirements of the unit. In some circumstances, they may be hired to replace staff who will leave but have not yet left. At other times, the staff vacancy may exist, but coverage will be needed for the unit until the orientee is able to assume full responsibility for patient care. In either case, the orientee's hours are in addition to the productive hours required for patient care. Based on analysis of turnover statistics and projections for future changes in staffing needs, it is possible to estimate the number of staff in various job categories who will be hired in the coming year.

Using the average number of weeks of orientation for each job category, the total annual orientation hours are calculated and converted to FTEs. This may be done on a departmental level, with all orientation expenses allocated to one cost center, or it may be determined by unit and added to each cost center budget. If orientation coverage has been included as part of the reported HPW or as part of the calculation for other worked hours, then it will not need to be added separately.

POSITION/HOURS BUDGET

The next step in personnel budget preparation is to convert FTEs into positions and hours. By comparing the currently authorized position and FTE complement to the projections, the nurse manager can identify where additions and deletions need to be made.

The Position Budget (Fig. 8–9) lists both the current authorized positions and the current authorized FTEs. Comparing this to the Personnel Budget Worksheet

---

FY 02

RESPONSIBILITY CENTER: 611 GENERAL SURGERY

CURR AUTH POSITIONS	POSITION TITLE	ST Hours	ST FTE	OT HOURS	OT FTE	TOTAL HOURS	TOTAL FTE
1	Nurse Manager	2,080	1.0	—	—	2,080	1.0
1	Clin Specialist	2,080	1.0	—	—	2,080	1.0
~~18~~ 16	Staff Nurse FT	*33,280* ~~27,040~~	*16.0* ~~13.0~~	*624* ~~1,040~~	*0.3* ~~0.5~~	*33,904* ~~28,080~~	*16.3* ~~13.5~~
~~8~~ 10	Staff Nurse PT	*10,400* ~~8,320~~	*5.0* ~~4.0~~	—	—	*10,400* ~~8,320~~	*5.0* ~~4.0~~
~~3~~ 2	LPN/LVN FT	*4,160* ~~6,240~~	*2.0* ~~3.0~~	208	0.1	*4,368* ~~6,448~~	*2.1* ~~3.1~~
~~1~~ 2	LPN/LVN PT	*2,496* ~~832~~	*1.2* ~~0.4~~	—	—	*2,496* ~~832~~	*1.2* ~~0.4~~
~~3~~ 4	Nsg Asst FT	*8,320* ~~6,240~~	*4.0* ~~3.0~~	624	0.3	*8,944* ~~6,864~~	*4.3* ~~3.3~~
3	Nsg Asst PT	1,248	0.6	—	—	1,248	0.6
4	Secretary FT	8,320	4.0	208	0.1	8,528	4.1
2	Secretary PT	1,664	0.8	—	—	1,664	0.8
2	Unit Aide FT	4,160	2.0	—	—	4,160	2.0
1	Unit Aide PT	832	0.4	—	—	832	0.4
~~42~~ 48 Total		*79,040* ~~69,056~~	*38.0* ~~33.2~~	*1,664* ~~2,080~~	*0.8* ~~1.0~~	*80,704* ~~71,136~~	*38.8* ~~34.2~~

CURRENTLY AUTHORIZED

$$\text{ST FTE} = \frac{69,056}{2080} = 33.2$$

$$\text{OT FTE} = \frac{2080}{2080} = 1.0$$

$$\text{TOTAL FTE} = \frac{71,136}{2080} = 34.2$$

CURRENTLY PROJECTED

$$\text{ST FTE} = \frac{79,040}{2080} = 38.0$$

$$\text{OT FTE} = \frac{1,664}{2080} = 0.8$$

$$\text{TOTAL FTE} = \frac{80,704}{2080} = 38.8$$

FIGURE 8–9. Position/hours budget worksheet.

(Fig. 8–8), we see that there is a net increase of 4.6 total FTEs, including overtime, requested in fiscal year 2002 (FY02) over those currently authorized. In addition, there will be a change in the distribution of these FTEs. Increases are projected for staff nurse full time (FT) and part time (PT), LPN/LVN part time, and nursing assistant full time.[1] A decrease is projected in the LPN/LVN full-time category. Although straight-time (ST) hours are increasing, overtime (OT) hours are projected to decrease.

Note that in the example the part-time positions vary in the number of hours assigned. The 10 part-time staff nurse positions may reflect 10 half-time (0.5 FTE) positions. The three part-time nursing assistant positions, however, obviously cannot be half-time positions but more likely represent positions of 0.2 FTE (8 hours per week) each. The one part-time unit aide position covers an average of 16 hours per week (0.4 FTE), equivalent to two of the nursing assistant positions.

Hours for full-time positions are calculated by multiplying the positions by the number of paid hours for one FTE, generally 2,080 hours. Hours for part-time positions are not calculated according to any standard but reflect the sum of the actual hours allocated to each individual position. Straight-time hours are divided by 2,080 to identify straight-time FTEs in each position category. Overtime hours are calculated by multiplying the overtime FTEs (from the personnel budget worksheet) by 2,080 hours. Overtime hours are listed with full-time FTEs, since they address hours over the full-time complement. Straight-time and overtime hours can then be totaled and divided by 2,080 hours to identify total FTEs in each position category. The positions and hours are then added to determine totals for the cost center and the hours converted to FTEs.

If the nurse manager has identified FTEs and hours to be allocated for float, per diem, or agency staff not regularly assigned to the unit, the FTEs required to cover these should be identified clearly in the budget as positions not available for recruiting and hiring.

SALARY BUDGET

Having completed the FTE and position budget preparation, the nurse manager is now ready to convert these into dollars. The employment cost budget includes several components: regular salaries, differentials and premiums, overtime, and fringe benefits. In calculating these, the costs associated with special programs designed as recruitment and retention incentives must also be considered. These programs can be costed and managed in a variety of ways, so it is imperative that the nurse manager become knowledgeable about the details of the organization's specific programs. Likewise, if all or part of the staff is part of a

---

[1]In most states this position is licensed practical nurse, or LPN. In several states this position is referred to as licensed vocational nurse, or LVN.

collective bargaining unit, the requirements and limitations covered by the employment contract must be well understood and factored into the employment cost calculations.

Regular Salaries

In projecting regular salaries for the employment cost budget, the nurse manager begins with current staff salaries. In the example shown in Figure 8–10, the nurse manager has been provided with a Salary Budget Worksheet, which lists

FY _02_

RESPONSIBILITY CENTER: 611 GENERAL SURGERY

JOB CATEGORY: STAFF NURSE PART TIME

NAME	FTE	SHIFT	BASE HOURLY RATE	BASE ANNUAL SALARY
Briggs, Martha	0.2	3–11	$23.03	$9,580
Coram, Amy	0.5	11–7	~~$22.69~~ *24.28*	~~$23,598~~ *25,253*
Douglas, Ida	0.5	7–3	$27.44	$28,538
Francis, Jamie	0.5	7–3	$19.47	$20,249
Howells, Robert	~~0.5~~ *0.8*	3–11	$24.79	~~$25,782~~ *41,250*
Martins, Mary	0.8	3–11	$29.25	$48,672
Ridley, George	0.5	7–3	$23.32	$24,253
~~Westbury, Vickie~~ *TERMINATE 4/15/01*	~~0.5~~	~~11–7~~	~~$20.79~~	~~$21,622~~
VACANT	*0.2*	*7–3*	*22.28*	*9,270*
VACANT	*0.5*	*11–7*	*19.47*	*20,248*
VACANT	*0.5*	*11–7*	*22.28*	*23,176*

Total This Job Class:

Positions ~~8~~ *10*

FTEs ~~4.0~~ *5.0*   Base Salary ~~$202,292~~ *250,489*

FIGURE 8–10. Salary budget worksheet.

for the part-time staff nurse category each employee currently in the cost center, their regular weekly hours expressed as FTEs, regular shift, hourly rate, and regular annual salary. The first step is to correct the information for each staff member to reflect what will be in effect at the beginning of the new fiscal year. Amy Coram, for example, will receive a merit increase before the beginning of the new fiscal year, and her salary is adjusted by the estimated amount of the increase. The revised annual salary is calculated simply as

$$\text{FTE} \times 2080 \times \text{Hourly rate} = \text{Annual salary}$$
$$0.5 \times 2080 \times \$24.28 = \$25{,}253$$

Robert Howells will be increasing his regular hours in the new fiscal year, and this is also corrected in the FTE column. The same formula will be used to correct his salary. Vickie Westbury will be resigning before the end of the fiscal year and so is deleted from the worksheet.

Since only 3.8 FTEs are now represented on the worksheet but 5.0 are projected for the new fiscal year, hours are identified and salaries estimated for the vacant positions. In estimating salaries for vacant positions, the nurse manager should estimate the probability of hiring new graduates versus experienced employees. In this cost center, the nurse manager is projecting that 1 of the 3 vacant positions will be filled by a new graduate at starting salary and 2 by experienced staff nurses. Again, the formula noted above is used to calculate the total annual salary. If FTEs have been budgeted for float, per diem, or agency staff, these costs are calculated separately since they are frequently paid at different rates from those paid to regular staff.

When salary budget worksheets have been completed for all categories of personnel, the results are added to obtain total straight-time salary expenses for the cost center.

Differentials and Premiums

Calculating the cost of differentials and premiums requires a clear understanding of the organizational policies that govern these additions to base salary. Differential and premium rates frequently vary among positions and therefore should be calculated individually for each job category.

Shift Differentials

Differentials are usually paid to staff who work the evening or night shift. These differentials may take the form of an hourly dollar amount, a percentage of base hourly pay for hours worked, or a monthly, quarterly, or annual lump sum. Calculating the impact of these differs but is simple.

If differentials are paid based on an hourly dollar amount, the calculation of the differential is made from the staffing pattern. Suppose, for example, that the staff nurse night differential is $2.50 per hour for all worked 11–7 hours. From the staffing pattern (Fig. 8–7), the manager has projected scheduling three staff nurses (24 hours) of coverage per night. Differential for staff nurses on the night shift can then be calculated at

Hours/night × 365 × Hourly rate = Total annual night differential
24 × 365 × $2.50 = $21,900

If the policy calls for a percentage of base hourly pay for hours worked, then the first step is to calculate the average hourly salary of the night staff nurses. If the night differential is 15% of base hourly and the average hourly rate of the night staff nurses is $20.00, then the differential is $20.00 × 15% = $3.00 per hour. This rate can then be applied to the formula described above.

If the night premium is a lump sum—for example, $1,000 per quarter or $4,000 per year per FTE—then the calculation takes the number of FTEs in the straight night shift position multiplied by the annual lump sum premium.

Weekend Differentials and Premiums

In most organizations, staff receive a differential or premium for working the weekend shifts. If this is an hourly rate or hourly percentage of base rate, then the total expense for the cost center can be calculated in the same manner as the shift differentials were calculated in the examples above. Again, the staffing pattern is the basis for determining the number of weekend hours generating the premium. The definition of eligible weekend shifts may include only Saturday and Sunday hours or may include some parts of Friday and Monday. Organizational policies must be consulted to determine this.

Holiday Premiums

Staff may receive a premium for working on certain scheduled holidays—Christmas or Labor Day, for example. The policies of the organization will govern the shifts for which the premium will be paid, as well as the rate at which these will be paid. The staffing pattern for the holiday is the basis for determining the number of hours of premium to be budgeted for the cost center. Multiplying total annual holiday hours by the holiday premium rate will yield the total annual holiday premium expense.

On Call Premium

In areas that require staff to be available to return to work if needed, staff are usually paid a premium to restrict their activities and be available for callback between scheduled shifts. This premium is usually some hourly amount, which is paid for any restricted hours excluding those during which the employee is called back to work. (If called back, the employee is paid regular or overtime hourly rates with appropriate differentials and premiums for the hours related to the callback. These hours were calculated earlier as part of the total FTE complement.) Calculation of the on call premium involves determining the number of on call hours required in a year, less the number of callback hours. If an operating room, for example, has two staff on call every night of the year on the 11–7 shift and two staff on call on weekends and holidays from 7 AM to 11 PM, then the total number of on call hours will be:

2 staff	×	365 days	×	8 hours	=	5,840 hours for 11–7 coverage
2 staff	×	104 days	×	16 hours	=	3,328 hours for weekend coverage
2 staff	×	9 days	×	16 hours	=	288 hours for holiday coverage
				Total	=	9,456 hours coverage

If, in addition, the manager has projected that the total callback hours in the year will be 832 hours and has calculated this as overtime hours in completing the personnel budget, then these can be deducted from the total coverage hours (9,456 hours coverage − 832 hours callback = 8,624 hours on call). Calculation of the total expense is hours on call multiplied by the hourly on call premium rate.

Overtime

Overtime payment practices are governed by the Fair Labor Standards Act (the federal wage and hour law). These are minimal regulations that may be enhanced by state law, organizational policy, or union contract. Therefore, overtime payment practices may vary among organizations. Minimally, overtime is paid to staff in eligible job categories for all hours worked beyond 40 hours in a week. Overtime for these staff is calculated at the actual average hourly rate for the period (including differentials and premiums) times 1.5 for all qualifying hours. Since it is difficult to predict which individual employees will in fact work the overtime hours budgeted for the cost center, the simpler method is to determine an average total hourly rate (including differentials and premiums) for the staff in a particular job category and use this to calculate the projected overtime expense.

Assume, for example, that the total straight time annual salaries for the 4.0 FTEs of full-time secretaries identified in Figure 8–9 has been calculated at $79,040 and the annual differentials and premiums at $11,446. Overtime costs can be calculated as follows:

Total annual salary	+	Total annual differentials/premiums	=	Total wages
$79,040	+	$11,446	=	$90,486

Total wages	÷	Total FTEs	÷	2080	=	Average total hourly rate
$90,486	÷	4.0 FTEs	÷	2080	=	$10.88/hour

Average total hourly rate	×	1.5	×	OT hours	=	OT costs
$10.88	×	1.5	×	208	=	$3,395

General and Merit Increases

Calculating salary expense for the new fiscal year has thus far been based only on current fiscal year salaries. The impact of projected general and merit increases must be identified in addition. The policies and practices of the organization will determine how these costs are to be included. Increases may be calculated on the total regular salary costs for the entire cost center, by job category or even by individual.

General and merit increases affect only the base salary rate and are not applied to costs of differentials and premiums that are hourly dollar amounts or periodic lump sum payments. However, the increases will affect premiums that are a percentage of base pay as well as overtime costs. These categories of expenses will need to be adjusted to reflect the anticipated increases.

Fringe Benefits

Fringe benefit expenses include the organization's share of the costs of FICA, health insurance, life insurance, and other benefits. These may be calculated as a percent of the total employment costs, with the specific percentages identified for the manager in the budget assumptions. In some organizations, the various fringe benefit costs are calculated by the personnel, payroll, or finance department, rather than by the individual cost center manager. In others, the human resource department or the finance department provide the assumptions or factors to use in calculating fringe benefits.

NONSALARY BUDGET

The nonsalary budget projects all direct expenses of the cost center, other than employment expenses. Generally, these expenses include medical services, supplies, or activities not individually charged to the patient (e.g., routine patient care items, nourishments, office and paper supplies, noncapital equipment, education and consultation costs, maintenance). In some circumstances, patient chargeable items—orthopedic implants, for example—may be initially charged to the cost center and then charged to the patient when used. In this case, the corresponding revenue is also reflected in the cost center's revenue budget.

Nonsalary expenses are allocated to individual accounts that group similar expenses within the cost center. In analyzing nonsalary expenses, it is important to identify specifically the costs included in each account. The chart of accounts will give a brief description of these costs, with more detail provided by reports generated through the finance department or through the department that provides the supplies or services (e.g., dietary, central supply, maintenance). These reports itemize the different components of the account expense, the volume or frequency of use, the cost per unit and extended cost (total units × cost per unit) for each component, and the total expense charged to the account.

The most useful reporting of nonsalary expenses relates both the volume or frequency of use and the expense to relevant indicators such as workload or number of staff. Statistical relationships frequently calculated for direct patient care related expenses, for example, may describe cost per discharge, cost per patient day, or cost per workload unit. Education cost may be expressed as expense per FTE or expense per position. As with other formulas, these must express logical relationships within like time frames.

The simplest method of calculating nonsalary expenses—and also, unfortunately, the least accurate—is to identify a total cost per unit of activity (patient day, workload unit, procedure, visit), multiply by the projected units of activity, and adjust for inflation. As we have seen, however, not all nonsalary expenses are related directly to activity. Educational expenses, for example, are more directly related to the number and mix of personnel, and maintenance expenses to the amount of specialized equipment or to the age and condition of the physical facility. The wheelchair purchased under noncapital equipment during the current year should not need to be replaced in the coming year, but additional IV poles may be required instead.

The key to budgeting nonsalary expenses, therefore, is to identify the most reasonable predictor within each account and to make expense projections based on that predictor. In some cases, more than one predictor may be needed. For example, assume that the delivery room's disposable linen account includes linen packs for vaginal deliveries and cesarean sections and scrub clothes packs for fathers attending deliveries. The predictor for the linen packs is logically the number of vaginal deliveries and cesarean sections projected. The predictor for the scrub clothes packs, however, may be the attendance at prepared childbirth classes, if this correlates more closely with the number of fathers attending deliveries.

In determining predictors for expense accounts, the emphasis must be on reasonableness. Theoretically, it may be possible to identify and project the cost of each item within an account. Some accounts, such as patient care supplies or pharmacy stock supplies, can incorporate tens or hundreds of different items. It is more practical for these accounts to group items according to the most likely predictor and identify separately only those items, if any, that generate a significant proportion of the expense within the account and are related to a different predictor or price variation. If suture prices are anticipated to increase by 15% and other patient care items by 10%, the operating room expenses will be significantly affected and the cost of sutures must be predicted separately. On patient care units where sutures are only occasionally used, the effect will be relatively small and sutures can be grouped with other patient care items.

In projecting expenses for accounts such as noncapital equipment or educational programs, a more direct approach is possible. Planning for the unit will include identification of specific equipment items that will need to be purchased. The manager can determine which seminars or conferences will be of value, the number of staff who will attend each, and the extent to which their expenses will be reimbursed. Other expenses, such as leased equipment, subscriptions and books, consultation services, and maintenance contracts, are also budgeted using this more direct approach.

Obviously, the manager needs to incorporate into the expense budget projections and costs related to the changes identified in the planning stage of the budget preparation. If the number of telemetry monitors on a medical unit is going to be increased, the cost of the monitors themselves will be part of the capital budget, not the operational budget. The expense related to EKG paper, however, is an operational expense, and one that will increase with the addition of the new monitors. This cost must be calculated and added to the operational budget. It is equally as important to describe those changes that have the potential to reduce expenses because of a change in practice, procedures, or products. Expenses for IV therapy, for example, would be reduced if plans include reducing the frequency of tubing changes, simplifying the taping procedure, or utilizing a less expensive administration setup.

Communication and coordination with related departments is also important in preparing the nonsalary expense budget. These departments will not only have necessary information on the cost of various items and activities, but they will also be able to identify operational changes that will affect unit expenses. If the pharmacy plans to implement system changes that require replacing a single page medication record with a multiple copy form, the cost of each record will increase significantly. The budget projection for forms must therefore reflect not only volume but also the increased unit cost of the medication record.

This coordination is particularly important if certain departments' charges to other cost centers are based on interdepartmental transfer of expenses. The print shop, for example, may house the duplicating machine and incur costs for the machine, paper, ink, and related maintenance. These expenses are then transferred to cost centers based on the number of copy pages made. The net result of the transfer should be zero (i.e., the amount credited to the print shop and the amount charged to the cost centers should be the same). Unless there is communication between the print shop and the cost centers, either or both budgets are likely to be misstated.

Most nonsalary expenses are calculated at projected volume times current cost and then adjusted for inflation. The forecasting techniques discussed in Chapter 6 may be useful in projecting the volume of a number of nonsalary items. The inflation factors are generally identified by management for broad categories (e.g., medical supplies, food, linen, drugs), and the most appropriate factor is selected for each expense category. Some expenses may be calculated directly—for example, contract maintenance according to the terms of the contract or education funds based on known registration fees for meetings and seminars.

REVIEW AND SUBMISSION

The next step in the budget process is to summarize the projected activity and resource requirements, revenues and expenses, for submission. At this point it is important to review these for the accuracy, appropriateness, and consistency of the total budget package.

Accuracy relates to the correctness of mathematical calculations. This can be done by reviewing each calculation. It is often helpful, however, to compare the results of the manager's calculations to a benchmark, such as the current budget or actual, to determine whether they are reasonable. Apparent inconsistencies may have a logical basis or they may be the result of errors in mathematical calculations.

For our sample cost center's revenue and expense budget (Fig. 8–11), the finance department has provided the year-to-date total of actual revenue and expenses and a 12-month projection for the current year. The projection is a straight-line projection, calculated by annualizing the year-to-date total actual (dividing the actual by the number of months represented—in this case 9—to derive an average per month and then multiplying that average by 12 months). This calculation assumes that the averages of the actual year-to-date totals will

RESPONSIBILITY CENTER: 611 GENERAL SURGERY

ACCOUNT NUMBER/ DESCRIPTION	FY 01 JANUARY YTD ACTUAL	FY 01 ANNUAL BUDGET	FY 01 PROJECTED ACTUAL	FY 02 BUDGET PROJECTION
311. Revenue				
010 Routine	($3,244,410)	($5,556,030)	($5,561,846)	(6,258,903)
020 Other	(27,590)	(47,893)	(47,297)	(45,832)
Total Operating Revenue	($3,272,000)	($5,603,923)	($5,609,143)	(6,304,736)
411. Salary Expense				
010 Salaries - Regular	$730,881	$1,292,966	$1,252,939	1,503,349
020 Salaries - Per Diem	2,758	0	4,728	0
030 Salaries - Overtime	40,128	62,288	68,791	48,565
040 Salaries - Differentials	97,995	170,419	167,991	188,606
050 FICA	61,285	107,316	105,060	124,778
060 Health Insurance	62,125	111,842	106,500	104,236
070 Pension	19,855	35,816	34,037	40,275
090 Other	17,228	29,092	29,534	33,826
Total Salary Expense	$1,032,255	$1,809,738	$1,769,580	2,043,635
611. Supply Expense				
010 Patient Care Supplies	$41,692	$62,023	$71,472	84,728
020 Office Supplies	1,907	3,070	3,269	3,225
030 Forms	3,111	5,560	5,333	5,041
040 Supplies Purchased	1,210	1,935	2,074	1,161
050 Equipment	1,553	2,903	2,662	5,548
060 Seminars/Meetings	1,163	2,258	1,994	2,580
070 Books	145	258	249	258
080 Equipment Rental	385	1,703	660	677
090 Miscellaneous	388	968	665	968
Total Supply Expense	$51,554	$80,677	$88,378	102,186
911. Interdepartmental Expense				
010 Central Supply	$ 7,828	$13,995	$13,419	13,327
020 Pharmacy	9,527	17,019	16,332	19,362
030 Linen/Laundry	16,046	28,678	27,507	29,331
040 Maintenance	977	4,515	1,675	1,935
060 Telephone	1,962	3,225	3,363	3,225
070 Photocopy	124	323	213	387
090 Miscellaneous	165	194	283	258
Total Interdepartmental Expense	$36,629	$67,948	$62,793	67,824
Total Operating Expense	$1,120,438	$1,958,363	$1,920,751	2,213,645

FIGURE 8–11. Sample revenue and expense budget worksheet.

continue through the end of the fiscal year. The assumption is questionable, but the 12-month projection provides a potentially helpful check against the budgeted figures. For example, consider the central supply expense in Figure 8–11. The budgeted expense is projected to be lower than the estimated annual expense for the current year. The unit activity—census, acuity, and workload—is projected to increase in the coming year, as shown in Figure 8–4, and the unit activity should be a reasonable predictor of the central supply expense. Unless the manager can explain why the expenses are anticipated to be lower than current projections, a detailed review of calculations should be done before the budget is submitted.

It is also important to review the budget plan once again in relationship to the budget assumptions, operational goals, and unit plan identified at the beginning of the process. The proposed budget should enable the manager and staff to implement the plan with a reasonable expectation of success. Budget plans that understate personnel requirements in relation to projected activity will not promote accomplishing the stated goals. The resources can be increased, the goals scaled back, or the systems and methods of implementation adapted to establish congruency. It is equally important for this review to identify any overstatement of requirements for resources. This may occur if operational efficiencies, related for example to changes in systems for delivering medications or processing orders, have not been incorporated into the budget plan. Submitting a budget plan that is intrinsically inconsistent or inappropriate for the expressed assumptions and goals creates significant difficulties in implementation. In addition, it leaves the manager's fiscal responsibleness open to question.

NEGOTIATION AND FINALIZATION

When all cost center budgets have been submitted, these are totaled to make up the operating budget for the organization. This initial budget is reviewed in relation to the operational objectives identified in the initial planning stages. If the objectives cannot be met under the projected budget, then adjustments must be made to assure operating effectiveness. It is at this point that the most difficult phase of budget preparation, the negotiation phase, occurs.

If the organizational objectives call for a greater profit margin than the proposed budget would yield, then the projections must be adjusted to increase revenue, decrease expense, or both. The degree to which operating revenue can be increased has usually been well-defined by this point in the process. If operating revenue is increased as a result of increased volume, related increases in expense must also be identified. Frequently, however, the focus is directed toward reducing expenses. To accomplish this, decisions must be made about the relative priority of programs, personnel projections, and equipment and supply needs among various departments and cost centers. This negotiation takes place at all levels in the organization, and cost center managers as well as department directors must be prepared to participate in the process.

In negotiating the budget, the manager will relate the projections to the plans and goals developed at the beginning of the budget process. The manager must be prepared to describe and justify the factors that determine the projections presented. The most effective justifications will be clear and concise and will include objective and reliable data. The level of understanding of the audience is also an important consideration: negotiation among nurse managers using the same PCS will require less explanation of activity projections than presentation to a budget committee whose members are unfamiliar with the concepts of acuity and workload. Because it may not be possible to implement all goals and projections, the manager must also be prepared to discuss the relative priority of these proposals and the potential impact of implementing or not implementing them. Finally, the manager must be able to evaluate the unit's goals and priorities in relation to those of other departments and the total organization. With limited resources available to the organization as a whole, staffing increases requested in support departments may have significant positive implications for the nursing staff and justify modifying or deferring nursing proposals.

Although decisions and approvals on budget proposals are the responsibility of senior management, these are influenced by the information presented through the negotiation process. Provided that managers are able to articulate clearly their projections and requirements, decisions can be made that promote organizational goals and objectives and that generate commitment and support.

After decisions and approvals have been communicated, the manager will adjust the cost center budget if necessary and prepare for implementation. Because the budget has been calculated for the fiscal year, it will be necessary to determine the allocation of the annual figures by accounting periods, sometimes called seasonalization of the budget. The simplest seasonalization method is to allocate units of service, hours, and dollars equally across all periods (i.e., divide the totals by 12 [or 13, if the organization has 28-day accounting cycles] and assume that the activity and resource utilization will be similar in each month).

Most organizations and units, however, experience seasonal variations in activity and in resource utilization. Admissions and attendant workload may be noticeably lower from mid-November through the first week in January. Workload, and therefore productive time requirements, may be similar in March and in July. However, nonproductive time may be much greater in July because of vacation scheduling. In addition, numbers of orientees may be greater during the summer months if the nursing department employs a significant number of spring graduates.

It is possible to manage these seasonal variations, even if the budget is spread equally across all months, using statistical relationships and historical trends. If the manager is scheduling staff to assure consistent available hours per workload, then fewer direct care hours will be paid over the winter holiday weeks and at other periods of decreased workload. This will provide an offset for those times in which the workload is greater than average. Knowing from analysis of historical data that increased orientation and nonproductive hours will be required in the summer months, the manager may limit the use of alternate sources of coverage earlier in the year in order to have additional hours available to use at a later date. It may also be possible to limit the number of prescheduled nonproductive hours that will be approved in any particular time period in order to distribute the actual use of nonproductive time more evenly throughout the year.

A more useful approach for the manager is to describe the most likely distribution of activity and need for resources expected during the fiscal year and to seasonalize the budget accordingly. Frequently, this method of seasonalization is used for the entire hospital and is based primarily on anticipated fluctuations in admissions or patient days. This seasonalization will usually approximate (although not necessarily mirror) the workload and direct care hours fluctuation. However, it may not relate as well to the nonproductive hours utilization. Based on historical data and unit practices, it is possible to project the expected variations in nonproductive hours utilization and to seasonalize the hours and salary budget using these projections. Simply calculate the percent of total annual nonproductive time used in each month (refer to the forecasting methods described in Chapter 6) and apply those percentages to the total nonproductive time budgeted for the coming fiscal year.

IMPLEMENTATION

At this point the manager will focus on the most important part of the process: implementation of the budget plan. As a plan, the budget describes anticipated outcomes for the unit and organization for the fiscal year. It is the responsibility of the nurse manager to initiate steps necessary to put the plan into effect and to provide leadership to the staff in achieving the goals articulated in the plan.

An important aspect of implementation relates to the management and utilization of the resources identified in the plan. For personnel, this means the translation of the annual FTE budget into shorter-range scheduling patterns that take into account variations around the averages identified in the budget, for example, weekday to weekend variations in workload or seasonal fluctuations in census or benefit time utilization. It also applies to the day-to-day and shift-to-shift staffing adjustments needed to meet changing patient care needs. For nonsalary expenses, this means developing or streamlining systems for acquiring and maintaining supplies and equipment.

Implementation also incorporates systems for monitoring actual experience against projected. One method is based on fixed budget analysis, which compares total actual FTE and expense utilization to the fixed budget. However, this approach does not account for the fluctuations in workload that are likely to occur during the budget year. A more useful monitor is based on a flexible budget approach and looks at the resources utilized in comparison to the changing workload. For the manager who has developed a budget based on targets for HPW, nonproductive factor, and staff mix, comparison of actual to expected experience on these parameters is more valuable. These targets are expressions of the relationship of resource utilization to workload. If the workload increases and the hours provided for each unit of work is constant, then the total care hours will increase but the HPW will remain the same. Similarly, if the workload decreases, the manager can be expected to adjust total care hours downward but still maintain the target HPW. To the extent that the identified relationships are maintained, the manager is following the budget plan and can explain and justify variances against the fixed budget. Monitoring actual performance against budget can also identify trends or variations that, if they persist over time, may require midcourse corrections to the original budget. The systems used in analyzing, monitoring, and controlling the administration of the budget are discussed in Chapters 13 and 14.

SUMMARY AND IMPLICATIONS FOR NURSE MANAGERS

In order to prepare the operational budget, the nurse manager must be familiar with the financial structure and reporting systems of the organization and with the data reported through these systems. These data are analyzed in conjunction with other known factors to define operational goals and to predict levels of activity and resource utilization. Nurse managers must understand the overall priorities and directions of the entire organization so that the budget plan is congruent with the organizational goals and objectives.

The actual preparation of the operational budget translates these goals and predictions into numbers. The activity budget identifies and quantifies the units of service or workload, which determines resource requirements. The revenue budget projects the income that will be generated by that activity.

The personnel budget identifies full time equivalents (FTEs) and positions. The workload is the basis for quantifying the productive hours needed, as well as allocating these hours by employee category and by shift. Calculating coverage required for nonproductive time is based on historical data and organizational policies. These hours are added to the productive hours to determine total FTEs, which are then described by hours and positions. The salary budget includes expenses for regular salaries, differentials and premiums, fringe benefits, and related employment costs.

Projections for the nonsalary budget are based on the most reasonable predictor for items or activities included in the different expense accounts and reflect the identified goals of the unit. Communication and coordination with related departments increases the accuracy of the budget projections.

Following negotiation and finalization, the nurse manager is responsible for the implementation and administration of the operating budget.

SUGGESTED READINGS

Barrett, C., and Schultz, M. (1997). Staffing the operating room: Time and space factors. *Journal of Nursing Administration.* 27(12), 27–31.

Benson, J.A., Michelman, J.E., and Radjenovic, D. (1996, December). Using information technology strategically in home care. *Home Healthcare Nursing.* 14(12), 977–983.

Cavouras, C.A., and McKinley, J. (1997, May). Variable budgeting for staffing analysis and evaluation. *Nursing Management.* 28(5), 34–36, 39.

Douglas, D.A., and Mayewske, J. (1996, February). Census variation staffing. *Nurse Management.* 27(2), 32–33, 36.

Edwardson, S., and Pejsa, J. (1993). A computer assisted tutorial for applications of computer spreadsheets in nursing financial management. *Computers in Nursing.* 11(4), 169–175.

Finkler, S.A. (1984). Electronic spreadsheets and budgeting: A case study. *Nursing Economic$.* 2(6), 116–174.

Finkler, S.A., and Ward, D.R. (1999). *Cost Accounting for Health Care Organizations: Concepts and Applications,* Second edition. Gaithersburg, MD: Aspen Publishers.

Graveley, E.A., and Murphy, M.A. (1995, September–October). Nursing informatics. Making financial management come alive. *Computers in Nursing.* 13(5), 217–220.

Hellman, E. (1991). Analysis of a home health agency's productivity system. *Public Health Nursing.* 8(4), 251–257.

Hernandez, C.A., and O'Brien-Pallas, L.L. (1996, September–October). Validity and reliability of nursing workload measurement systems: Review of validity and reliability theory. *Canadian Journal of Nursing Administration.* 9(3), 32–50.

Hlusko, D., Weatherly, K., et al. (1994). Computerization of a nursing financial management system using continuous quality improvement as a framework. *Computers in Nursing.* 12(4), 193–200.

Irvin, S.A., and Brown, H.N. (1999, July–August). Self-scheduling with Microsoft Excel. *Nursing Economic$.* 17(4), 201–206.

Jacobs, S.M., and Pelfrey, S. (1995). Decision support systems: Using computers to help manage. *Journal of Nursing Administration.* 25(2), 46–54.

Kasper, D. (1986). The credibility of patient classification instruments. *Patients & Purse Strings.* F.A. Schaffer. New York: National League for Nursing.

Keeling, B. (1999). How to allocate the right staff mix across shifts, Part I. *Nursing Management.* 30(9), 16–17.

Keeling, B. (1999). How to allocate the right staff mix across shifts, Part 2. *Nursing Management.* 30(10), 16–18.

Kirby, K.K., and Wiczai, L.J. (1985). Budgeting for variable staffing. *Nursing Economic$.* 3(3), 160–166.

Kirk, R. (1986). *Nurse Staffing and Budgeting—Practical Management Tools.* Gaithersburg, MD: Aspen Publishers.

Malloch, K., and Conovaloff, A. (1999). Patient classification systems, Part 1: The third generation. *Journal of Nursing Administration.* 29(7/8), 49–56.

Malloch, K., Neeld, A., et al. (1999). Patient classification systems, Part 2: The third generation. *Journal of Nursing Administration.* 29(9):33–42.

Mills, M., Roman, C., and Heller, B. (1995). *Information Management in Nursing and Health Care.* New York: Springhouse.

Pelfrey, S. (1997, March). Managing financial data. *Seminars for Nurse Managers.* 5(1), 25–30.

Porter-O'Grady, T. (1987). *Nursing Finance: Budgeting Strategies for a New Age.* Gaithersburg, MD: Aspen Publishers.

Saba, V., and McCormick, K. (1995). *Essentials for Computers for Nurses,* Second edition. New York: McGraw-Hill.

Samuels, D.I. (1997). *The Healthcare Financial Management & Budgeting Toolkit.* Chicago: Irwin.

Sarnecki, A., Hass, S., et al. (1998). Design and implementation of a patient classification system for rehabilitation nursing. *Journal of Nursing Administration.* 28(3), 35–43.

Sengin, K.K., and Dreisbach, A.M. (1995, February). Managing with precision. A budgetary decision support model. *Journal of Nursing Administration.* 25(2), 33–44.

Simpson, R.L. (1997, September). CIOs and trends in health care computing. *Nursing Management.* 28(9), 20–21.

Storfjell, J., Allen, C., et al. (1997). Analysis and management of home health nursing caseloads and workloads. *Journal of Nursing Administration.* 27(9), 24–33.

Swansburg, R.C. (1997). *Budgeting and Financial Management for Nurse Managers.* Boston: Jones & Bartlett Publishers.

Villemaire, M., and Lane-McGraw, C. (1986). Nursing personnel budgets: A step by step guide. *Nursing Management.* 17(11), 28–32.

Ward, W.J., Jr. (1994). *Health Care Budgeting and Financial Management for Non-Financial Managers: A New England Healthcare Assembly Book.* Westport, CN: Auburn House Publishers.

Wild, J., and Imbrogno, L. (1996, July). Market changes create need for practice budgets. *Healthcare Financial Management,* 50(7), 77–78.

9

Revenue Budgeting

The goals of this chapter are to:

discuss sources of revenues;

explain the importance of prices and volume in revenue budgeting;

clarify why revenues are often ignored in nursing budgets;

discuss when revenues should be considered in nursing budgets;

provide examples of revenue budget calculations;

discuss revenues from managed care organizations;

define capitation;

explain the impact of capitation on risk;

provide an example of how capitation rates can be calculated; and

define risk-sharing pools and discuss their use.

INTRODUCTION

The last chapter discussed preparation of a nursing unit budget. However, it focused primarily on the expense side of that budget. Operating budgets consist of both revenues and expenses. This chapter focuses on issues related to revenues. Revenues are the amount the organization earns in exchange for the services it provides. Revenues are critical for every organization.

Revenues must be adequate to cover all the costs of providing services during the current year. Additionally, revenues should be great enough to provide a profit. This is true whether the organization is a for-profit or not-for-profit organization. Profits are used to expand the type of services offered, expand the volume of services offered, and to replace buildings and equipment. Both inflation and technological advances often cause new capital acquisitions (see Chapter 10 for a discussion of capital budgeting) to be more expensive than those they replace. Profits earned each year help the organization to have sufficient resources for replacements and expansion.

There are many different sources of revenues that are relevant to nurses. Typically one thinks of patient revenues. These are amounts that are received either directly from patients or from third parties, such as insurance companies. They are payments for health care services provided. However, in various nursing situations there are a wide variety of other revenue sources. Swansburg has listed some sources of nursing revenue as:

grants, continuing education, private practice, community visibility, health care students and staff, HMOs, city health departments, industry, unions, third-party payments, professional corporations, and nurse-managed centers[1]

and that list is far from exhaustive.

In a growing number of situations, nurse managers are required to prepare revenue budgets and are held accountable for revenue. This chapter begins with a discussion of some basic issues and addresses a number of questions related to revenues. What are they? How are they earned? Why are they often ignored in discussions about nursing budgets? When should they be considered? Next the chapter moves on to a discussion of the calculations of revenues, as it relates to nursing.

The chapter concludes with a discussion of issues related to managed care revenues, with a particular emphasis on issues related to revenues from capitation arrangements. That section provides an introduction to managed care concepts, including risk. The role of risk pools in revenue budgeting is also addressed. An example of how capitation rates can be determined is provided.

THE REVENUE BUDGET

The operating budget for any organization consists of a revenue budget and an expense budget. In many situations nurses have been held accountable for revenues. For example, traditionally the director of the operating room has been charged with earning a profit, based on having revenues that exceed costs. Units or departments that have revenue budgets are called *revenue centers* in health care. They are often called *profit centers* in other industries. However, in most cases, nurse managers are given authority over expenses only. Units or departments that do not have a revenue budget are called *cost centers* or *expense centers*.

Why Aren't All Nursing Units Revenue Centers?

In most industries, including health care, managers are generally responsible for expense centers. Imagine buying a car. Perhaps you go to a new car dealer and buy a car for $25,000. Suppose that the dealer in turns pays $23,000 to the manufacturer. How should the manufacturer view the $23,000 of revenue it received? In order to make the car there was an engine department, a bumper

---

[1]Russel C. Swansburg, *Budgeting and Financial Management for Nurse Managers,* Jones and Bartlett Publishers, Boston, 1997.

department, a door department, a steering wheel department, and other departments. Should each of those departments be revenue centers or just expense centers? In your mind, how much of the $25,000 you paid was for the engine? How much for the bumper? In turn, when the dealer bought the car, how much was it paying for each component?

In reality, as a buyer, you viewed the purchase as one lump sum. You probably did not divide the car into the pieces made by the various departments, assign a value to each piece, and make sure that the total of the pieces came to exactly the $25,000 you were paying. Neither did the dealer when it paid $23,000. Therefore it is difficult for the manufacturer to divide up its $23,000 of revenue by department. The important issue for the manufacturer is to produce high-quality parts efficiently. Each department is given an expense budget based on what it should cost to efficiently manufacture the parts made by the department. As long as the total cost of all the parts is less than the $23,000 the dealer paid to the manufacturer, the manufacturer is making a profit. This is fairly typical of most organizations. Revenue is not assigned to individual managers, departments, or units.

In any health care organization that receives a lump-sum payment for each patient, it makes sense to avoid setting up revenue centers. In many health care organizations, nursing is like the engine department. It is critical to the final product. The car being manufactured cannot run without an engine. Many health care providers cannot provide treatment to patients without nurses. However, if patients pay on a flat basis, such as a fixed DRG payment regardless of resources consumed, it is difficult to decide how much of the total payment is for nursing as opposed to other services.

However, not all patients pay a flat amount for their care. There are still many situations where patients are charged for x-rays, lab tests, and pharmaceuticals. Why not charge for nursing services as well? Historically, the division into revenue and expense centers was based on differential consumption. If all patients consumed exactly the same amount of a resource provided by a department, it was considered to be an expense center. If different patients consume different amounts, the department was established as a revenue center. For example, some patients have an operation and some do not. Of those who have an operation, some have a long, costly one, while others have a short, relatively inexpensive one. As a result, the operating room was established as a revenue center, charging a different amount to different patients.

In contrast, consider the security guard standing at the front door of the hospital. The guard protects the entire organization, its employees, its patients, and their visitors. It is difficult to argue that one patient consumes more benefit from the guard than another. The security guard will therefore be considered to be part of an expense center. All the costs of expense centers will be aggregated and charged to the patient in a lump sum, such as a daily room charge.

Some departments provide differential services, but it is just not worth the cost and effort of measuring and assigning those services. For example, different patients consume different amounts of laundry. But it would be expensive to track exactly how many sheets and towels are used by each patient. Instead, the laundry department is an expense center.

Nursing units were historically treated the same as the laundry! Yes, different patients do consume different amounts of nursing resources. However, it was costly to track that differential consumption. Exactly how much service is consumed by each specific patient? It would be expensive to hire an accountant to follow each nurse and keep track of how much of the nurse's time was used to provide care to each patient.

Today, however, the health care industry is making rapid progress in the area of computerization. Nurses could scan their ID card whenever they provide care to a patient, and computers could track the different amount of nursing care received by different patients. So it is now becoming feasible to charge different patients different amounts for the nursing services that they receive. Movement toward making nursing a revenue center in hospitals has been slow. Finance has been resistant to change. However, there does finally seem to be some movement toward making the nursing portion of health care revenues more explicit. Both Maryland and Maine now have laws requiring separation of nursing on hospital bills.[2] This could be the beginning of a trend that would substantially extend the nurse manager's involvement and responsibility for revenues.

When Are Nurse Managers Responsible for a Revenue Budget?

Despite the slow movement to nursing revenue centers in hospitals, there are many situations in which nurse managers are already responsible for developing revenue budgets, and these situations are likely to increase rapidly in the first decade of this century. In some cases these opportunities will occur in hospitals, where nurses are already responsible for revenue budgets for the operating room, recovery room, labor and delivery, and some other departments. However, hospitals should not be the focus, as their role in providing health care services has been diminishing. The last decade saw a clear shift away from hospital inpatient care to provision of care on an outpatient basis. This shift has created growing opportunities for nursing to have revenue responsibility.

In outpatient settings, nurse managers are often responsible for the revenue budgets of outpatient surgery units, clinics, community health centers, and home care agencies. In many cases, nurse entrepreneurs need to prepare revenue budgets for their own clinical practice, consulting practice, or other type of venture. Nurse educators may be responsible for tuition revenues. Nurse researchers are responsible for grant revenues. The situations where nurses must prepare and manage revenue budgets are extensive and growing.

---

[2]Swansburg, *ibid.*, p. 26.

The Elements of a Revenue Budget

The basic elements of a revenue budget are simple—price and volume. The revenue budget essentially consists of the price charged for each service provided by the unit, department, or organization multiplied by the number of units of service provided. The complications involved in a revenue budget are estimating the volume of services to be provided, deciding on the prices to charge, and estimating how much of the total amount charged will actually be collected.

Consider a simple example. Suppose that the Best Clinic treats patients on a cash basis. That is, patients pay for their treatment in cash as the treatment is provided by the clinic. If 10 patients are expected to be treated, the charge to each one is $100, and all amounts are collected, the revenue will be:

$$\$100/\text{patient} \times 10 \text{ patients} = \$1,000 \text{ of revenue.}$$

Even this simple first look at revenue is complicated. How did the organization decide to charge $100? How did it decide that 10 patients were likely?

Prices or Rates

A number of different types of prices are used in health care. Organizations set a price or charge for their services. However, some payers pay a percent of the charge that is less than 100%, based on a contractual agreement. Other payers pay a flat amount per case, regardless of the amount charged. Hospitals are sometimes paid on a per diem basis or a per discharge basis. The per discharge payment may be adjusted for diagnosis or might be a broad average payment regardless of patient type. Some payers just reimburse the organization for the costs that have been incurred in providing care. Home care can be reimbursed on a flat amount per visit or could be paid a flat amount per patient regardless of the number of visits required. Under capitation, discussed later, the health care provider is paid a flat amount per member regardless of whether the member consumes any health care resources at all!

For ongoing organizations, the finance department may provide the nurse manager with information about the prices (often called rates) that will be charged for each service. In such cases the manager is primarily responsible for estimating the future number of each type of patient to be treated and for multiplying the volume of each service times the given prices, to arrive at the revenue budget. The main difference between this and the $1,000 of revenue for Best Clinic discussed above is the fact that there typically will be many different kinds of patients with different prices, and the manager must be as accurate as possible in estimating the future volume of each type of patient.

In some cases, however, the nurse manager will be responsible for setting prices. This is often referred to as *rate-setting*. Prices can be *market-based*, *cost-based, mark-up based,* or negotiated. Market-based prices are those that are set based on a survey of what others in the community are charging for the same services. If you charge substantially more than others are charging, you may lose your customers. Some organizations intentionally set prices below the competition in an effort to stimulate business. The success of strategies to undercut the competition or to charge above the market (and make more profit per patient) depend largely on how sensitive buyers are to price.

Many individuals will shop around to buy a car, seeking the lowest price for what is essentially the exact same product. For example, if a specific model car from a specific manufacturer is sold by three different dealers in the area, the customer may shop for the best price from among the three dealers. What if a gall bladder operation can be obtained from three different doctors at three different hospitals? The customer is less likely to view the product as being identical. Shopping may be based more on the reputation of the surgeon or hospital than on the price.

Suppose that a nurse manager starts a home care agency in an area that already has two home care agencies. Will potential customers consider the service to be identical and therefore look for the lowest price? The nurse entrepreneur can decide to compete by charging less than the competition. Or the manager might decide simply to market the service as being better in some way (higher-quality nurses, more caring attitude, longer visits). Or the manager might decide simply to charge the market price and take a lot of discharge planners out to fancy dinners to gain referrals.

Alternatives to market-based prices are cost-based or mark-up based prices. Cost-based refers to charging exactly your cost. By cost we typically mean average cost. There are many instances where law or regulation require such prices. For example, a state might mandate that home care agencies charge Medicaid exactly the cost of providing care. Mark-up based prices are those where the manager determines the cost of care and sets the price a certain percentage above cost. For example, if a visit costs $40 to provide, an organization with a 20% markup would charge $48 for the visit (i.e., $40 + [20\% \times $40]$).

It is also becoming more common for health care providers to negotiate rates with insurance companies. The negotiation can result in a variety of different payment approaches, such as flat fees, percent discounts, or payments per episode.

Suppose that the Best Clinic, using a market-price strategy, sets its price at $100. Does that mean that the clinic will collect $100 for each patient? In reality, patients do not usually arrive with cash in hand. More often they have insurance. Some insurers will pay the full $100. But that is extremely rare. Many insurers only pay a specific amount for a particular service. Others demand a percentage discount. Often prices paid by insurers are the result of a protracted negotiation. A complete revenue budget must take into account the fact that health care providers do not usually collect the full amount charged.

For example, Blue Cross might say its members can only be charged $60 for the clinic's service. If you want to accept a Blue Cross patient, you cannot charge them more. So, in preparing a revenue budget, it would be necessary to estimate the percent of patients who are insured by Blue Cross and calculate their revenue as being $60 rather than $100. Another insurer might negotiate a percentage discount rather than a specific price for each service. Suppose that some of the clinic's patients are insured by Prudential and that the clinic's agreement with that insurer calls for them to pay 80% of charges. The amounts that the clinic agrees to give as discounts are called *contractual allowances*. Best Clinic's revenue budget might look like Table 9–1. Total net revenue is $860, rather than the $1,000 revenue originally calculated for the 10 patients.

Some of the clinic's patients might be Medicare or Medicaid patients. Assume that Best Clinic has one of each. Suppose that Medicaid regulations call for it to pay the cost of care and that the cost of each visit is $55. The allowance for the Medicaid patient is $45. Suppose further that Medicare has a fee schedule that calls for it to pay $70 for this type of patient. The allowance for the Medicare patient is $30. The revenue budget would now appear as is seen in Table 9–2. Note that the total net revenue is $785.

At this point it is clear that health care organizations often collect substantially less than the amount they charge for services. One reason that health care providers charge so much for health care services is because so many customers receive discounts. This is exacerbated by the fact that some customers do not pay their charges at all! Some patients will not be able to pay for their care because they don't have the financial resources. Others may just not be willing to pay.

In the former case the organization may decide to treat the patient as a charity case. In such instances the organization will either charge a lower amount or nothing at all. Suppose that one of the patients treated has no insurance and is poor. Best Clinic decides to give the patient a 75% discount. In that case, the gross revenue from that patient will be only $25. We do not include care that is being given as charity as part of gross revenues. It is a gift rather than a charge that is not collected. The cost of that care, however, will be included in the expense budget.

Some patients have the resources to pay for care but never pay. This occurs in

TABLE 9–1. *Best Clinic Revenue Budget for the Year Ending December 31, 2001*

Patients by Payer	Gross Revenue	Contractual Allowance	Net Revenue
2 Blue Cross patients	$ 200	$ 80	$120
$100 × 2 = $200 gross revenue			
$100 – $60 = $40 allowance per patient			
$40 × 2 patients = $80 allowance			
3 Prudential patients	300	60	240
$100 × 3 = $300 gross revenue			
$100 × 20% = $20 allowance per patient			
$20 × 3 patients = $60 allowance			
5 Other patients	500	0	500
Total	$1,000	$140	$860

TABLE 9–2. Best Clinic Revenue Budget for the Year Ending December 31, 2001

Patients by Payer	Gross Revenue	Contractual Allowance	Net Revenue
2 Blue Cross patients	$ 200	$ 80	$120
$100 × 2 = $200 gross revenue			
$100 – $60 = $40 allowance per patient			
$40 × 2 patients = $80 allowance			
3 Prudential patients	300	60	240
$100 × 3 = $300 gross revenue			
$100 × 20% = $20 allowance per patient			
$20 × 3 patients = $60 allowance			
I Medicaid patient	100	45	55
I Medicare patient	100	30	70
3 Other patients	300	0	300
Total	$1,000	$215	$785

two different ways. Some patients do not have insurance and simply fail to pay part or all of their bill. Many patients do have insurance but are required to pay a portion of the charge—perhaps 20% or 30%. That portion is called a co-pay or co-payment. If a patient fails to pay the co-pay portion, the insurance company often will not pay that amount either. When patients do not pay amounts that have been charged to them, the amounts not paid are referred to as *bad debts*. Bad debts may arise from self-insured patients who do not pay their bills or from the co-pay share of insured patients. Organizations should bill promptly, send monthly statements, and use collections agencies if necessary to collect as much of the money owed to them as possible. Assume that Best Clinic has one *self-pay* (uninsured) patient whose bill is not paid.

Table 9–3 shows the net revenue for the clinic. Note that the bad debt is included in net revenue and then subtracted separately as an expense. Accounting rules for reporting the financial results of an organization require bad debts to be treated as expenses rather than revenue reductions. Bad debts are isolated this way to highlight them. Some organizations do a better job and some a worse job of collecting amounts owed to them. Seeing the bad debts as a separate item helps the reader get a sense of how well a particular organization has done in this area.

It is important to note that Best Clinic only expects to collect $610 for providing care to the 10 patients (Table 9–3). Even though there were 10 patients who each received a $100 service, only $925 was charged in total (because of the charity care) rather than $1,000. The final amount collected was $610 because of allowances and bad debts. Unless the manager is careful to go through this computation, there may be a mistaken assumption that the organization has much more money available to spend on providing care than is actually the case. It is critical to estimate the actual amounts that will be collected for each patient as carefully as possible. This means spending time trying to determine the likely rate of bad debts (often from historical experience), reviewing contracts with insurers to determine payment rates, and even considering things such as discounts given to credit card companies for patients who charge their bills.[3]

Volume Estimates

Even if the amount collected per patient is meticulously considered, the revenue budget still depends heavily on estimates of volume. Volume can be estimated using the forecasting techniques that are discussed in Chapter 6. Note that it is not sufficient to estimate total patient volume. The volume of each type of patient or procedure for which there is a different charge must be estimated. This may entail estimation of home care visits by nurses versus aides. Or perhaps a manager will need to estimate patients, patient days, treatments, hours, procedures, and tests. Some degree of flexibility is required to forecast based on

---

[3]If a patient charges a $100 bill for health care services on a credit card, the credit card company will typically pay the provider anywhere between $95 and $98. The difference between the $100 charge and the amount the credit card company pays is a fee to cover the costs and some of the profits of the credit card company.

TABLE 9–3. *Best Clinic Revenue Budget for the Year Ending December 31, 2001*

Patients by Payer	Gross Revenue	Discounts and Contractual Allowances	Net Revenue
2 Blue Cross patients	$200	$ 80	$ 120
$100 × 2 = $200 gross revenue			
$100 – $60 = $40 allowance per patient			
$40 × 2 patients = $80 allowance			
3 Prudential patients	300	60	240
$100 × 3 = $300 gross revenue			
$100 × 20% = $20 allowance per patient			
$20 × 3 patients = $60 allowance			
1 Medicaid patient	100	45	55
1 Medicare patient	100	30	70
1 Charity self-pay patient (75% discount)	25	0	25
1 Bad debt self-pay patient	100	0	100
1 Other self-pay patient	100	0	100
Total	$925	$215	$ 710
Less Bad Debt Expense			−100
Net Revenue Less Bad Debts			$ 610

type of patient or type of procedure or test, depending on the specific requirements of a particular situation.

In preparing the revenue budget, it is extremely important to consider all possible sources of revenue or support. In addition to patient charges for services, these sources might include ancillary activities such as gift shops or restaurants, endowment income, gifts, or grants. Clearly, the final revenue budget will be more complex than Table 9–3, showing revenues not only by type of payer but also by different types of patients or procedures and including information about other types of revenue.

Table 9–4 presents a somewhat more sophisticated example for an outpatient organization that provides both same-day surgery and a variety of clinic services. However, even this example is simplified, as it only breaks patients down into same-day surgery versus clinic groups, as opposed to a more detailed breakdown by type of surgery, type of visit, procedure, or tests. In Table 9–4 the first column on the left indicates the different revenue sources, listing the different types of patients by payer, and other revenue sources. The next column, column A, Quantity, indicates the forecast volume level for each revenue source. In this

TABLE 9–4. Surgery and Clinic Revenue Budget for the Year Ending June 30, 2002

Revenue Source	(A) Quantity	(B) Rate or Charge	(C = A 3 B) Gross Revenue	(D) Average Net Charge	(E = C 3 D) Revenue Net of Discounts and Allowances
Same-Day Surgery					
Private Insurance	1,000	$1,500	$1,500,000	75%	$1,125,000
Medicare	600	1,500	900,000	80%	720,000
Medicaid	400	1,500	600,000	60%	360,000
Self-Pay	500	1,500	750,000	70%	525,000
Clinic Patients					
Private Insurance	3,000	250	750,000	75%	562,500
Medicare	1,800	250	450,000	80%	360,000
Medicaid	1,200	250	300,000	60%	180,000
Self-Pay	1,500	250	375,000	85%	318,750
Gift Shop	7,000	17	119,000	99%	117,810
Donations	400	200	80,000	100%	80,000
Subtotal			$5,824,000		$4,349,060
Less Bad Debt Expense					– 112,500
Net Revenue Less Bad Debts					$4,236,560

example, 1,000 same-day surgery patients with private insurance are expected. There are anticipated to be 7,000 purchases from the gift shop and 400 donations.

Moving to column B, Rate or Charge, the full charge on average for each type of service is indicated. For example, the average same-day surgery charge is expected to be $1,500. Obviously, a more realistic budget would show different types of surgery patients and different charges for each type. In column B we also see that the average purchase at the gift shop is $17 and the average donation to the organization is $200.

Column C, the Gross Revenue, can be found by multiplying column A by column B. This represents the total of all charges by the organization to its patients, as well as gift shop charges and donations.

Column D, the Average Net Charge, represents the average percent of the full charge that is collected. For example, if private insurance payments typically average 75% of the full charge, then Column D shows 75%. Note that the percentage shown for self-pay patients in this column reflects contractual allowances but not bad debts, which appear later in the exhibit.

The percentage shown for the gift shop reflects the fact that the organization provides a 10% discount for purchases by employees. If employees account for 10% of all purchases from the gift shop, that would result in an average discount of 1% across all gift shop sales (i.e., a 10% discount to employees who make up 10% of all purchases = 10% × 10% = 1% discount on all sales on average).

Column E is simply column C multiplied by column D. This represents the amount expected to be collected. At the bottom of this column we see that bad debts are shown as $112,500. This represents 10% of all amounts charged to self-pay patients (i.e., [$750,000 same-day surgery + $375,000 clinic] × 10%). The 10% typically would be based on historical bad debt experience. Note in Table 9–4 that although Surgery and Clinic expects to have gross charges of $5,824,000, they only expect to collect $4,236,560 for the services provided for the year.

Environmental Scan

In predicting revenue for the coming year, managers should consider many issues. Managers need to be concerned not only with what they might want to do but also with other factors such as the economy, inflation, growth, employment, interest rates, competition, and so on. Managers should undertake a common-sense review of the likely impact of the economic environment on the organization. Just as an environmental scan is essential for budgeting in general, the information from the scan should be applied to the revenue budget.

Even a change in the proportion of patients covered by each type of insurer is a significant event. Consider what would happen to Surgery and Clinic in Table 9–4 if an economic downturn forced a number of patients with private insurance to shift to Medicaid. In the exhibit, Medicaid pays a much lower percent of charges than private insurance. Such a shift could have a dramatic impact on total revenues collected by the organization. Note that the number and types of patients would remain the same; therefore the costs would remain the same. But a shift in payer mix can dramatically change both the revenues and overall fortunes of the organization, and managers must anticipate and consider the impact of such changes.

REVENUES FROM MANAGED CARE

The last decade of the twentieth century saw tremendous growth in the area of *managed care*. In an environment highly focused on controlling the costs of providing health care services, managed care organizations (MCOs) flourished. A managed care organization is any organization that tries to control the use of health care services to provide cost-effective care. MCOs try to eliminate provision of care that is not needed or is not cost-effective. The debate that often surrounds managed care relates to how we define care that is not cost-effective.

Sometimes it is easy to spot cost-effective solutions. Suppose that a mother and newborn are physically well and could be discharged from the hospital after two days. However, it is desirable to check the infant for jaundice on the third day. Should the mother and infant be kept in the hospital for a third day, or should a nurse practitioner go to see the mother and infant in their home on the third day? The cost of the home visit is substantially less than the additional day in the hospital. Assuming that clinical outcomes are equally as good if the mother and infant are discharged after the second day, if they are insured by a MCO they will likely be sent home after two days. The result is lower cost with no decline in outcomes.

However, there are many ethical problems that arise from the definition that many MCOs use for cost-effective care. What if a test is needed to determine if a patient has a problem that is serious but highly unlikely. Perhaps the test costs $5,000 and would produce a positive result in only 1 out of 1,000 people tested. That means that if the test were performed on 1,000 people it would probably find one person with the illness. The thousand tests would cost a total of $5,000,000. Managed care would probably deem that test not to be cost-effective and would refuse to pay for it. In contrast, before the advent of managed care, if a physician ordered the test, many insurance companies would have paid for it. Is it right to deny payment for that test? That is a moral dilemma with no easy answer.

Capitation versus Fee-for-Service

Prior to managed care almost all care was provided on a *fee-for-service* basis. Fee-for-service means that there is a charge for each type of service provided. Patients or their insurance companies paid based on the specific services they consumed. If patients had a lab test, they were charged for the lab test. If patients had a home care visit, they were charged for the visit. Patients consuming more services were therefore charged more than patients consuming fewer services. Managed care proponents argue that the fee-for-service system encouraged overprovision of services. If the health care provider earns more money as more services are provided, why not provide a lot of services, whether needed or not?

The last sentence might outrage some. Who is some big insurance company to decide what services are needed and what services are not? But the reality is that some abuses likely did exist. Some patients did receive more lab tests or home visits than were absolutely necessary. And to some extent it's hard to determine what is really necessary. Would patients who receive home care visits once a day benefit it there were two visits a day instead? Probably. But how much would they benefit? Would the extra benefit be worth the extra cost of the additional visit? These are difficult questions to address. What we can say is that the assumption (correct or incorrect) that fee-for-service leads to some overprovision of services was one factor leading to the development of capitated payment.

Capitation is a flat payment per covered member (sometimes referred to as per covered life) regardless of the amount of care provided. Capitation agreements are contractual agreements between two parties for the provision of some defined set of health-related services in exchange for a flat periodic payment per patient. The purchaser of the services is the managed care company, and the seller is the health care provider. Although the most common capitated contracts are between MCOs and physicians or hospitals, such contracts can also be established with a variety of health care organizations run by nurses, such as home care agencies or community health centers.

A nurse could contract with a MCO to provide certain services to its members for a premium payment per member per month. The MCO would provide a list of covered members and would pay a flat monthly amount regardless of how much care the members consume. In many months the nurse will receive a payment for some members who do not consume any care at all, as well as for other patients that consume lots of care. One should not look at the profit or loss for any specific member. It is necessary to consider the total of the capitated payments received for the month for all members, in contrast to the total amount of services provided to all covered members that month.

Although capitated payments to nurses may not yet be extremely common, they do exist. For example,

One approach to managing care on a capitated basis is the Community Nursing Organization (CNO). Under a Medicare demonstration project, four CNOs receive capitated Medicare payments to provide a range of services to approximately 10,000 frail elderly patients in their homes and communities. The CNOs, which are nurse-managed, provide home health, physical therapy, occupational therapy, and speech-language therapy services, as well as medical equipment and supplies and ambulance services, along with preventive services. Initial data suggest that the CNOs may provide an important means of reducing utilization of higher-cost services while providing a range of needed services to the frail elderly.[4]

---

[4]Personal e-mail communication from David Keepnews, September 28, 1999.

Many MCOs do not use capitation for all their contracts. Instead they may negotiate a discount from normal fees. In those cases, revenue is still paid on a fee-for-service basis (although the fee may be discounted), and the discussion related to revenue earlier in the chapter applies. Capitation, however, is a dramatically different form of payment.

From the viewpoint of the MCO, capitation is beneficial because there is no incentive for providers to overserve patients. If a home care patient receives extra visits, there is no extra payment received by the agency. So there is no reason to deliver unneeded care. From the perspective of the provider, capitation provides a predictable revenue stream. Daily ups and downs in the flow of patients do not impact on the regular monthly receipt of capitation payments. You get paid whether the managed care members get sick or not.

It is also sometimes possible to negotiate payments in advance of the provision of services. A new nurse entrepreneur, just starting out and with many expenses, can work out an arrangement to receive capitated payments at the beginning of each month. That money can be used to pay rent and salaries. It provides some revenue stability to the practice.

Capitated payment also has the potential to simplify paperwork. Each month the provider gets a list of covered members. When a member comes for treatment, the provider often collects a minimal co-payment from the member (perhaps $10) on the spot. The only other payment is the monthly capitation.

The essence of the concept behind capitation is that it shifts risk to the provider of care. Under fee-for-service, the patient, employer, or insurance company is totally at risk. The more health care services the patient consumes, the more the patient or insurer pays. Capitation, however, puts the provider at risk. The more health care services consumed by a covered patient, the worse off the provider is. This creates a situation in which the provider benefits from keeping the patient healthy. Preventive care is less costly to the provider than curative care, so providers are more likely to provide services that keep patients healthy. Also, all providers have an incentive to use the lowest cost-efficacious treatment. Rather than providing more care to the patients you have, the way to increase revenue moves to having more covered members.

Money Flows Under Capitation

In most capitated systems the primary payment comes from the purchaser of health insurance. This is generally the employer and employee, who share the cost of the premium. The insurance company, often an HMO, keeps part of the premium and uses the rest to pay for health care services. The two largest groups to receive payments are hospitals and physicians.

The key to revenues under capitation are the capitation rate and the number of capitated members. Suppose that a home care agency contracts with a MCO to provide all home care visits needed for $12 per member per month (PMPM). If the MCO has 250 members who will be covered by the contract, then the monthly revenue will be:

$$\$12 \text{ PMPM} \times 250 \text{ members} = \$3,000$$

and the annual revenue will be:

$$\$12 \text{ PMPM} \times 250 \text{ members} \times 12 \text{ months/year} = \$36,000$$

The key to increasing revenue in a capitated environment is to get more covered members. This could either come from gaining a greater share of the members signed with one MCO or by signing additional contracts with other MCOs. Bear in mind that since fixed costs will not change (rent on physical facilities, salary for an office manager, etc.), volume of members (and therefore the total amount of capitated revenue) becomes critical to success. As long as the capitated payments exceed variable costs, more members lead to better financial outcomes.

Developing Capitated Rates

As a provider of health care services, setting the capitation rate is critical. Often a contract is signed committing the provider to accept the agreed-upon rate for at least a year. If the rate is set too low, the organization will lose money on patients throughout the year. Setting capitated rates is much more complicated than ordinary price-setting. The reason is that capitated rates depend critically on utilization.

In a fee-for-service payment situation, one tries to compare the price of a particular service to the cost of providing that service. For example, suppose that the average cost of providing a home care visit is $38 and the fee charged is $45. One can therefore anticipate a profit on each visit. However, in a capitated situation the payment is the PMPM, regardless of the number of visits for each patient. In negotiating a capitated rate, it is critical to evaluate the population covered and the likely utilization rate for that population. For example, an elderly population will obviously have far more home care visits than a younger population.

The starting point in determining a capitation rate is identification of the exact services to be covered by the contract. Next, the provider must obtain estimates of the utilization of each service offered. Utilization rates should be adjusted for actual population demographics. Costs should be estimated and converted to PMPM equivalents. It is helpful to set the marginal cost (i.e., incremental or additional cost) for the services to be provided as the lower limit and the fee-for-service charges as the upper limit for rate negotiations. Calculating the PMPM cost of each component on a charge, average cost, and marginal cost basis provides the manager with solid information to enter a negotiation. These elements for determining a capitation rate are discussed in the following paragraphs.

There is usually easy agreement over the services to be provided. The MCO wants to protect itself by having contracts to provide the services its members will need. So it will clearly specify what it wants to buy. In some cases, however, if there is great uncertainty about the cost of a service or the utilization of the service, there may be a *carve-out.* That is a service that would normally be provided but is excluded. For example, if liver and heart transplants are expected to be expensive and rare in a population, then a provider of surgical services (e.g., a hospital) might exclude, or carve out, those two services from a contract to provide all hospital surgical care. If a patient needs a carved-out service, it would be provided on a fee-for-service basis.

Determination of expected utilization is more complex. A good place to start is with historical demand data. For example, assuming that a home health agency has already been providing services, it can use its own records to estimate the typical frequency of visits. Unfortunately, most providers can ascertain the visit frequency only for those patients who have at least one visit, treatment, admission, or other episode of care. What about all the members of the general population who do not seek any care during the year? Estimating utilization of capitated populations is difficult because the payment covers all members, whether they receive any care or not. Furthermore, the population covered by the managed care contract may be more or less likely to require care than the organization's historical patient base.

Although the MCO may offer its perspective on the amount of care that is needed for the population, one must consider that the managed care company has a vested interest in underestimating required care. The managed care company wants to pay the lowest rate it can. Often it is necessary to employ the services of an actuarial firm. Such a firm can examine the covered population, consider historical utilization rates for that population, adjust for utilization rates for the particular geographic region, and adjust for gender and age of the covered population.

Once the services to be provided have been determined and the utilization rates have been estimated, the next element in the process is for the provider to determine the fee-for-service charges, average costs, and marginal costs for the services to be provided under the managed care contract. The charges are needed because that is the amount that the provider would ideally like the MCO to pay. If the agreed-upon capitation rate provides as much money as charges would have provided, then the contract is bringing in additional patients and additional revenue at prices as good as are currently being earned.

Average cost represents a middle ground. In the short run, a rate based on average costs would make the provider better off. If some costs are fixed, as they undoubtedly are, then the additional patients would improve the short-term profits of the provider. Marginal costs represent the minimum that should be accepted. If the capitated price provides less than the marginal cost, the provider will actually be financially worse off because of the contract with the MCO.

MCOs will offer a price stated as a PMPM. This is because employers pay premiums on a monthly basis, based on the number of insured employees for the month. As job turnover occurs, employers eliminate some individuals from health insurance coverage and add others. The MCO will in turn eliminate some individuals from the payments made to the provider each month. Therefore, cost should be converted to PMPM equivalents.

Setting a Capitation Rate–An Example

Assume that you are the manager of a home care agency. You are currently negotiating a capitated rate with a MCO. Your charges for visits are currently $60 for a visit by an RN and $40 for a visit by an aide. Based on the history of the agency with noncapitated patients, plus information provided by an actuary, you have the following expectations regarding utilization by members of the MCO[5]:

1.2 RN visits per member per year
3.0 aide visits per member per year

To provide the visits, you will need additional nurses and aides. The number of nurses and aides depends on productivity levels. Suppose you expect the following number of visits per employee:

1,400 patient visits per RN per year
1,000 patient visits per aide per year

and suppose further that the annual salaries, including benefits, for nurses and aides are:

Annual compensation $50,000 per RN
Annual compensation $15,000 per aide

The direct labor cost for the visits can be calculated PMPM as follows:

RN Visits

Average cost per visit = $50,000/1,400 = $35.71 per visit
Per member per year = $35.71 × 1.2 visits per
                       year = $42.85
PMPM rate   = $42.85 ÷ 12 months
                    = $3.57 PMPM

Aide Visits

Average cost per visit = $15,000/1,000 = $15.00 per visit
Per member per year = $15.00 × 3 visits per year = $45.00
PMPM rate   = $45.00 ÷ 12 months
                    = $3.75 PMPM

---

[5]The data used in this example are hypothetical and do not reflect true utilization rates or costs for any home care agency.

Each visit requires some supplies. Assume that the supply cost per visit is $5. This can be converted to a supply cost per member per month as follows:

Supplies

$5 per visit × 4.2 visits = $21.00

$21 ÷ 12 visits per year = $1.75 PMPM

In addition, there will be support staff working for the agency. In some cases such staff may be fixed, while in other cases it may be variable. For example, the cost of the office manager will not vary with the number of visits. But other staff members are needed to schedule patient visits. The more patients, the more staff hours needed for such activities. Assume that the agency has found that it needs one-tenth FTE of a support staff member for each FTE nurse or aide and that support staff members earn $20,000 on average. Such support staff will be considered to vary with the number of nurses and aides and therefore with the number of members. Support staff that do not vary with the number of visits will be included in other overhead, as shown below.

Number of RNs per member = 3.0 visits/1,400 visits per RN = 0.00214
Number of aides per member = 1.2 visits/1,000 visits per aide = 0.0012
Total nurses and aides per member = 0.00214 + 0.0012 = 0.00334
Support staff = 0.00334 × 0.1 support staff per nurse or aide
= 0.000334 support staff personnel per member
Support staff cost = 0.000334 × $20,000 = $6.68 per member per year
Support staff cost PMPM = $6.68 ÷ 12 months = $0.56 PMPM

Note how cumbersome the calculation becomes because of the small fractions. Utilization rates are often stated by thousand members to avoid dealing with small fractions. If the support staff calculation had alternatively been done per thousand members, it would appear as follows:

Number of RNs per 1,000 members = 3.0 visits × 1,000 members ÷ 1,400 visits per RN
= 2.14 RNs per 1,000 members
Number of aides per 1,000 members = 1.2 visits × 1,000 members ÷ 1,000 visits per aide
= 1.2 aides per 1,000 members
Total nurses and aides = 2.14 + 1.2 = 3.34 nurses and aides per 1,000 members
Support staff = 3.34 × 0.1 support staff per nurse or aide
= 0.334 support staff personnel per 1,000 members
Support staff cost = 0.334 × $20,000 = $6,680 per 1,000 members per year
Support staff cost PMPM = $6,680 ÷ 1,000 members ÷ 12 months = $0.56 PMPM

Notice that whether the calculation is performed on a per member basis or per

1,000-member basis, the PMPM result is exactly the same. Assume that all other costs, such as fixed staff, rent, and electric work come out to $3 PMPM.

Based on the above information, a PMPM based on average costs can be calculated as follows:

	PMPM
RNs	$ 3.57
Aides	3.75
Supplies	1.75
Support staff	0.56
Other overhead	3.00
Average cost PMPM	$12.63

It was noted earlier that the manager should calculate rates based on charges, average cost, and marginal cost. We have just calculated the average cost as being $12.63. Earlier it was noted that the charges for the agency are $60 for an RN visit and $40 for an aide visit. This can be converted to a PMPM as follows:

1.2 RN visits per member × $60 per visit ÷ 12 months = $ 6.00 PMPM
3.0 aide visits per member × $40 per visit ÷ 12 months = $10.00 PMPM

Total charge for RN and aide visits = $16.00 PMPM

The marginal cost of the visits can also be determined. The RNs, aides, supplies, and support staff will all increase if the contract is signed. The other overhead is fixed and will be incurred in any event. Therefore, the marginal cost of providing the additional visits is $9.63 per member per month (i.e., $12.63 average cost − $3.00 other overhead). We can now compare the three measures:

	Charge	Average Cost	Marginal Cost
Per member per month	$16.00	$12.63	$9.63

This comparison provides the manager with critical information needed to enter PMPM capitation rate negotiations. The goal is to negotiate a revenue as close to the $16 PMPM charge as possible but in no case to lower than the $9.63 marginal cost. Once the rate has been agreed on, the revenue from the agreement is simply the capitation rate multiplied by the number of members covered by the agreement.

Incentive Risk Pools

Managed care contracts often also include incentive arrangements to minimize overall costs. For example, suppose that all providers are capitated, except for hospitals. Assume that hospitals are paid on a discounted fee-for-service basis by the MCO. How can the MCO encourage providers to avoid unnecessary patient hospitalizations? A common arrangement is the use of inpatient services *risk pools*. Risk pools consist of some money that has been withheld from each provider. The withheld amount is eventually paid to the provider if utilization achieves certain targets.

For example, suppose that the home care agency discussed above negotiates a $13 PMPM capitation rate from a managed care provider for 2,000 members. The agency is entitled to revenue of $26,000 per month ($13 PMPM × 2,000 members). However, the MCO is concerned about the incentives created by capitation. It worries that the agency might try to save money by not providing all the visits needed, since the agency receives the same $13 PMPM regardless of the number of visits provided.

Failure to provide visits when needed might result in a patient being rehospitalized. This is a poor outcome for the patient and costly for the MCO. To avoid this the MCO might withhold 10% of the capitated payments until a year-end reconciliation is performed. That amount is combined with money withheld from other providers to create a risk pool. The agency would only receive $23,400 each month ($26,000 × 90%). At the end of the year, the agency would get back some or all of this amount, based on actual hospital utilization versus an expected level of hospital utilization. If hospital utilization is unexpectedly high, the risk pool is used to pay the hospital and there may be nothing left in the pool to pay the agency. The agency can lose the entire 10% that had been withheld. But if hospital costs are very high, the MCO will be liable for any costs that the risk pool cannot cover. So both the providers and the MCO are at risk to lose some money if utilization is higher than expected. This is referred to as *risk-sharing.*

It should also be noted that in some cases withhold arrangements may lead to poorer care. For example, to keep hospital utilization low, physicians or nurse practitioners might fail to admit patients who actually need hospital care. Some would argue that MCOs are not really worried about quality of care at all. From that perspective risk pools are established solely to save money for the MCO by discouraging patient admissions and other costly forms of care. Nurse managers involved in managed care negotiations must always consider the implications of the contract for the quality of care to be provided to their patients.

SUMMARY AND IMPLICATIONS
FOR NURSE MANAGERS

Revenues are the amount the organization earns in exchange for the services it provides. Revenues are critical for every organization. Revenues must be adequate to cover all costs of providing services during the current year. Additionally, revenues should be great enough to provide a profit. Profits are used to expand the type and volume of services offered and to replace capital equipment.

In some situations nurses are not given revenue responsibility because their actions cannot affect the revenues of the organization. This would be the case in a situation in which all patients pay a fixed fee regardless of services received. More commonly, however, nurses have not been given revenue responsibility because historically it was difficult to assess the amount of nursing resources consumed by different patients. Computer technology is removing this barrier, and it is becoming more feasible to charge different patients for the differing amounts of nursing services they receive. Nurse managers should continue to push for revenue responsibility.

The basic elements of a revenue budget are simple—price and volume. The revenue budget essentially consists of the price charged for each service provided by the unit, department, or organization multiplied by the number of units of service provided. The complications involved in a revenue budget are estimating the volume of services to be provided, deciding on the prices to charge, and estimating how much of the total amount charged will actually be collected. Nurse managers who are responsible for the revenue of their unit, department, or organization should be actively involved in estimating or at least understanding these factors.

The last decade of the twentieth century saw tremendous growth in the area of *managed care*. A MCO is any organization that tries to control the use of health care services to provide cost-effective care. In some cases MCOs pay in much the same way as other payers, often negotiating a discount from standard fees or charges. In some cases, however, MCOs pay providers based on capitation.

Capitation refers to paying a set amount for each covered member, regardless of the amount of care consumed. From the viewpoint of the MCO, capitation is beneficial because there is no incentive for providers to overserve patients. From the perspective of the provider, capitation provides a predictable revenue stream. Nurse managers need to understand their costs in order to negotiate effective capitation rates. They should also attempt to negotiate advance monthly payments, if their organization frequently has trouble meeting its monthly expenses that must be paid in cash.

Nurse managers should always be cautious when working on capitated arrangements. In such arrangements the MCO shifts risk to the provider. If for whatever reason patients consume more resources than expected, it is the provider who will lose money as a result. Many providers buy insurance to protect themselves from severe losses resulting from unexpectedly high patient utilization rates.

The capitation payment, called the PMPM rate, must cover all costs and profits for the organization related to the covered members. The starting point in determining a capitation rate is identification of the exact services that are to be covered by the contract. Next, the provider must obtain estimates of the utilization of each service covered. Utilization rates are generally stated per thousand members. Utilization rates must be adjusted for actual population demographics. Costs must be converted to PMPM equivalents. It is helpful to use the marginal cost for the covered services as the lower limit and fee-for-service charges as the upper limit for rate negotiations.

Once the PMPM has been determined, it can be multiplied by the number of covered members to determine the organization's revenue from the MCO. The key to increasing revenue in a capitated environment is to get more covered members. Special care should also be paid in negotiating risk pools. Risk pools represent portions of the PMPM rate that are held back and may not be paid if utilization rates or costs for specific types of care exceed a set amount.

SUGGESTED READINGS

Boland, P, editor. (1996). *The Capitation Sourcebook*. Berkeley: Boland Healthcare.

Cleverley, W.O. (1997). *Essentials of Health Care Finance*, Fourth edition. Gaithersburg, MD: Aspen Publishers.

Gapenski, L.C. (1999). *Healthcare Finance: An Introduction to Accounting and Financial Management*. Chicago: Health Administration Press.

Merisalo, L.J. (1999, September). Seek specifics to avoid pitfalls of contracting nuances and vagaries. *The Managed Care Payment Advisor*. 3(3), 1–5, 11.

Spitzer-Lehmann, R., editor. (1994). *Nursing Management Desk Reference: Concepts, Skills & Strategies*. Philadelphia: W.B. Saunders.

Swansburg, R.C. (1997). *Budgeting and Financial Management for Nurse Managers*. Boston: Jones & Bartlett Publishers.

Ward, W.J., Jr. (1994). *Health Care Budgeting and Financial Management for Non-Financial Managers: A New England Healthcare Assembly Book*. Westport, CN: Auburn House Publishers.

Zelman, W.N., McCue, M.J., and Milikan, A.R. (1998). *Financial Management of Health Care Organizations: An Introduction to Fundamental Tools, Concepts, and Applications*. Malden, MA: Blackwell Publisher.

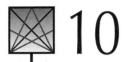

10

Capital Budgeting

The goals of this chapter are to:

define capital budgeting;

explain why there is a separate accounting process for capital budgets;

discuss the generation of capital budget proposals;

introduce the concept of the time value of money;

explain the concept of relevant costs for capital budgeting;

recognize the role of politics in capital budgeting decisions;

generate an understanding of the benefits of formal decision models for capital project evaluation; and

explore the factors involved in evaluating capital budget items.

DEFINITION OF CAPITAL BUDGETING

Capital budgeting is the name commonly used for planning the acquisition of long-term investments. These investments can range from investments as small as the acquisition of a new IV pole to projects as large as the complete rebuilding of a hospital at a new location.

The key element in capital budgeting is that the building or piece of equipment being acquired has a lifetime that extends beyond the year of purchase. Anything that the organization builds or buys and starts to use in one year that will still be useful in future years is considered to be a capital item. Capital budget items are treated separately from the regular operating budget process. Each year, each unit or department lists all items with a multiyear life separately from operating budget expenses. These capital items go through a separate review and approval process. If approved, these capital acquisitions are accounted for separately from regular operating budget expenses.

Once the organization has completed its program budgeting process (see Chapter 7), any program changes such as the addition of a new service should be communicated to all departments that will be affected by that program change. This will allow the departments to consider the implications of the program change on both their capital and operating costs. If the program change requires a department to provide services that require multiyear investments, those proposed acquisitions would become part of the department's capital budget. The capital budget will also contain any other requests for purchases of multiyear items for the continued support of existing services.

Capital budget items are often referred to as *capital assets*. They are also referred to as *long-term investments, capital investments, capital acquisitions,* and *capital items.* In all cases, the "capital" is used to signify the fact that the item's life extends beyond the year of purchase. Capital budget items generally are purchased to replace older items of a similar nature, to improve productivity (substituting equipment for more expensive labor), to improve quality of care (often addition of newer technology), or to provide needed equipment for a new service or expand an existing service. A variety of other reasons to acquire capital assets will also arise from time to time, such as for equipment that will improve employee safety.

WHY HAVE CAPITAL BUDGETS?

Long-term investments are worthy of special attention for several reasons. First, capital items receive particular scrutiny because they often are significant in amount. Unlike day-to-day supplies that have relatively minor costs, capital investments frequently involve significant amounts of cash, all tied up in a single investment decision.

For example, heparin locks appear in the operating budget, and ICU monitors are part of the capital budget. Suppose that the nursing department purchases 50 heparin locks from a new supplier and is completely dissatisfied with their quality. Even if it has to throw the locks away, the loss is limited. On the other hand, if 10 new monitors are purchased for the ICU, at a price of $80,000 per monitor, there is an $800,000 investment. If it turns out that the monitors do not provide the information required and have to be replaced immediately, the financial loss is obviously much greater. The more expensive the acquisition, the more closely the proposed purchase needs to be examined.

Not only is it necessary to assess the immediate capabilities of capital acquisitions because of their large dollar cost, but it must also be recognized that their multiyear lives mean that the organization is committing to these items for a long time. For example, disposable gloves are part of the operating budget. Renovating space is part of the capital budget. If one brand of disposable gloves starts to decline in quality over time, the organization can shift to a different supplier. If the nurses' stations throughout a nursing home are totally renovated and it is then determined that there are quite a few inconvenient features about the new stations, the units will likely have to live with those inconveniences for 10 years or longer. The longer the commitment represented by an acquisition, the more carefully the decision to buy it must be scrutinized.

As a consequence of the high cost and long-time commitment to many capital budget items, it is important to examine alternatives when developing capital budget proposals. Just as with Zero-Base Budgeting for a complete program, reviewing alternatives is critical when evaluating capital assets. What would happen if an old piece of equipment is not replaced? Will it break down? If it does, what effect will that have on patient care? What if it is replaced with a cheaper model or one with less capacity? What benefits would there be if it is replaced with a model with more capacity? Reviewing a variety of alternatives will help to insure that resources are not spent unnecessarily and that the unit or department does not regret its decision after a year or two.

In considering why the capital budget is distinct from the operating budget, however, the high cost and lengthy time commitment required by capital acquisitions are not in themselves sufficient reasons to justify the completely separate and duplicative budgeting process that capital budgeting represents. Alternative approaches could still be satisfactorily reviewed. If high cost and long-time commitment were the only issues, a manager would be justified in arguing that these items should be included in the operating budget but reviewed carefully. After all, nursing personnel are included in the operating budget and they represent millions upon millions of dollars of cost each year. Why create the whole separate process of capital budgeting?

The third and critical reason that a separate capital budgeting process exists relates to the multiyear nature of capital assets. They are only partly used up in any one year, and in any one year the organization earns only part of the revenues that the capital assets generate over their useful lifetimes.

The expenses included in an operating budget for a specific year represent the cost of the services the organization provides in that year. Operating budget revenues for any year are the amounts of money that the organization is entitled to receive in return for providing services in that year. In the case of capital assets, the amount spent to acquire the asset exceeds the amount used up in one year, since the asset lasts more than 1 year. Some of the capital asset remains available to provide services in the future. And the revenues that are received as a result of the investment will be earned over a number of years.

If capital items are included in the annual operating budget, substantial confusion will arise. The purpose of the operating budget is to compare the revenues and expenses for one year. Including the acquisition cost of multiyear assets in the operating expense budget would make the costs of providing services appear to be misleadingly high. It would cause the budget to convey a distorted picture of the organization's financial viability. By mixing expenses that are just costs of a single year with the acquisition cost of capital items, the receipts in the first year will often not cover the cash outlay, and therefore, few capital projects might seem affordable. Investments must be viewed over their entire lifetime to make fully informed decisions. A way is needed to show the carryover benefit of long-term investments into subsequent years. Capital budgets provide the means to accomplish this.

In the capital budgeting process, a plan is made for acquiring capital assets. All, some, or none of the items requested by a department in its capital budget proposal will be approved and subsequently acquired. For those items that are approved, a depreciation schedule will be developed. Depreciation is a means to allocate a share of the capital item's cost over a period of years. Suppose that the organization buys an $80,000 monitor and that it is anticipated that the monitor will be used for 10 years before being replaced. The organization will allocate a part of the $80,000 cost into the each of the 10 years of the monitor's useful life by *depreciating* it at a rate of $8,000 per year for 10 years. The $80,000 cost of the capital item will be included in the capital budget once. Each year, $8,000 will be included in the operating budget as an expense. This reflects the fact that one tenth of the capital item is being used up each year to provide that year's services. Each year an appropriate share of the cost of the monitor becomes a part of the operating expense budget. Thus the capital budget is linked to the operating budget through the annual depreciation charges for the capital items that have been acquired.

HOW MUCH DO CAPITAL ASSETS COST?

Capital assets are often quite expensive, as was discussed earlier. However, high cost is not a required element for an asset to be a capital asset. The only requirement is that the capital asset must be able to provide useful service beyond the year it is first put into use.

If a nursing unit acquires a ball-point pen for $.89 and starts to use that pen 1 week before the end of the fiscal year, the pen is technically a capital asset if it is still functioning during the first week of the next fiscal year. From a theoretical point of view the pen clearly meets the multiyear definition of a capital asset.

However, in order to keep accounting records accurate, the cost of capital assets must be depreciated, and a depreciation charge must be assigned to the operating budget for each year during the useful life of the asset. It does not seem practical to have a staff of accountants keeping track of each ball-point pen purchased. The accounting cost would exceed any benefit gained.

As a result, most organizations set a minimum dollar limit on capital assets. Items that have a low cost will be treated as part of the operating budget even if they have a multiyear life. For instance, most health care organizations have a minimum cost requirement of anywhere from $300 to $2,500 in order for an item to be included in the capital budget. Anything below the cutoff is treated as a routine operating expense.

In fact, cutoffs of $500 or $1,000, commonly seen in many hospitals, are far below the $3,000, $5,000, or $10,000 cutoffs that are observed in many other industries. Why do hospitals maintain fairly low dollar cutoffs for which items will be treated as capital assets and which items will not? The answer has to do at least partly with government reimbursement. The Medicare system historically paid a flat DRG payment for each Medicare patient discharged. Thus, if a hospital provides a patient with extra lab tests or more hours of direct nursing care, there is no additional payment for those extra resources provided.

However, that flat payment was for operating costs. Medicare made an additional payment to hospitals to cover a portion of their capital costs. Suppose that a hospital has a $1,000 cutoff for capital assets. A $750 refrigerator for a nurses' station will be treated as an operating cost. No additional Medicare payment would be received to pay for the refrigerator. If the same hospital had maintained a $500 cutoff for capital items, the refrigerator would be over that threshold. It would be considered a capital asset. In this case, in addition to the DRG operating payment, Medicare paid the hospital an additional amount to cover a portion of the $750 cost of the refrigerator. This is referred to as a cost pass-through. Thus, hospitals had a definite financial incentive to keep their capital asset cutoff as low as possible. The result is that more of their acquisitions were categorized as being capital costs, and they received more total Medicare reimbursement for the same group of patients than would otherwise be the case. However, Medicare has been phasing out reimbursement based on the cost of capital equipment. Therefore it would not be surprising to see hospitals raise their capital cutoff levels in the early years of this decade.

GENERATING CAPITAL BUDGET PROPOSALS

The starting point in the capital budgeting process is generating proposed investments. In the case of nursing, such proposals may occur either directly or indirectly. The manager of a nursing unit may desire some remodeling of the unit. The nurse manager in a home health agency may propose acquiring several company cars to reduce travel time between patients (assuming public transportation is currently being used). The nurse manager in the coronary care unit or the operating room of a hospital may suggest acquiring a particular piece of equipment. These are examples of direct capital budgeting proposals. It will be up to the nurse manager, with the assistance of financial managers, to prepare the capital budget.

Many indirect proposals will also affect nurse managers. For example, the pharmacy may suggest adding a new piece of equipment that will automate the reconstitution of a particular drug. Not only will there be a saving in the pharmacy in terms of reduced technician time required in preparing the drug for reconstitution, but there will also be a savings in nursing time, if the nurses currently do the actual reconstitution of the drug on the floor. In such cases, the pharmacy will be performing the majority of the analysis, but the nurse manager will be called upon to help determine the potential impact upon the nursing budget.

Figure 10–1 presents an example of the type of worksheet a nurse manager would use to list capital proposals. (See the Appendix at the end of this book for an example of the specific instructions that a nurse manager might receive with a form of this type.) The first column represents the manager's priority ranking for

CAPITAL BUDGET WORKSHEET

FY_____

COST CENTER_____

PRIOR. #	TYPE CR/RE/RU AS/AN	EQUIP. QTY	DESCRIPTION	UNIT COST	EXTENDED COST	COMMENTS

FIGURE 10–1. Capital budget worksheet.

the request. The most important acquisition would be ranked number 1. The second column indicates the type of capital item being requested. These include construction or remodeling (CR), replacing an existing item (RE), replacing and upgrading an existing item (RU), an item that is an addition to similar existing items and adds to their capacity (AS), or an additional item that is not currently available in the unit (AN).

Developing the list of proposals is the first step in the capital budgeting process. There are a variety of issues that will typically lead to proposals for capital budgeting. Some capital projects are obvious. When the roof starts to leak, it had better be repaired. Hopefully, however, perhaps the roof can be prevented from leaking. The long-range plan of the organization should require that capital expenditures be made on a systematic basis. Reroofing is one example. Replacing all the hospital beds is another. The maintenance department of the hospital will often be the cost center that has to deal with such routine, although infrequent, capital expenditures. In many hospitals, bed replacement is a nursing department responsibility. Such replacement should not be done in a haphazard way.

The nursing department should take the approach of systemizing capital expenditures. For example, suppose that each nursing station has a refrigerator. The refrigerators can be added to the capital budget proposal (Fig. 10–1) when they break down. That is an unfortunate approach because it will either result in a nursing station being without a working refrigerator for a number of months or an unexpected and unbudgeted expenditure for a new refrigerator. An alternative to this would be a formalized approach to generating capital budget proposals.

Basically, such a formalized approach requires managers to maintain a list of all capital items for which they are responsible. If a nurse manager is responsible for 15 refrigerators, among other capital items, then a plan should be established. The plan may be to replace all 15 refrigerators every fifteenth year. If one assumes that most refrigerators will last between 14 and 18 years, this may be a reasonable approach. One problem with this approach is that it places the entire cash outflow in a single year. An alternative would be a staggered system, in which one refrigerator is replaced every year. The cash flow to buy refrigerators will remain pretty much the same each year, and equipment will not be getting very old because the organization is constantly replacing the older items. On the other hand, the organization will not get volume discount if it buys just one refrigerator each year.

Whichever approach is taken, listing all capital items will draw attention to the replacement of many routine items before they wear out and break down. To generate all appropriate capital proposals, managers should go beyond simply listing the items and showing their projected replacement date. Managers should think about and encourage all nurses in their department to consider the following: Is the cost of care too high? Is there something we could do to reduce the cost of care? Is the quality of care acceptable? What could be done to improve the quality of care? Is the capacity adequate?

Many of the suggestions that result from those questions impact on both the operating budget and the capital budget. There is a tendency for individuals to complain that things are not done the way they should be. Having a mechanism for suggestions can result in benefits in several ways. First, it lets individuals get the complaints off their chests, which makes them feel better. Second, if changes are instituted, the nurses will be happier because they will not have to put up with whatever they were complaining about. Third, they will tend to be more motivated in their work if they are in a responsive environment. Finally, the suggestions will help the organization run more efficiently and provide higher-quality cost-effective care.

A number of proposals will be generated through this overall process. For nonfinancial managers, the difficult issues of capital budgeting rarely concern the generation of capital investment proposals. Such proposals will be generated. The key issue is whether or not the proposals merit the investment. It is the evaluation of the proposals that poses the most difficult problems.

EVALUATION OF CAPITAL BUDGET PROPOSALS

The evaluation of capital budget proposals is often carried out by financial managers. However, it is useful for nurse managers to understand the elements of the evaluation process. Such an understanding will provide the nurse manager with additional insight about the capital budget process. This in turn will help nurse managers prepare capital budget proposals, including a strong supporting justification for the expenditure.

Data Generation

The first step in the evaluation process is to collect data about the project. Specifically, information must be collected about how much cash will be spent or received each year over the life of the investment or project. The difference between the cash received and the cash spent in any given year will be referred to as the *net cash flow* for that year.

The typical capital investment has a negative net cash flow in the first year or several years because more money is spent on the acquisition than is being received from its use. The cash flow often becomes positive in subsequent years.

The nurse manager can generally seek the aid of financial managers of the organization for the specific estimates of cash inflows and outflows. Cash inflows can be particularly difficult, since the entire billing process is normally handled outside of the control of the nurse manager. On the other hand, with respect to estimating costs, the nurse manager is more likely than any financial manager to be able to estimate what resources will be needed when. The payroll and purchasing departments will be a great aid in converting the raw resource information into dollars based on projected salaries and prices. This estimating process should be done separately for each year that the capital asset is expected to provide useful service.

It is not adequate simply to estimate the total amount to be spent and total receipts over the lifetime of the investment. This ignores something called the *time value of money.* When cash is received or spent is just as important as how much is received or spent. For example, suppose that the organization was considering two alternative investments in photocopy equipment for the Department of Nursing Services. Both projects will require a total cost of $10,000 for the machine, and both will have identical copying capabilities. It seems as if the two offers are identical.

Suppose, however, that the organization has to pay $10,000 for one machine at the time of purchase, but the other offer is an installment purchase requiring five annual installments of $2,000 each. If the organization were to accept the first alternative, its expenditure would be $10,000, all in the first year. If the machine has a 5-year life expectancy, then the operating budget for each of the next 5 years would include a prorated depreciation cost of $2,000. If it goes with the second alternative, paying installments of $2,000 per year, the operating budget will again show a $2,000 cost for each of the next 5 years. Are the alternatives equal?

The answer is definitely and emphatically no! In the case of the first project, all $10,000 is paid at the start. In the second project, only $2,000 is paid immediately, allowing the organization to hold onto the other $8,000. This $8,000 can be invested in interest-bearing savings accounts. Each year when it's time for the next payment, the organization will be able to keep the interest earned. This interest can be spent on more capital assets or perhaps on nursing staff increases. Clearly, the organization is better off if it can hold onto most of the $10,000 and pay for the photocopy machine gradually over time. This is a carryover from the philosophy of program budgeting—capital budgets should examine alternatives and their trade-offs. It is not enough simply to evaluate whether the department can afford a photocopy machine. Capital budgeting should examine alternative machines and alternative payment plans, such as buying outright versus installment purchase. When payments occur is critical to the outcome of the analysis.

In estimating the cash flows, care must also be taken to include relevant and exclude irrelevant cash flows. For example if the organization is a proprietary (for-profit) concern, then it should consider the impact of any investment on income taxes. It may well be that two different investments, both providing the same health care services, will have totally different tax implications. In the above photocopy machine example, suppose that there was a third alternative to lease the machine for 5 years. There are a number of tax laws aimed specifically at the issue of leasing. It may well turn out that, depending on the organization's specific situation, there are significant tax benefits if the equipment is leased rather than purchased or vice versa. If the tax consequences of a capital investment are ignored, the manager might select the wrong alternative.

It is important to note that the relevant cash flows concerning a project are the *incremental* cash flows. Incremental refers to the amount that the organization's cash would change if the project is undertaken versus if it is not undertaken. The incremental flows are the change in the total amounts received and the change in the total amount spent because of the acquisition of the capital asset.

If the manager is trying to determine the cost of adding a new piece of equipment, it is necessary to include in the incremental costs the purchase cost of the equipment and of any additional supplies and labor needed. If the equipment uses a lot of electricity, then that cost should be included as well. Suppose, however, that if the equipment is acquired, administrative overhead will be assigned to that equipment through the cost allocation process. For example, a portion of the salary of the organization's chief executive officer might be allocated to the unit. This is an irrelevant cost in deciding whether to purchase the equipment. This cost will be incurred by the organization whether it buys the equipment or not. Even though the organization's accountants may assign some of that administrative cost to the unit using the equipment, the cost should not be included when determining whether or not the organization should acquire the equipment. The manager needs to be able to determine whether the added costs of having the new equipment can be covered by the added revenues. If the organization would incur the administrator's salary cost in any case, then it should not require the new equipment to bear a share of that cost as a prerequisite for approving the acquisition.

The other side of the coin is that all incremental costs should be considered. For instance, suppose that several nurses will be needed to care for patients treated by the equipment. Suppose further that the equipment is used only during the day and that the nurses using the equipment are paid regular daytime wages. Because of shortages of available nurses, however, assigning nurses to work with patients using this equipment results in an increase in overtime for nurses elsewhere in the hospital. Without the machine, the hospital would not have had to pay those overtime costs. In this case, even though the nurses directly working with the equipment are not collecting overtime, the additional overtime costs incurred by the hospital should be considered a part of the operating costs of the proposed investment in the machine.

Sometimes the incremental costs may be indirect. Consider the home health agency that wants to buy cars for several of their nurse employees so that time spent waiting for public transit can be spent on more visits to patients. Politically, the purchase of cars for some of the nurses may mean that an agency car will have to be acquired for at least the chief executive officer of the agency and perhaps several other top-level managers as well. If so, then the decision of whether or not to acquire cars for the nurses or home aides must include all the cars that otherwise would not have been purchased, even those that are not directly used to improve service to the patients.

Choosing Among Capital Assets

Sufficient resources are not usually available to allow an organization to acquire all the items it desires. The capital budget facilitates choices that have to be made in the allocation of the organization's resources. In describing proposed capital expenditures, the nurse manager provides a priority ranking (Fig. 10–1). It is also appropriate to justify each requested purchase by giving a description of the item, its cost, its impact on operating expenses and revenues, and the justification for acquiring it. See Figure 10–2 for an example of a justification form for a capital asset acquisition.

The justification should be thorough and should specifically indicate the consequences if funding for the item is not made available. Equipment costs include not only purchase price but also shipping and installation costs. Construction costs should be reviewed by the planning and engineering departments. In all cases, vendor estimates or proposals should be included if possible. The impact on operating costs should include salaries, fringe benefit costs, maintenance costs or maintenance contracts, utilities, supplies, and any interdepartmental impacts. Incremental revenue to be generated by the capital asset, if any, should be described and estimated to the greatest extent possible.

The capital budgets for all departments are evaluated in light of available cash. An investment that seems to make a lot of sense to a clinical department manager may have to be deferred for one year, or indefinitely, simply because the organization does not have enough cash to make the purchase. Cash budgeting is discussed in Chapter 12.

In choosing among alternative capital proposals or even in evaluating just one proposed item, managers need to determine whether the amount of money to be spent is justified by the anticipated economic return. Decision making can be substantially improved by having a system for evaluating capital acquisitions that considers the economic ramifications of the decision. Rational decision making calls for formalized, systematic, quantifiable evaluation. Such evaluation must consider not only the financial impact of decisions but also the clinical impact. The overall goals of providing medical services call for providing high-quality care; this must be a critical element of the manager's thinking. Unfortunately, quality of health care is not easily measured.

The dilemma of achieving high quality at low cost is not one that can easily be solved. Neither economists and accountants nor health care providers have found a way to reconcile completely the costs of investments with both the dollar revenues the investments generate and the improved quality benefits. Certainly, if an investment will improve quality and generate adequate revenues to cover its cost, there is no problem. Difficulty arises if the costs of an investment exceed the potential dollar revenues, but there are quality-of-care issues that make the investment desirable. Does the organization go ahead with the investment or not?

There is no easy answer to this question. One thing became clear in the 1980s. The tremendous growth of the health care sector put serious strains on the national economy. As a result, throughout the 1990s, more and more pressure was put on the health care sector to slow its cost increases. This pressure continues today. Therefore, it is likely that there are going to be severe limits on total revenues available to health care organizations. Health care organizations will not

CAPITAL JUSTIFICATION FORM

FY_____.

COST CENTER_____   PRIORITY ITEM #_____

Description of item or project:

Justification:

Construction Costs:

Fees   _____

Construction   _____

Contingency   _____

  Total   _____

Date of Estimate_____

Equipment Costs:

Purchase Price   _____

Installation   _____

By_____

Impact on Operational Expenses:

Impact on Revenues:

FIGURE 10–2. Capital justification form.

be able to afford to make investment decisions based solely on the informal knowledge that the investment will improve quality. That approach, which has been a common one in the health sector, will start to threaten the survival of many health care institutions. The increasing prominence of managed care will exacerbate this situation.

At the other extreme, it must be recognized that traditionally politics has had a great deal to do with acquiring capital assets. Often, the decisions have not been made on the basis of economic analysis, financial return on money invested, or even on the impact on quality care. Decisions have been made on the basis of political clout. However, under financial pressure from managed care organizations, it has become clear that politics, while a reality, must be tempered with economic logic.

As a result, health care organizations are more and more frequently starting to use formal mechanics of project evaluation that parallel the capital budgeting methodology used in the vast majority of *proprietary* industries. These formal methods provide the economic basis for capital budgeting decisions. These methods are described in the Appendix at the end of this chapter.

This use of formalized, quantitative approaches to capital investment evaluation should not and does not rule out decisions that ultimately defy the economic results. The formal modeling of capital budgeting is mechanical. The methods described in the Appendix to this chapter are sophisticated mathematical approaches capable of providing precise predictions about the economic viability of an investment. Finance officers will use these methods by applying them to the capital budget proposals that nurse managers develop and the data for the evaluation that nurse managers generate. However, as with most mathematical models, these methods are totally devoid of judgment and incapable of addressing the human impact of a decision. They look at the dollars and cents.

You are responsible for contributing the common sense to the decision. Never accept a model's result as a dictate. Consider it only as advice. The formal approaches of capital budgeting can advise you regarding the strict economics of an investment. A manager must take all factors into account when making a final decision regarding the investment.

What the formal model can accomplish, however, is formal recognition of trade-offs. If the organization decides to make an investment even though the long-run prospect is a loss of money, that decision clarifies two issues. First, there is recognition that a loss will occur and that the organization is willing to bear that loss to gain some qualitative benefit for the organization or its patients. Second, there must be recognition that a profit will have to be earned elsewhere to offset that loss. Without the availability of a profit elsewhere, going ahead with a losing project may be suicidal to the continued existence of the organization.

Even long-term financial suicide may be deemed to be a better outcome than to provide inferior care. This is a decision that the management of the organization must make. By combining capital budgeting efforts by clinical managers with modeling by finance, one can determine the likely impacts of making the investment. It is then up to the clinical managers to work together with top management to arrive at decisions that are in the long-run best interests of the organization, its patients, and its employees.

SUMMARY AND IMPLICATIONS
FOR NURSE MANAGERS

Capital budgeting refers to planning for the acquisition of resources that are useful beyond the year in which they are purchased. Such capital items require special attention because they usually cannot generate enough revenue in the year they are acquired to appear to be financially feasible. Since they generate revenues over a period of years, their costs should be allocated over a similar period of years. This requires evaluation of the acquisition in a separate plan, called a capital budget. Each year's share of the total cost of a capital asset is allocated to the operating budget for that year in the form of a depreciation charge.

To determine whether or not the organization can afford the item or project, revenues and expenses must be compared over the lifetime of the asset. Operating budgets focus only on the portion of revenues and expenses that relate to 1 year. It is the role of capital budgeting to examine the long-term financial implications of resources with multiyear lives. Many capital items do not generate any revenue. The costs of these items should also be spread over their useful lifetime in order to understand the implications of the spending.

Capital budgets evaluate the impact of resources over long-time periods. Because of this, the money spent on the resources cannot be directly compared with the revenues received from using the resource. Dollars earned in the future are not worth as much as dollars spent today because of the time value of money. That is, the money spent on a capital asset could have been earning interest. The revenues received from the project should be great enough to cover that interest cost as well as to return the amount invested. Present value methods that allow comparing future amounts to present amounts are available and are discussed in the Appendix to this chapter.

The first step in capital budgeting is to generate proposals for capital acquisition(s). The next step is to collect cash flow information, detailing the amount and timing of cash receipts and cash payments. The final step is to evaluate the cash receipts and payments. While this should be done using the formalized approaches of analysis discussed in the Appendix, it is also critical to keep in mind that only clinical managers can have a full perspective on the actual benefits to be received from an investment. Often, these benefits are patient care related, rather than being profit-oriented. While it is vital that nurse managers consider the financial implications of their proposals, it is also vital for the health care manager to consider noneconomic issues, such as impact on quality of care.

It may be in the interest of organization to sacrifice some economic benefits for increased noneconomic benefits. Bear in mind that capital budgeting techniques are merely tools. You should always know the economic implications of your decisions, but you do not have to make your decisions based solely on economics.

In the cases where a proposal is found to fail on the grounds of economic merit, the nurse manager has two potential choices. One choice is to decide that the capital item is not important enough to fight for if it is not economically advantageous for the institution. The other choice is to decide that the purchase is in fact vital and worth fighting for. In that case, you should be prepared to offer a clear statement concerning the benefits to be gained from the investment, as well as why you feel the benefits are worth the cost.

SUGGESTED READINGS

Anderson, J.R., George, H.W., and Perrin, R.A. (1991, May). Capital equipment management planning and control. *Journal of Healthcare Materiel Management.* 9(4), 24, 26, 28.

Hogan, A.J. (1987, February). Capital expenditure planning: The value of information to hospitals. *Hospital & Health Services Administration.* 32(1), 21–37.

Cleverley, W.O. (1997). *Essentials of Health Care Finance,* Fourth edition. Gaithersburg, MD: Aspen Publishers.

Gapenski, L.C. (1997). *Financial Analysis and Decision Making for Healthcare Organizations: A Guide for the Healthcare Professional.* Chicago: Irwin Professional Publishers.

Magiera, F.T., and McLean, R.A. (1996, Fall). Strategic options in capital budgeting and program selection under fee-for-service and managed care. *Health Care Management Review.* 21(4), 7–17.

McLean, R.A. (1996). *Financial Management in Health Care Organizations.* Albany: Delmar.

Neumann, B.R., Clement, J.P., and Cooper, J.C. (1997). *Financial Management: Concepts and Applications for Health Care Organizations.* Dubuque, Iowa: Kendall Hunt Publishing.

Newbould, G.D., and Carroll, J.J. (1986, December). Inflation, risk, replacement, closure: Concerns in capital budgeting. *Healthcare Financial Management.* 40(12), 64–68.

Pelfrey, S. (1991, March). Financial techniques for evaluating equipment acquisitions. *Journal of Nursing Administration.* 21(3), 15–20.

TerHark, D., and Diaz, J. (1990, April). A spreadsheet for capital equipment financial modeling. *Medical Laboratory Observer.* 22(4), 71–73.

Ward, W.J., Jr. (1994). *Health Care Budgeting and Financial Management for Non-Financial Managers: A New England Healthcare Assembly Book.* Westport, CN: Auburn House Publishers.

Zelman, W.N., McCue, M.J., and Milikan, A.R. (1998). *Financial Management of Health Care Organizations: An Introduction to Fundamental Tools, Concepts, and Applications.* Malden, MA: Blackwell Publisher.

Quantitative Methods for Capital Budgeting

The goals of this technical appendix are to:

provide specific techniques for evaluating capital budget proposals;

explain time value of money in detail;

describe discounted cash flow analysis;

discuss time value of money calculation mechanics; and

discuss the role of profits for not-for-profit health care organizations.

Several different models for capital budgeting will be discussed in this Appendix. These are the payback approach, the present cost approach, the net present value approach, and the internal rate of return approach. Capital budgeting often takes the perspective that current expenditures are offset by future cash receipts. The heart of the analysis is whether the future cash receipts are great enough to justify the current outlays financially. This Appendix will also recognize that in health care many capital acquisitions cannot be directly matched against future revenues. Therefore, a part of the following discussion will revolve around outlays for alternative capital items aimed at accomplishing a particular goal. Methods will be presented for determining the least costly approach.

THE PAYBACK APPROACH

Once all the appropriate cash receipts and cash expenditures have been estimated, the payback approach can be used as a quick-and-dirty estimate of whether the project is feasible financially. The payback approach evaluates how long it will be before the organization receives an amount of cash receipts from the investment that equals the amount of cash put into the investment.

As short a payback period as possible is preferred. For example, if the organization invests $1,000 today and gets cash receipts of $300 in the first year, $700 in the second year, and $500 in the third year, the payback period would be two years. On the other hand, if the cash receipts were $200, $400, and $900 for the three years respectively, the payback period would be three years. Although the total amount received is $1,500 in both cases, the organization has recovered its $1,000 investment during the second year in the first case but not until the third year in the second case.

There is some intuitive appeal to this approach. The longer the organization has to wait before it recovers the amount it has invested, the more risky the investment. If the organization has to wait many years until it breaks even on an investment, there is the risk that something may happen that was not anticipated. Although some investments are not very risky (e.g., a refrigerator for the nurses' station), technological obsolescence is a common problem in health care that creates significant risk. On any medical equipment, there is the risk that it will have to be replaced before it wears out.

This problem is an especially difficult one because it is often not possible to predict technological change accurately. If the organization knows that a piece of medical equipment could last for 10 years but will be obsolete in five years, then it can just anticipate that it will have a five-year life. But if it anticipates a five-year life and the equipment becomes obsolete in three years, there will be a problem. Therefore, investments that quickly pay back the initial invested amount are relatively safer.

The payback method does have some severe weaknesses, however. The problems with the payback method are that it ignores what happens after the payback period is over and it ignores the time value of money. Suppose that one machine would last for 10 years while another machine would last for only five years. Suppose further that the price for the latter machine is slightly lower. It may well be that the second machine will have a shorter payback period because of its lower price. The first machine, however, will continue to be useful for an extra five years. The payback approach is so concerned with risks over time that it pays relatively little attention to the future and ignores events after the payback period.

Further, the timing of payments within the payback period is not of particular concern under this method. Suppose that the organization spends $1,000 to acquire a piece of equipment, and under one alternative it receives $100 in the first year, $100 in the second year, and $800 in the third year. Under another alternative it still spends $1,000 to acquire the equipment, but it receives $800 in the first year, $100 in the second year, and $100 in the third year. According to the payback method, these two alternatives are equal.

In fact, they are not equal. By receiving $800 in the first year, the second alternative is superior. In the first year, the second alternative returns $700 more than is provided under the first alternative. That $700 can be put in the bank to earn interest in the two intervening years.

Suppose further that the first alternative made payments of $100, $100, and $800 for the three years as described. Now suppose the second alternative made payments of $800, $100, $99, and $1 over a four-year period. The first alternative would be deemed to be superior because it has a shorter payback period, three years as opposed to four years. Yet considering the interest earned on the $800 received in the first year under the second alternative, the organization is better off under the second than under the first method, even though the payback is longer.

These problems are serious. As a result, the payback method is often used for a first appraisal—a quick-and-dirty evaluation of the project. If a proposed investment cannot pay back its cost within a reasonable period—certainly not longer than the useful life of the investment—then on strictly economic grounds, it should be rejected (although it may be accepted anyway because of qualitative merits). If an investment passes the payback test, more sophisticated evaluation is still needed to determine if a specific proposal is acceptable or to help select from among alternatives.

THE TIME VALUE OF MONEY

The three remaining approaches for evaluating capital budgeting proposals require formal acknowledgment of the implications of the time value of money. Money paid or received at different points in time is not equally valuable. One would always prefer to receive money sooner and pay it later. By receiving money sooner, one can use the money for current needs or can invest it. If the money is used for current needs, then less money will need to be borrowed from the bank and the organization can avoid interest payments. If the organization already has enough money so that it does not have to borrow from banks, then it can invest the money in an interest-bearing account. Either way, by paying money later or receiving it sooner the organization is financially better off. It can either earn interest or avoid having to borrow money and pay interest.

In its simplest form, there does not appear to be much of a problem with the time value of money. If the organization receives a $100 payment from a patient today, it is better off than if it does not receive that payment for a year. At the very least, it could put the money in a bank account earning 5% interest. At the end of the year it would have $105 rather than $100.

Therefore, when a nurse manager looks at alternative investment opportunities, there must be consideration of not only how much the organization will put in and how much it will get out but also of when the money will be spent and received. For example, if a nursing unit invests $100 in a new machine and receives $155 over its five-year lifetime, is it financially better or worse off than if it had put the money into a five-year bank account with 10% interest?

That happens to be a complex question, much more so than may appear on the surface. The money invested in the bank earns 10% interest, and 10% of $100 is $10. For five years, one may think that the organization would earn five times $10, or a total of $50 in interest. In that case it would have $150 from the bank versus $155 if it bought the machine. But that is not correct. The money in the bank will earn 10% *compound* interest. Most banks compound interest at least once a year and often more frequently than that. Compounding means that the amount of interest that is earned during each compounding period is calculated and added to the initial amount. In the subsequent periods, interest is earned not only on the initial investment but also on any interest previously earned.

In this example, assuming compounding once a year, $10 in interest on the $100 invested in the bank account would be earned by the end of the first year. At that point there will be $110 in the bank—the original investment plus the interest earned. During the second year interest earned will be 10% of $110, or $11. During the third year, interest earned will be 10% of $121 (the $110 from the beginning of the second year plus the $11 interest earned in the second year). By the end of five years, the bank account will have $161. In this case, it appears that from a strictly financial view keeping the money in the bank is better than buying the machine after all.

However, this is not necessarily true. As was noted earlier, this is a complex problem. If the $155 from the use of the machine is received at the end of the fifth year, the bank investment is better, but if that $155 is received during the five years, some of it will be available to be invested in another project or in a bank and thus earn additional receipts. The timing of cash receipts is crucial. As you can imagine, this makes for some complex calculations. The next section discusses these calculations.

DISCOUNTED CASH FLOW APPROACHES

The more sophisticated approaches to capital budgeting take into account the time value of money. Such methods are referred to as discounted cash flow models. *Discounting* is the reverse of compounding of interest. One hundred dollars today would be worth $161 in five years with 10% compound interest, as noted earlier. In just the reverse process, $161 received five years from now would be worth just $100 today if one were to discount the interest earned in the five intervening years. Discounted cash flow techniques are designed to take future cash flows and discount the interest to find out what those flows would be worth today. The cash inflows and outflows can then be compared to cash outlays today to determine if a project is worthwhile financially.

The two most common discounted cash flow models are *net present value* and *internal rate of return*. Before these specific models can be discussed, it is necessary to delve more deeply into the mechanics of calculating the time value of money.

Suppose that two investments are being considered. One investment requires an outlay of $10,000 today; the other requires an outlay of only $7,500. Over the life of the investment, the operating costs will be $3,000 per year for five years for the first alternative but $3,600 per year for the second alternative over the same five years. This might be the situation for the purchase of several air conditioners. Which alternative is less expensive?

Note that there is no revenue in this example. Often in health care the focus is on cost-efficient ways to accomplish an objective. In this case, different types of air conditioners are being compared. Over the five-year life of the air conditioners, the organization will have spent $10,000 plus $3,000 per year for five years, or a total of $25,000 for the first alternative. The second type of air conditioner is less expensive to buy but is not as fuel efficient. It will cost $7,500 plus $3,600 per year for five years, or a total of $25,500. Which alternative is cheaper? The first project requires the organization to spend $500 less over its lifetime. But it does require it to spend $2,500 more at the beginning. That $2,500 could have been earning interest, thus offsetting some of the extra operating costs.

A way is needed to compare dollars spent at different times. Then one would be able to consider not just how much cash is involved but also when it is received or spent. Rather than solve the problem of the air conditioners now, put it aside for the time being. Let us focus attention on the methodology for dealing with cash flows at different times. Then it will be possible to return to the problem of the air conditioner investment later in this Appendix.

Time Value of Money Calculation Mechanics

The key to capital budgeting calculations is to be able to evaluate cash coming and going at different times. The amount of money spent or received today is referred to as the present value (PV). The interest rate is referred to as i%. The number of interest compounding periods is referred to as N. The compounding process is straightforward. Multiply the interest rate (i%) times the initial investment (PV) to find the interest in the first year. Add that interest to the initial investment. Then multiply the interest rate times the initial amount invested plus all interest already accumulated to find the amount of interest for the second year. If the investment were expected to last for 40 years, this simple process would become tedious.

To make matters worse, cash flows (both in and out) often take place monthly. Therefore, for a greater degree of accuracy regarding how much cash is available for use at any time, use i% as a monthly interest rate, N as the number of months, and do compounding on a monthly basis. For a 40-year project, this will require 480 monthly calculations.

However, formulas have been developed that ease the process. The most fundamental of these formulas is:

$$FV = PV \, (1 + i\%)^N$$

This formula allows a one-step determination of the future value (FV) of some amount of money (PV) invested today at an interest rate (i%) for a period of time equal to N. (This formula will not be derived here. Those interested are referred to any of the basic accounting or finance texts listed in this chapter's references.) Many modern handheld business calculators have this and other time-value-of-money formulas built in. A nurse manager who wants to know what $100 would grow to in five years at 10% interest would input into a calculator that the PV = $100, i% is 10, and N is 5. Then pressing the calculate button would provide the resulting FV.

Calculators are also relatively simple to use if one wishes to compound more frequently than once a year. When compounding occurs more frequently, one is dealing with a greater number of shorter periods. For example, to compound monthly, instead of N being equal to 5 for a five-year period, it would be equal to 60, the number of months in five years. The interest rate cannot be 10%, because that would imply that 10% was earned each month for the 60 months. Therefore, it will be necessary to divide 10% by 12 to get the monthly interest rate for the 60 months. Thus, i% = 10%/12, and N = 60. In order to make these conversions for quarterly, monthly, or even daily compounding, simply multiply the number of years by the number of quarters, months, or days in a year and divide the interest rate by the same number.

So far this discussion has focused on finding out how much an amount of money held today would grow to in the future. It is also important to be able to take an amount of money to be received in the future and determine what it would be worth today. That requires reversal of the compounding process. This reversal is called discounting, and the interest rate used in the calculation is called the *discount rate.* In the above example, if one expected to receive $161 five years in the future, the calculator could be given the FV = $161, i% = 10, and N = 5 and readily solve for the equivalent present value amount, which is $100. That is equivalent to saying that at a 10% compound interest rate, one would have to put $100 aside today in order to receive $161 in five years.

What if it is expected that some money will be received or spent every year rather than all at one time in the future. For instance, what is the value today of receiving $100 every year for the next three years? One way to solve this problem would be to take the PV of $100 to be received one year from now, plus the PV of $100 to be received two years from now, plus the PV of $100 to be received three years from now.

Obviously, this has the potential to be a tedious process. Any time payments are to be made or received and the payments are exactly the same in amount and evenly spaced in time, those payments are referred to as an annuity. (Business calculators generally have a key or button marked PMT. This stands for periodic annuity payment.) Although many people are familiar with annuities as being annual payments of round amounts of money, any amount paid over and over at even periods of time forms an annuity.

To calculate the PV of $100 received every year for three years, one would calculate that the PMT = $100, N = 3, and i% = 10. The calculator can then determine the PV. Note that FV does not enter into this calculation because there is not one single future value but rather a series of payments, all considered by the term PMT.

The Present Cost Approach

To return to the problem raised earlier, recall that there are two potential air conditioners. One will cost $10,000 and will have operating costs of $3,000 per year for five years. The other air conditioner will cost $7,500 and will have operating costs of $3,600 per year for five years. The problem of choosing one or the other concerns the fact that the total cost of the first alternative is $25,000, while the second alternative costs $25,500, but the one with the lower total cost has the higher initial cash outlay.

In today's dollars, the first alternative is $10,000 plus the present value of an annuity of $3,000 per year for five years. The second alternative is $7,500 plus the present value of $3,600 per year for five years. The appropriate interest rate to use is the subject of some controversy. For now, simply assume an interest rate of 10%. The problems concerning the selection of the interest rate are discussed later in this Appendix. At N = 5 and i% = 10, the PV when PMT is $3,000 is $11,372. When the PMT is $3,600, the PV is $13,647. Together with the initial outlays, the PV of the first alternative is $21,372 and for the second alternative it is $21,147. Therefore, other things equal, the second alternative would be chosen.

This method is the present cost approach. It considers the present value of the costs of alternative projects accomplishing the same end. Assuming that both projects are just as effective in terms of accomplishing the desired outcome, the alternative with the lower present value cost is superior. This approach is rarely used in most industries because it totally ignores revenues. It starts from the presumption that the project or investment is going to be made and simply determines which alternative will have the lowest effective cost over its lifetime. Most industries are very concerned with the profitability of the project.

Health Care Organizations and Profitability

In order to examine profitability, one must use either the net present value or the internal rate of return approach. Proprietary organizations in the health care industry are particularly interested in using these methods. They are potentially valuable, however, even for the not-for-profit part of the health care industry. There are many reasons that a not-for-profit organization must actually earn a profit on some of its programs, services, or investments.

Why should a not-for-profit organization want to make a profit? That seems paradoxical. The term not-for-profit, however, merely means that the main purpose of the organization is not to make profits. However, it does not mean that the revenues of the organization cannot exceed their expenses. Such profits are needed to offset losses on various services. They are also needed for replacing buildings and equipment and expanding the number and types of services offered.

Inflation and technological change compound this problem. If the organization bought a patient monitor 10 years ago for $50,000, a new one may well cost $100,000. To be able to buy the new one without borrowing money, the organization would have to have made a $50,000 profit during the life of the machine it is replacing. The cash to buy the new, more expensive equipment must come from somewhere.

The bottom line is that the organization must consider whether at least some investments will be profitable to offset losses and for future investment needs. Furthermore, since resources are limited, it must be able to do more than determine if a project is profitable; it must have a method to choose the best project from among a number of profitable alternatives.

Therefore, the net present value and internal rate of return approaches are important for all health care organizations. These methods, like the present cost approach, are discounted cash flow methods because they analyze cash flow information by discounting back to the present amounts to be spent or received in the future. Both methods aid in choosing the best project from a group of alternatives.

The Net Present Value Approach

The net present value (NPV) method of analysis determines whether a project earns more or less than a stated desired rate of return. That rate of return is the interest rate used in the calculations of the time value of money. Recall that the interest rate for finding the PV of money received in the future is referred to as the discount rate. In NPV this rate is often referred to as the hurdle rate or required rate of return. The starting point of the analysis is the determination of this rate.

The Appropriate Discount Rate

The key factor in present value calculations is the interest rate chosen. Yet there is no general consensus on the rate that should be used, especially in the not-for-profit sector. Earlier it was noted that one of the key reasons to consider the time value of money is that money could be kept in an interest-earning account. Therefore, one would not want to get involved in a project that did not earn at least that rate.

Most health care organizations do not have the luxury of large amounts of money in the bank. If the money is not needed for this particular project, there certainly are other pressing needs for which the money will be used. In fact, most health care organizations usually have a certain amount of long-term borrowing. Therefore, it has often been suggested that the appropriate discount rate be the cost of obtaining the funds needed for the project.

This in itself brings up a number of problems. Some funding comes by way of contributions, while other funds are borrowed at high rates from banks or through the issuance of bonds. This can lead to inconsistent decisions. Poor projects (from an economic viewpoint) may be accepted in years when contributions are high because the cost of the contributed funds used for the project is zero. On the other hand, fairly good projects might be rejected if contributions are particularly low one year.

It is generally agreed that any particular project's inherent merits should not be based on where the funding for that particular project will come from. Therefore, there should be some average rate commonly applied to all projects. The next question concerns whether that common rate should average the cost of borrowing money with the zero cost of contributed funds. This question has no clear-cut answer. On the one hand, one might argue that if all projects can earn a weighted average of the cost of funds, then the organization can survive financially. On the other hand, it means that projects will be accepted that would be rejected if there were no contributions.

For example, suppose that a hospital could borrow $9,000,000 at a 10% rate and that it receives contributions of $1,000,000. The interest cost on the borrowed money is $900,000/year, and on the contributions the interest cost is zero. The combined cost for the $10,000,000 total would be $900,000, or an average rate of 9%. If this average is used as a hurdle rate, then the organization will accept projects with a projected return of 9% or more. It would, for instance, be willing to accept a project with a 9.5% return, since it would more than cover its cost. The objection to this is that a for-profit business would have rejected a 9.5% project because it would presumably have no contributions. The 9.5% return is less than the 10% cost of borrowed money. Therefore, from a purely financial standpoint, it is not a good investment.

The contention is that even not-for-profit organizations should make wise resource allocation choices. This requires them to act as if they were a for-profit organization. The counter to this argument is that a not-for-profit organization by its very nature is willing to undertake unprofitable ventures because of its desire to provide some benefit to society. Furthermore, the contributed funds did not come from individuals hoping the hospital would only spend money when it can make a profit. They were contributed to cover losing operations.

It is advocated here that projects first be evaluated from a strictly economic approach. Can the project bring in enough money to cover the cost if it had to borrow money to finance it? Such projects can all be undertaken, assuming that the organization has the personnel available to institute them, since they will not place a drain on the financial resources of the institution.

With respect to the projects that cannot meet this criterion, they can be evaluated on the basis of what they contribute to the organization and its patients relative to the money it has to spend on them. This results in a more socioeconomic approach. Projects that will yield a return less than that required from an economic viewpoint can be subsidized by those projects that earn more than the cost of the borrowed funds needed to support them, plus the money from contributions. Thus, the 9.5% project would not be automatically accepted, since it does not surpass the 10% hurdle rate, based on the cost of borrowed funds. It would have to compete with all other projects that earn less than the hurdle rate, based on its qualitative social merit.

The nurse manager will not have to make major decisions regarding appropriate discount rates. The financial officers of the organization have undoubtedly gone over this problem in detail and made some policy decision. If the budget process is extremely efficient in your organization, then the discount rate will be included in the set of assumptions that was prepared as part of the budget foundations process. In such cases, the discount rate will be readily available. Many health care organizations are less sophisticated, and it would be necessary to call upon your financial officers to get an appropriate rate.

NPV Calculations

Once the hurdle rate is determined, the NPV method can be used to assess whether a project is acceptable. The NPV method compares the present value of a project's cash inflows to the present value of its cash outflows, as calculated at a particular hurdle rate. If the present value of the money coming in exceeds the present value of the money going out, then the project is earning a rate of return greater than the hurdle rate. In equation form, NPV can be defined as follows:

$$NPV = PV \text{ inflows} - PV \text{ outflows}$$

If the NPV is greater than zero, the inflows are greater than the outflows when evaluated at the hurdle rate. If the NPV is less than zero, then the organization is spending more than it is receiving. If the NPV is exactly zero, the inflows are equal to the outflows, and the project is earning exactly the hurdle rate. In most cases, it will be financial managers rather than nurse managers who perform the actual calculations. Nevertheless, nurse managers should understand the evaluation process that capital projects are subjected to prior to approval.

To find the NPV, first sum the PVs of the cash received in each year. Then find the sum of the PVs of the cash spent each year. Then compare the sum of the PVs of the inflows to the sum of the PVs of the outflows.

For example, suppose that the hospital is considering adding a new wing. There is an initial cash outflow of $10,000,000. Assume that the money for the wing could be borrowed at 10%. Suppose that the operating cash expenses (including information about the costs relating to nursing, which you have contributed to the analysis) and the cash revenues for each of the 20 years of the useful life of the wing are as shown in Table 10–1. Without considering the timing of the cash flows, a total of $16,570,000 is being spent, and $35,435,192 is being received. The project appears to be very profitable. Note, however, that a large amount of money is spent at the beginning of the project, while revenues are earned gradually over the 20 years.

By using present value methodology, the present value of each cash flow can be calculated, then the present values of the inflows and the outflows can be summed. The result is that the total PV of the inflows is $12,622,639, while the PV of the outflows is $12,506,777. The NPV, equal to the PV of the inflows less the PV of the outflows, is $115,862. Since this is greater than zero, the project is earning more than 10% and is acceptable. However, it is not nearly as profitable as it appeared at first glance.

Even though the net present value is positive, that does not necessarily mean that the organization will go ahead with the project. It may have limited resources

TABLE 10–1. *An Example of Project Cash Flows and Present Values*

	Cash Flow		Present Value (PV)	
	Cash Expenses	Cash Revenues	Cash Expenses	Cash Revenues
Start	$10,000,000		$10,000,000	
Year 1	200,000	$ 1,000,000	181,818	$ 909,091
2	230,000	1,020,000	190,083	842,975
3	250,000	1,081,200	187,829	812,322
4	270,000	1,146,072	184,414	782,783
5	270,000	1,214,836	167,649	754,318
6	280,000	1,287,726	158,053	726,888
7	290,000	1,364,990	148,816	700,456
8	310,000	1,446,889	144,617	674,985
9	310,000	1,533,703	131,470	650,440
10	320,000	1,625,725	123,374	626,787
11	330,000	1,723,269	115,663	603,995
12	345,000	1,826,665	109,928	582,032
13	355,000	1,936,265	102,831	560,866
14	370,000	2,052,440	97,433	540,472
15	380,000	2,175,587	90,969	520,818
16	390,000	2,306,122	84,875	501,879
17	400,000	2,444,489	79,137	483,628
18	410,000	2,591,159	73,742	466,043
19	420,000	2,746,628	68,673	449,096
20	440,000	2,911,426	65,403	432,765
Totals	$16,570,000	$35,435,192	$12,506,777	$12,662,639

and not be able to undertake all projects in a given year, even if they all earn better than the hurdle rate.

Alternatively, projects may exist that conflict. For example, suppose that the organization is considering using a site either for a traditional new wing, a new co-op care wing, or medical office space. Assuming that the land can be used for only one of these three uses, a conflict will exist if all three projects have an NPV greater than zero. Another method of capital budgeting, called internal rate of return, is designed to utilize a ranking system to help make a choice among competing projects. It should be noted, however, that the ranking will be based on strictly economic calculations, and managerial judgment will be needed to make any final decisions. There may well be qualitative or political aspects that will affect the ultimate choice. Nevertheless, even if these other aspects are important to the final decision, it is appropriate to make the economic comparison so that the organization's management can fully understand the trade-offs that are being made.

The Internal Rate of Return Approach

The principal objection to the net present value approach is that it does not indicate the specific rate of return that a project is earning. It simply indicates whether the proposed investment is earning more or less than a specified rate of return. This creates problems if there are several projects that exceed the hurdle rate. This is especially true when the projects conflict or if there are insufficient funds to undertake all projects with a positive NPV. The internal rate of return (IRR) method is a mathematical formulation that sets the present value of the inflows equal to the present value of the outflows. This equation holds true only at the exact interest rate that a project is earning. If the equation is solved for the interest rate that makes it hold true, then that is the rate of return that the project is earning.

Although the mathematics for calculating the internal rate of return are complex, a calculator or computer can be used to determine the interest rate that any project earns. Unfortunately, IRR mathematics are complex. This is particularly true when the cash flows are not the same from year to year. To solve the problem when the cash flow is different each year requires a trial-and-error approach. There is really no better method for finding the internal rate of return than by trying a variety of rates of return until the one rate that makes the PV of the inflows equal to the PV of the outflows is found. While this would be a tedious operation by hand, there are some business calculators and many computer programs that can do this process for you.

Project Ranking

One of the advantages of the IRR method is that it allows the organization to list all the projects being considered and rank them in order from the highest return on investment to the lowest. The IRR method tells the specific interest rate that each project is expected to return. Even if the organization is not-for-profit, it must consider the fact that the projects with the highest return on investment, or rate of return, will provide the largest amount of cash coming into the organization in the future. This cash can in turn be used to allow for additional projects to be undertaken. By listing projects in order from the highest rate of return to the lowest, this ranking makes the project selection process far easier.

Calculators that compute time value of money calculations can be purchased for a relatively small sum—in the $30 range. The computations can also be performed easily using a spreadsheet program such as Excel or LOTUS 1-2-3.

SUMMARY

Capital budget proposals can be evaluated by several methods. The first of these is the payback approach, which is a rather unsophisticated model that is useful for a first assessment of the capital item but is flawed by the fact that it ignores the time value of money.

Discounted cash flow techniques are accurate. These approaches include the present cost, net present value, and internal rate of return methods. All these discounted cash flow techniques account for the time value of money. The present cost approach is useful for comparing alternative ways to accomplish the same goal. The method does not evaluate revenues. Both the net present value and internal rate of return methods determine whether the cash inflows are adequate to justify the cash outflow, from a strictly economic point of view. The internal rate of return method additionally allows for a ranking of projects by rate of return on investment. This method is somewhat more complex to use than net present value.

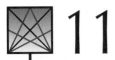

11
Performance Budgeting

The goals of this chapter are to:

introduce the concept of performance or outcomes budgeting;

describe the Management by Objectives (MBO) approach to budgeting;

identify weaknesses in traditional measures of output and performance;

create an awareness of the importance of focusing on goals and measuring the accomplishment of goals;

outline the specific technical steps of performance budgeting;

provide an example of performance budgeting; and

identify potential output measures for use by nursing in performance budgets.

INTRODUCTION

The extreme financial pressure faced by health care organizations in recent years has resulted in substantial budget cuts. Managers are having to find ways to make do with less. A major concern in this environment is that the quality of patient care is likely to suffer. There is a growing call for evaluation of the outcomes of health care organizations. Budgeting can help managers by focusing to a greater extent on the results that departments and organizations achieve. This process, called *performance* or *outcomes budgeting,* is the topic of this chapter.

Performance budgeting is a technique that evaluates the activities of a cost center in terms of what the center accomplishes, as well as the costs of that accomplishment. It is an approach to budgeting specifically designed to evaluate the multiple outcomes of cost centers rather than a single budgeted output, such as the number of home care visits. Performance budgeting provides a mechanism for gaining a better understanding of the relationships between financial resources and the level and quality of results.

Traditionally, budgets focused primarily on the resources used by a department or cost center. There is detailed information on the number of nurses working in a unit and their pay rate. Supplies, educational seminars, and publications are all carefully considered. However, all these are inputs. They are the resources the unit needs to achieve its objectives. Unfortunately, there has been little focus on objectives. What are the goals of the unit? What is it trying to achieve? Cost centers often define their goals only in the simplest terms, such as the number of visits, patient days, or procedures. Performance budgeting shifts the focus from the resources the unit plans to use to the various things it is trying to accomplish.

The first step in performance budgeting is to define the objectives or areas of accomplishment for the unit or department. These are called performance areas. Some examples of performance areas are quality of care, nursing satisfaction, patient satisfaction, productivity, and innovation. The second step is to identify the operating budget costs for the cost center being evaluated. In a nursing unit these costs include items such as the salary for the unit nurse manager, salaries for clinical staff, education costs, and supplies. The third step is to determine what percentage of available resources should be used for each performance area. The fourth step is to assign the budgeted costs for the center to the individual performance areas on the basis of those percentages. The fifth and final step is to choose measures of performance for each performance area and to determine the cost per unit of workload based on those measures.

MANAGEMENT BY OBJECTIVES (MBO)

One of the forerunners of performance budgeting was Management by Objectives (MBO). MBO is a budgeting technique in which a supervising manager and subordinate manager agree on a common set of objectives that will be used as a basis for the measurement of performance. This process requires more than simply developing an operating budget and agreeing to work toward attaining it. MBO programs require that there be a set of specific, measurable goals for each manager. These goals represent the performance of the manager, rather than just the performance of the unit.

A principal reason for introducing MBO was that many organizations were dictating budgets to their department managers. Such an approach gained little support. Managers felt that the budgets were unattainable and reflected little recognition of the realities faced by the department. The MBO approach is one that guarantees more active participation by the manager. There are clear incentive benefits of such an approach. On the other hand, there is a big time commitment on the part of the supervisor and the manager to work out a sensible, meaningful set of objectives.

MBO is a potentially useful approach. For those organizations not yet ready for performance budgeting, it provides a middle ground. It allows for better measures of performance, without the major time and effort commitment of performance budgeting. Performance budgeting starts where MBO leaves off. It recognizes the need to specify performance in terms of more than simply the typical department cost and general output measure. However, performance budgeting goes beyond

MBO in that it allocates a portion of the unit or department operating budget to each of the objectives.

WHEN IS PERFORMANCE BUDGETING APPROPRIATE?

In any organization that has multiple goals and objectives, performance budgeting may be useful. Performance budgeting allows the organization to define the various elements of performance that are important. It can then assess managers and departments based on their accomplishments in terms of those elements. Each department can have its own set of performance or outcomes criteria. Most existing budget measures focus on simple criteria, such as the number of patient days. Such measures are incapable of getting at issues such as quality of care per patient day or cost per unit of quality of care.

When nursing budgets are cut or inadequately increased for changes in patient acuity, wage rate increases, or other factors, there is often an expectation by top management that at least the same amount of work will be performed. Often this is an unreasonable and unrealistic expectation. While it is true that the number of patients or patient days may be cared for with a smaller budget, the amount of care given may not be the same. Performance levels and outcomes are likely to deteriorate. Unfortunately, rarely is there a linkage between the budget or amount spent and the amount of care provided, other than one simplistic measure such as the number of patient days.

If a nursing unit can care for 10,000 patient days in a year with a budget of $2,000,000, what happens if the budget is slashed to $1,750,000? If the unit still provides 10,000 patient days of care, traditional budgeting makes it appear that costs are down and output is unchanged. In reality, it is highly unlikely that outcomes are unchanged. Quality of patient care is likely to have declined along a number of dimensions. However, a traditional operating budget, focusing on the number of patient days, is unlikely to capture any of the changes that have occurred. A performance budget can help measure those changes.

THE PERFORMANCE BUDGETING TECHNIQUE

Determining Key Performance Areas

Nurse managers attempt to achieve a number of different objectives. Nursing units attempt to provide high-quality care. They attempt to satisfy patient needs and desires. They attempt to control costs. If you do not define clearly the performance that you hope to achieve, you cannot measure your success. The key is to develop a set of performance areas for measurement.

In developing performance areas, one should consider a variety of questions, such as: What important goals should be measured? What elements of a unit's performance are within the control of the nurse manager, and what elements are not? How should the nurse manager most productively spend working time? How should the nursing staff most productively use their time? How can the performance of a nursing unit be evaluated?

In addressing these questions, it is necessary to categorize the major elements of the manager's and unit's job or function. For example, consider a nurse manager of a 30-bed unit. Some effort should go toward assuring a high level of patient care. Some effort should go to staffing the unit, some to controlling unit expenses, some to improving productivity, some to improving patient and staff satisfaction, and some to innovation and long-range planning. These are some key performance areas for the manager and unit. There may well be other important outcome areas that are not listed here. A performance budget for a nursing home or ambulatory care organization might well have a different set of performance areas than those used by a hospital-based nursing unit. Managers must establish performance areas based on their own unit or department's specific circumstances.

Technical Steps in Performance Budgeting

Identifying the performance areas for a cost center is the first step in performance budgeting. The second step is to identify the existing line item budget for the cost center being evaluated. In a nursing unit, this budget includes the cost of items such as the salary for the unit nurse manager, salaries for clinical staff, education costs, and supplies.

The next step is to define how much of the resources represented by each line item are to be devoted to each of the performance areas. This requires that the manager develop a resource allocation model. This process forces the manager to think about what elements of the job are really important and how important they are.

If, for instance, patient satisfaction is very important to the organization, the manager must consider whether an adequate amount of time and effort is being devoted to achieving patient satisfaction. The resource allocation for the performance budget explicitly notes the specific portion of the nurse manager's time, staff time, and other resources that should be spent on assuring patient satisfaction.

It is up to the nurse manager to decide how to allocate resources among the various processes that are associated with the desired outcomes. How much of the resources should be focused on quality of care? How much on staffing? A percent of the total effort should be assigned to each of the performance areas. The manager's allocations will likely not be the same for management time, staff time, and other resources. Each resource is allocated based on differing needs. For example, unit nurse managers might allocate 5% of their own time, 35% of clinical staff time, and 90% of supplies to direct patient care. A chart or table should be developed that shows the performance areas and the percent of each line item cost being allocated to each performance area.

The allocation of resources to different performance areas should be based on explicit decisions related to organizational priorities. However, when a performance budget is first introduced, it is easier to make allocations based on historical information. This information can be gathered by having all personnel keep a log of their time for several weeks or can be based on their best guess of how they use their time. Once the performance budget is developed, more information will be available to the manager, and explicit choices can be made to reallocate resources in a more useful manner.

Once the percent of each resource to be used to achieve each performance area has been decided, a calculation must be made to determine how much money has been budgeted for each performance area. This can be done by taking the percent of each line item allocated to each performance area and multiplying it by the total amount of money in the budget for that line item. For instance, if the nurse manager's salary is $50,000 and 10% of the manager's working time is spent on improving quality of care, then $5,000 is calculated ($50,000 × 10%) as being spent on quality. If the staff nurses for the unit earn $500,000 in total and they spend 5% of their efforts on improving quality, there is another $25,000 ($500,000 × 5%) being allocated to quality improvement. The nurse manager can total all the costs for each performance element. In this case, a total of $30,000 has been budgeted for improving quality of care.

The final step is to choose measures of performance for each performance area, budget a specific numerical objective for each area, and determine the budgeted cost per unit of each objective based on those measures. For instance, suppose that the nurse manager chooses to measure quality of care improvement based on the number of medication variances. Suppose further that the performance budget calls for reducing the number of medication variances for the unit by 30 instances. Since $30,000 has been allocated to improve quality, it can be said that $1,000 has been budgeted per medication variance eliminated. The next year the same amount of money might need to be budgeted just to maintain the level of care.

This approach may be sufficient, if eliminating medication variances is a sufficient measure of an overall quality improvement. On the other hand, more than one measure for quality may be needed in order to gain the quality improvements that are sought. Just as it is important to select appropriate areas of performance that the manager wanted to consider, it is also critical to select good measures of performance to allow the manager to see how well things are being done in each critical performance area.

Note that the performance budget specifies an amount of an outcome to be accomplished. For example, it might budget a certain specific number of fewer medication errors. The performance budget also specifies the inputs to be devoted to achieve that outcome. A certain amount of nurse time is budgeted for accomplishing the reduction in medication errors. Thus, goals are matched with resources needed for their accomplishment. The process of performance budgeting can be clarified with an example.

PERFORMANCE BUDGET EXAMPLE

The first step in developing a performance budget is to determine the performance areas that the nurse manager intends to use. The following is one possible set of performance areas:

- Patient care
- Quality of care improvement
- Staffing
- Cost control
- Increased productivity
- Improved patient satisfaction
- Improved staff satisfaction
- Innovation and long-range planning

The second step is to get the cost information for the unit from the operating budget. Converting operating budget information into a performance budget will give a clearer focus of how the unit spends the budgeted amount of money. The operating budget already gives information such as the number of full-time equivalents (FTEs) by skill level. However, those are inputs rather than outcomes. The performance budget will provide information about results rather than just inputs. Suppose, hypothetically, that the line item operating budget for a nursing unit is $1,000,000 for the coming year, as follows:

Nurse manager	$ 50,000
Clinical staff salaries	800,000
Education	20,000
Supplies	40,000
Overhead	90,000
Total	$1,000,000

The third step is to determine the percentage allocation of operating budget resources to performance areas. The allocation of the nurse manager's time to performance areas might be as follows:

Quality of care improvement	15%
Staffing	15%
Cost control	20%
Increasing productivity	20%
Improving patient satisfaction	10%
Improving staff satisfaction	5%
Innovation and long-range planning	15%
Total	100%[1]

---

[1]This simplified example treats the nurse manager's time as if it were all directly under her control. A more realistic calculation might set aside an amount of time such as 20% for administrative mandated activities.

By developing the allocation to areas of performance, a plan is provided for how the nurse manager should spend her time and of what areas are deemed to be either the most important or else the most in need of her efforts.

There is no reason to believe that all resources within a department or unit should necessarily be allocated in the same fashion. The time allocation for clinical staff might be as follows:

Direct patient care	30%
Indirect patient care	30%
Quality of care improvement	5%
Cost control	5%
Increasing productivity	2%
Improving patient satisfaction	5%
Other	23%
Total	100%

The allocation of time for direct patient care seems low, but this is misleading. Since this budget is ultimately based on total unit costs, it includes nonworked time for sick leave, vacation, and holidays. It also includes worked time off the unit, such as inservice education days. These items might account for most of the Other time. Furthermore, a substantial portion of the time spent in quality of care improvement and improved patient satisfaction may in fact be additional direct patient care time, with a specific focus on those two goals. Therefore, this allocation might imply that about half of nurses' time on the unit is spent on direct patient care.

To develop a full performance budget for the unit, it also will be necessary to determine how education, supplies, and overhead resources relate to the performance of the unit. Suppose that a reasonable expectation for the role of education in a given year is as follows:

Quality of care improvement	20%
Cost control	20%
Increasing productivity	20%
Improving patient satisfaction	10%
Improving staff satisfaction	10%
Innovation and long-range planning	20%
Total	100%

Supplies used by a nursing unit are primarily clinical supplies for direct patient care and, to a much lesser extent, administrative forms and other administrative supplies. Suppose that a reasonable expectation for the role of supplies is as follows:

Staffing	2%
Cost control	2%
Direct patient care	90%
Indirect patient care	5%
Other	1%
Total	100%

There is no uniquely correct way to allocate overhead, since much of it is assigned to a nursing unit in an arbitrary manner. Ultimately, performance budget measures will be used to assess the cost of devoting resources to a particular activity, such as improving quality of care. Since overhead is not likely to vary based on how much effort the manager and clinical staff devote to improving quality of care on the unit, it is reasonable to assign the unit's overhead all to direct patient care. However, this too is an arbitrary allocation, and alternative approaches are possible.

Direct patient care	100%

The above percentage allocations are summarized in Table 11–1. Every line-item category within the original operating budget has had a percentage assigned to performance areas based on what the manager decides is a reasonable allocation of resources.

The original operating budget can now be assigned to performance areas, as is seen in Table 11–2. This table takes the total cost for each line item in the operating budget and multiplies it by the percentages in Table 11–1 to determine the budgeted cost for each performance area for each line item. For example, Staff Salary is budgeted at a total of $800,000 (Table 11–2, Total column). Of this amount, 5% is allocated to quality of care improvements (Table 11–1, Quality column, Staff Salary row). As a result, 5% of $800,000, or $40,000, is allocated to quality of care improvements (Table 11–2, Quality column, Staff Salary row).

The total budgeted cost of each of the performance areas can be assessed. It is expected that the nursing unit will spend $51,500 in total on quality improvement efforts (Table 11–2, Quality column, Totals row), $8,300 on staffing, $54,800 on cost control, and so on. In Table 11–2, compare the *bottom row*, which gives the total for each key performance area, with the *Total column*, which gives the total by line item from the original operating budget. The original operating budget appears to be primarily a fixed budget over which the unit has little control. It shows only the amount to be spent on each input resource consumed. However, the bottom row shows that implicit choices are being made about the allocation of the operating budget resources to different priority areas. Each column in Table 11–2 tells the amount of money budgeted for each performance area. The manager does in fact have at least some ability to modify how these resources are spent. It could be decided that relatively greater efforts should be made in one

TABLE 11-1. Summary of Percentage Allocation to Performance Areas

					Performance Areas						
Cost Item	Quality	Staffing	Cost Control	Productivity	Patient Satis.	Staff Satis.	Innov.	Direct Care	Indirect Care	Other	Total
Nurse Manager	15%	15%	20%	20%	10%	5%	15%	0%	0%	0%	100%
Staff Salary	5%	0%	5%	2%	5%	0%	0%	30%	30%	23%	100%
Education	20%	0%	20%	20%	10%	10%	20%	0%	0%	0%	100%
Supplies	0%	2%	2%	0%	0%	0%	0%	90%	5%	1%	100%
Overhead	0%	0%	0%	0%	0%	0%	0%	100%	0%	0%	100%

TABLE 11-2. Allocation of Expenditures to Performance Areas

					Performance Areas						
Cost Item	Quality	Staffing	Cost Control	Productivity	Patient Satis.	Staff Satis.	Innov.	Direct Care	Indirect Care	Other	Total
Nurse Manager	$ 7,500	$7,500	$10,000	$10,000	$ 5,000	$2,500	$ 7,500	$ 0	$ 0	$ 0	$ 50,000
Staff Salary	40,000	0	40,000	16,000	40,000	0	0	240,000	240,000	184,000	800,000
Education	4,000	0	4,000	4,000	2,000	2,000	4,000	0	0	0	20,000
Supplies	0	800	800	0	0	0	0	36,000	2,000	400	40,000
Overhead	0	0	0	0	0	0	0	90,000	0	0	90,000
Totals	$51,500	$8,300	$54,800	$30,000	$47,000	$4,500	$11,500	$366,000	$242,000	$184,400	$1,000,000

particular area and less in another. Knowing that $51,500 is budgeted for quality, $47,000 for patient satisfaction, and $366,000 for direct patient care is much more valuable information than knowing that $800,000 is budgeted for staff salaries. The focus has shifted from inputs to performance.

Note, however, that a performance budget has still not been fully developed. The allocation of operating budget to performance areas (Table 11–2) is a valuable plan that provides an indication of whether the unit is planning to proceed in the most appropriate manner. It does not go far enough, however. It is not specific in terms of quantifying the goals for each performance area.

Table 11–3 presents the next step—the actual performance budget. In Table 11–3, the performance areas have been moved from the top row to the left side of the table. The difficult task of choosing a performance measure and quantifying the budgeted level for each performance area must be addressed.

Health care organizations try to produce improved health. Since this cannot be measured directly in most cases, proxies such as the number of patient days of care are used. Performance budgets add additional proxies to assess the accomplishment of the organization's goals. In Table 11–3 it is seen that a budget can be developed that gives information about such items as the budgeted cost to attain a reduction in patient care planning errors. In this example, the budgeted cost is $5,150 for each 1% drop in the rate of failure to comply with patient care plan procedures (Table 11–3, Average Cost column, Quality Improvement row). The next section addresses the issue of developing proxies for performance measurement.

DEVELOPING PERFORMANCE AREA MEASURES

To be able to create a performance budget that will be as useful as possible, there must be specific ways to measure accomplishments in each performance area. Some of the measures developed for the different performance areas will appear to be crude proxies at best. However, patient days is itself a crude proxy for the process of providing health care, which in turn is a proxy for improved health. Yet patient days is a useful measure. Over time, performance budgeting will improve as better proxies are suggested and incorporated into the technique. What are some potential output measures for evaluating the results of a nursing unit? Each of the performance areas likely has some associated key activities that can be budgeted and measured.[2]

It will take a fair amount of thought to come up with a good set of performance areas and measures of performance. For example, are patient complaints an appropriate measure of patient satisfaction with the nursing unit?

---

[2]The measures described are a mix of both process and outcome measures. They also overlap to some extent. Eventually, performance budgeting may be refined to a point where such problems can be overcome.

TABLE 11–3. *Performance Budget*

	Type of Activity	Description of Output Measure	Amount of Output Budgeted	Total Cost of Activity	Average Cost
Quality Improvement	Patient Care Planning	Patient Care Plan Compliance	10% Reduction in Failure Rate	$ 51,500	$5,150/Percent Drop in Failure Rate
Staffing	Daily Staff Calculations	Number of Daily Calculations	365 Daily Calculations	8,300	$22.74/Per Daily Calculation
		Reduction in Paid Hours per Patient Day	.2 Paid Hours per Patient Day		$4,150/.1 Hour Reduction
Cost Control	Reduce Cost	Reduction in Cost/Patient Day	$8/Patient Day	54,800	$6,850/$ Reduction
Increase Productivity	Revise Procedures Work More Efficiently	Reduction in Total Unit Cost per Direct Care Hour	$3 Reduction per Direct Care Hour	30,000	$10,000/$ Reduction
Increase Patient Satisfaction	Respond to Needs	Complaints	10% Reduction in Complaints	47,000	$4,700/1% Reduction in Complaints
Increase Staff Satisfaction	Respond to Needs	Turnover	25% Reduction in Staff Turnover	4,500	$180/1% Reduction in Turnover
Innovation & Planning	Planning Sessions	Number of Meetings	12 Meetings	11,500	$958.33/Meeting
Direct Care	Direct Patient Care	Hours of Care	10,000 Hours	366,000	$36.66/Direct Care Hour
Indirect Care	Patient Charting	Number of Patient Days	7,300 Patient Days	242,000	$33.15/Patient Day
Other				184,400	
Total				$1,000,000	

If the patients complain about nurses, is it because the quality of care or attention to patients is not what it should be or simply that the patients are reflecting their general mood related to their illness? However, *increases* in the rate of complaints may well be a meaningful performance measurement.

Quality of Care

The quality of care measure will be addressed first, since quality always presents a particular measurement challenge. Earlier, the use of medication variances was suggested as one possible measure for the change in quality of care. Another possible approach is to focus on the patient care plan as a quality indicator. If staff are not skillfully developing patient care plans, ultimately patient care may suffer. Therefore it is possible to measure the quality of nursing by how well plans are developed. Measurement can be based on the *percent* reduction in the number of incomplete care plans, or it can be based on the *number* of incomplete care plans. Many nursing units already measure the quality of their patient care planning. However, with performance budgeting, not only is the quality measured but the measurement is also associated with the expected cost of improving compliance.

In the first row of Table 11–3, it can be seen that Quality Improvement is one performance area being budgeted for. The measure used for this performance area will be the percent reduction in incomplete patient care plans. A 10% reduction is budgeted. As Table 11–2 showed, $51,500 is devoted to this area of the budget. Therefore it is expected that each percent reduction in incomplete plans will cost $5,150. This represents the total $51,500 to be spent in this area divided by the volume of output expected, in this case, $51,500 divided by a 10% reduction equals $5,150 per percent.

This approach recognizes that improvements in performance cost money. It is insufficient simply to dictate that a nursing unit improve its patient care planning without providing additional resources to accomplish this end. Can this unit lower its failure rate even more? Yes, it probably can. However, the performance budget provides explicit information that improved patient care planning requires more attention from the nursing staff. Such additional attention requires real additional resources in terms of increased staffing. If additional staffing is not provided, the only way to improve patient care planning is to devote a greater percent of the staff's efforts to compliance in this area (unless productivity can be increased). However, this will mean devoting less time to other areas.

It is possible that a unit is satisfied with its patient care plans. The nurse manager of the unit does not believe that it is worth a substantial effort to improve its patient care planning. However, even maintaining a given level of quality requires staff attention. Thus the performance budget might show a goal of no change in the number of incomplete plans. An explicit portion of the performance budget would still be allocated to the quality area, to achieve that steady state.

What happens if the overall budget for the nursing unit is cut? The performance budget allows determination of areas in which resources should be cut. If a choice is made to cut resources in an area that affects quality, it would not be surprising to detect later that the number of incomplete patient care plans is increasing. The performance budget would show how the cuts to the unit are expected to affect the various performance areas. Budget cuts must explicitly be assigned to the performance areas to be cut. Rather than expecting no impact of budget cuts, explicit choices are made, and the unit can demonstrate what outcomes are likely to deteriorate as a result of the budget cut.

Staffing

A nursing unit manager must make many staffing decisions throughout the year, as well as manage vacations, holidays, sick leave, and busy and slow periods. In Table 11–3, it is assumed that daily calculations are made for staff adjustments. This requires some managerial time each and every day.

Calculations by the unit manager to adjust unit staffing could conceivably be made weekly or just once a month. If staffing were only adjusted monthly, extra staff might be assigned all month long so that there would be adequate staff for busy days. Less frequent work on staffing would save managerial time but would likely result in higher staffing costs. Monthly calculations would only require the unit to devote about $250 of management resources to staffing annually instead of the $8,300 annual cost when staffing is adjusted daily. However, the cost of extra nursing staff might offset the savings. The performance budget serves a useful function by making explicit the costs of daily calculations.

The performance budget can also show the benefits of daily calculations. Suppose that it is expected that by adjusting staffing daily, seven days a week, to the desired staffing level for the actual workload, it is possible to reduce the overall average paid hours per patient day by 0.2 hour (12 minutes). Presumably, by monitoring staffing needs closely, it is possible to avert unneeded overtime, excessive use of agency nurses, or periods of overstaffing. If the 0.2 hour per patient day reduction is achieved by calculating staffing daily, $8,300 of the departmental budget will be devoted to staffing calculations. However, if the nursing unit has an average census of 20 patients, there would be a savings, on average, of four paid nursing hours per day (20 patients × 0.2 hour per patient day), or 1,460 nursing hours per year. The cost of 1,460 nursing hours would far outweigh the $8,300 investment in daily calculations to adjust staffing.

For example, suppose that the average nurse wage on the unit is $30 per hour. The total wage savings is $43,800. A return on investment can be calculated by dividing the savings of $43,800 by the cost of $8,300, or 5.28. In other words, $5.28 is saved for every dollar spent by doing staffing adjustments daily.

Cost Control

The purpose of cost control is to reduce or restrain increases in the organization's costs. For health care providers paid under a prospective payment system, such as capitation or diagnosis related groups (DRGs), reduced costs per patient directly improve the organization's financial health. The performance measure for cost control in Table 11–3 focuses on a reduction in the cost per patient day. The activity, reduce cost, really represents a goal rather than a description of specifically how the nurses in the unit are to go about accomplishing the goal. However, the budget shows a clear commitment in this area: $54,800 is allocated specifically to accomplishing this end. Referring to Table 11–1, it is possible to see how much of the cost control effort is expected to come from the nurse manager's time, how much from the staff, how much from formal education, and so forth. In this example, each staff nurse is expected to spend 5% of the time, or about two hours per week, specifically focusing on cost reduction. This could mean eight hours at a continuing education program once per month. It does not necessarily mean that each week each nurse will spend two hours on cost control.

In Table 11–3, it can be seen that the performance budget calls for a cost reduction per patient day of $8. The cost of the efforts in this area are budgeted to be $54,800. Most of this comes from requiring the staff to make a specific effort to find ways to contain costs. When the $54,800 budgeted cost for cost control is compared with the budgeted cost reduction of $8 per patient day, for each dollar saved in cost per patient day it will cost the unit $6,850.[3] That seems rather high. Perhaps the unit is spending more on this activity than it is worth. In some cases the performance budget may make explicit the fact that the unit is spending more to accomplish some end than it is worth.

However, care must be exercised in interpreting the performance budget. If $6,850 is spent to save a dollar per patient day, there must be a consideration of how many patient days there are likely to be. If the unit's average census is twenty, there will be 7,300 patient days during the year (20 patients per day × 365 days in a year), and the savings at $1 per patient day would be $7,300, or slightly more than the $6,850 cost. If the census is 28, the savings would be substantial. If the census is 14, the efforts to save money are costing more than they are saving.

Cost control is a general goal. While the cost per patient day is a rough proxy intended to measure success with respect to that goal, it may be that the cost control efforts are also saving money by getting patients discharged sooner. The shorter length of stay decreases overall costs. To determine the true payback for cost control efforts, it would be necessary to combine the savings from the

---

[3]$54,800 ÷ $8 per patient day = $6,850 per patient day. Typically we find the cost per unit, such as the cost per percent reduction in turnover or the cost per percent reduction in incomplete patient care plans. This is similar to finding the cost per patient day or the cost per discharge.

reduced cost per patient day with the savings from the shorter length of stay. The same $54,800 effort for cost control will be working toward both of those ends. For this reason, although it is more complicated, it is often worth using several different measures of performance to more completely assess the unit and its accomplishments. This is discussed below, in the Multiple Measures section of this chapter.

Increased Productivity

The desired productivity outcome is for the unit to accomplish more with the same or less resources. Procedures may need to be revised to help the staff accomplish this. While it is difficult to specify exactly how this can be accomplished, it is not difficult to establish how to measure success. Assume that the organization is concerned about the cost of direct hours of care per patient day. If the total budgeted cost for the department is divided by the total direct patient care hours, a cost per direct care hour can be determined. It will probably be necessary to do occasional special studies to measure, on average, how many direct patient care hours are being provided.

Performance can then be assessed by the reduction in the overall unit cost per direct patient care hour. Such a reduction would indicate either a reduction in total costs or an increase in direct care hours. This approach has a big advantage over simply looking at the cost per patient day. If the cost per patient day declines, this could mean that patients are getting less care during each day. With this measure, cost of care is directly linked to the number of hours of direct care.

Is it worth it for the unit to allocate $30,000 of resources to attempt to reduce the cost per direct care hour? This comes out (see Table 11–3) to a cost of $10,000 for each $1 reduction in the cost per direct care hour. The answer depends on how many direct care hours are provided. Over time, bedside computer terminals will likely become more sophisticated and more widely used. That will allow direct patient care hours to be easily obtainable information, making this approach practical, as well as informative.

Patient and Staff Satisfaction

The key approach to satisfaction is to be responsive to the needs of individuals. Some health care organizations use a formal instrument for collecting data on patient satisfaction. That would be a good tool to use for performance budgeting. However, even if the organization is not that sophisticated or is unwilling to spend the money on data collection that a formal instrument requires, performance budgeting can still be useful. One simply needs to be a bit more creative in establishing the measurement proxies.

For example, to measure patient satisfaction the number of complaints could be counted. It may be true that some complaints are unreasonable or are about things that are not controllable. Many dissatisfied patients may not complain.

However, some reduction in the number of complaints may be a way to go about measuring improvement in patient satisfaction. As with other areas, it must be determined how much improved patient satisfaction it is hoped can be generated and whether the cost of the improvement is acceptable relative to the expected level of improvement.

Staff satisfaction might also be measured in terms of complaints. However, turnover rates might be a better indicator. If the hypothetical numbers in the example were correct, then taking actions to increase staff satisfaction that require $4,500 of total cost would be worthwhile, since it would cost only $180 for each 1% reduction in staff turnover on the unit. This is likely to be a small cost compared with the cost of recruiting and orienting new staff.

Innovation and Planning

Sometimes it is difficult to measure performance. Innovative activity is one example. Proxies for performance in this area tend to be particularly weak. On the other hand, one of the most important things that a manager can do is to be innovative and to foster innovation. By making innovative activity explicitly a part of the performance budget, the necessity of devoting energies to this area can be recognized even if the proxies available to measure performance are weak.

One measure of innovative activity and accomplishment is the number of procedure changes introduced based on recently published research. Another is the number of meetings related to change. The fact that meetings are taking place is probably an indicator that activity is going on in this area. Are the meetings themselves the end goal? No. Do more meetings necessarily mean that more is being accomplished? No. They do, however, provide some sense of the degree of innovative activity.

It is also beneficial to see how expensive meetings are (see Table 11–3). When managers and staff are aware of the cost per meeting, there is likely to be more serious work done, in less time, with fewer meetings.

Although meetings are used in Table 11–3, it is clearly a measure of process rather than of actual innovation. The number of useful innovative ideas generated might be a better measure. And certainly some formal system of rewards should be developed to give employees an incentive to generate innovative ideas.

Direct Care

The measure suggested for performance evaluation in this area is the direct care cost per direct care hour. Lowering the cost per direct care hour can be achieved either by increasing the number of hours produced for the same cost or by lowering the costs for a given number of direct care hours. This is not the total unit cost per direct care hour. Rather, it considers the total cost for only the hours of direct care provided, divided by the hours of direct care. This will generate information on the cost per hour of the direct care. If this cost can be lowered, it often implies that less overtime or fewer agency nurses are being used. Another common way to achieve this goal is to substitute less skilled caregivers (e.g., unlicensed assistive personnel) for RNs or to substitute less expensive RNs for more experienced, expensive RNs. Although these approaches may decrease costs, they may also adversely affect patient outcomes.

Indirect Care

Indirect care is more difficult to measure than direct care because it comprises a wide variety of activities, such as charting and communication with physicians. One approach is to measure the cost per patient day for these indirect activities. Reducing the cost per patient day for indirect activities is likely to indicate improved efficiency, unless the quality of the activities deteriorates. However, if there is a series of quality performance measures, such as patient care planning, adverse patient events, and other checks on quality, such deterioration would probably not go unnoticed.

Other

Some activities do not lend themselves to quantification and analysis. It is preferable to reduce the portion of the budget used for "other" purposes by as much as possible. However, to the extent that it exists, there is no simple way to measure performance with respect to the use of resources devoted to these activities.

This discussion is not meant to be comprehensive. Rather, it presents some examples of how specific measures can be associated with various performance areas. It is necessary for the nurse manager to manage staff closely to ensure that they follow the performance budget as closely as possible. If staff are included in the process of preparing performance budgets, they are more likely to strive to achieve the budgeted targets. One indication of the success of the performance budget approach is the extent to which the unit achieves its performance budget goals.

MULTIPLE MEASURES

In most of the above cases, one measurement was used for each of the various performance areas. This is not always an optimal approach. For example, the percent of patient care plans that are incomplete is not the only measure of quality available to nursing units. Adverse events such as medication errors or the number of patient falls could also be measured. As performance budgets become more sophisticated, it would not be unreasonable for the $51,500 allocated for quality to be subdivided. Perhaps half of the quality efforts will be related to patient care plans, one quarter to reducing patient falls, and one quarter to reducing the number of medication variances. In that case, the $51,500 in the performance budget would be subdivided into $25,750 for patient care plans, $12,875 for reducing patient falls, and $12,875 for reducing medication variances. The budgeted cost per fall prevented and the budgeted cost per medication variance avoided could be calculated in the same way as the budgeted cost for reducing failures to comply with patient care plan procedures was calculated earlier.

This multiple measure approach is clearly superior to use of one measure for each performance area. Since it is likely that the nurse manager will be trying to improve quality in many areas, assigning all $51,500 to one area is likely an overstatement of the cost per unit of performance in that area. It also ignores other important activities. Some quality improvement activities such as providing research-based care may improve several areas of quality, while other approaches such as a staff development program on decreasing medication errors may be specific to one area.

Suppose that the quality outcome area is subdivided and it is determined that ten medication variances can be eliminated by focusing some specific attention in that area. Suppose further that it would cost $12,875 to do this. The cost per medication variance eliminated would be $1,287.50. Is this too much to spend on this problem? Perhaps it is so low that even more should be spent to try to eliminate additional medication variances. The key is that this approach allows the manager to quantify the financial impact of many activities that are done now without any specific cost-effectiveness measurement. With this method it is possible to assess whether the results in a given area warrant the resource investment in that area.

In some cases, rather than allocating the cost to several different areas, it simply makes sense to aggregate the benefits yielded by the unit's efforts. For example, in the case of cost control, there may be efforts to reduce the cost per direct care hour, reduce supply costs, and also reduce the average length of stay. In real-life situations, it is probably hard to determine how much staff effort goes to reduced length of stay and how much effort to reduced direct hours per day. One solution is to calculate the benefits from both shorter length of stay and reduced direct hours per patient day and combine them. Thus the total benefits can be compared with the total costs.

SUMMARY AND IMPLICATIONS FOR NURSE MANAGERS

There is a wealth of information to be gained from performance budgeting. It is a tool that is likely to improve both the planning and control processes in hospitals substantially. Performance budgeting represents a proactive approach to management. This approach follows a basic concept of budgeting: managers prepare a *plan* and attempt to manage according to that plan.

The starting point in performance budgeting is to determine the key performance areas. Next the operating budget is used to determine resources available. There is no conflict between the operating budget and the performance budget. They should work together. The operating budget focuses primarily on input resources. How much is going to be spent on RNs, how much on aides, and how much on supplies? The performance budget focuses on both processes and outcomes. How much is being budgeted to improve quality, how much to provide direct patient care, how much to innovate?

As health care organizations move forward in managerial sophistication, they must move beyond the focus on inputs and begin to focus on performance. Financial pressure to be more efficient can easily lead to deterioration in the quality of care provided. However, cuts in resources do not have to affect performance in a random or arbitrary manner. Performance budgeting can show where resources are being used. Movement toward a measurement focus on the cost of the goals of the nursing unit can allow the manager to make choices and to allocate scarce resources wisely among alternative possible uses.

Performance budgeting is time-consuming and challenging. In some cases, the allocation of money to goal achievement will be inexact or arbitrary. However, it has tremendous potential value in health care organizations. Performance budgets can allow for an indication of the level of quality of care expected in a planned budget. They can *explicitly* show quality decreases that are likely if budgets are cut without corresponding reduction in patient days. It is likely that as part of the evolution in budgeting, this is an approach that will gain ever wider use.

SUGGESTED READINGS

Castaneda-Mendez, K. (1997, July–August). Value-based cost management: The foundation of a balanced performance measurement system. *Journal of Healthcare Quality.* 18(4), 6–9.

Ditmyer, S., Keopsell, B., Branum, V., et al. (1998, June). Developing a nursing outcomes measurement tool. *Journal of Nursing Administration.* 28(6), 10–16.

Finkler, S.A., and Ward, D.R. (1999). *Cost Accounting for Health Care Organizations: Concepts and Applications,* Second edition. Gaithersburg, MD: Aspen Publishers.

Groah, L. (1996, January). Evaluating financial outcomes in perioperative services. *Seminar of Perioperative Nursing.* 5(1), 23–31.

Hill, B.A., Johnson, R., and Garrett, B. (1998, July/August). Reducing the incidence of falls in high risk patients. *Journal of Nursing Administration,* 18(7/8), 24–28.

McKeon, T. (1996). Performance measurement: Integrating quality management and activity-based cost management. *Journal of Nursing Administration.* 26(4), 45–51.

Reed, L., Blegen, M.A., and Goode, C.S. (1998, May). Adverse patient occurrences as a measure of nursing care quality. *Journal of Nursing Administration.* 28(5), 62–69.

Rizzo, J. (1993, July). Flexible and performance budgeting for the nursing unit. *Hospital Cost Management and Accounting.* 5(4), 1–8.

Roey, K. (1997). *Managing Outcomes, Process, and Cost in a Managed Care Environment.* Gaithersburg, MD: Aspen Publishers.

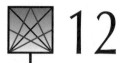 # 12

Cash Budgeting

The goals of this chapter are to:

introduce the concept of a cash budget;

distinguish between revenue and expense, and cash inflows and outflows;

clarify the importance of cash flow;

explain the role of nurse managers in cash management;

describe the elements of cash management;

outline the steps in cash budget preparation; and

provide a cash budget example.

WHO'S RESPONSIBLE FOR CASH BUDGETING?

Cash budgeting is not a direct nursing responsibility. The financial officers of the organization must be aware of the timing of the organization's *cash receipts* and *cash payments*. In order to respond to this responsibility, these financial officers will prepare cash budgets that predict when excess cash will be available and when the cash balance is likely to become negative if specific actions are not taken. Nevertheless, all managers should understand the relationship between the various budgets in the organization. Cash budgeting is as vital as program, capital, and operating budgets are to the survival and well-being of the organization. The nurse manager should have a reasonable understanding of cash budgets and the cash budgeting process. It is often cash budget problems that force a need for modifications in the budgets that nurse managers prepare. This increases the need for the nurse manager to have a basic understanding of the elements of cash budgeting.

THE CASH BUDGET

A substantial part of this book has focused on the operating budget and its control. The operating budget is concerned with the revenues and expenses of an organization. Revenues and expenses should not be thought of as being the same as the cash receipts and cash payments. For most organizations, revenues and expenses are not recorded in the accounting records at the time cash is received or paid. Revenue, for example, is usually recorded when patients are billed. It may be weeks or months before the patients or a third-party payer such as Medicaid pays the bills. Furthermore, capital expenditures often require substantial cash outlays at the time a capital item is acquired.

The operating budget is defined in terms of revenues and expenses. This allows for an assessment of whether the planned operating budget implies an expected surplus, break-even situation, or loss. Determining whether a surplus or loss is expected is critical information for management decision making. To a great extent, this calculation of whether the results of normal operations of the organization are likely to result in a surplus or loss is seen as information more valuable than knowing when the revenues will actually be received in cash or when the expenses will have to be paid in cash. As a result, the operating budget focus is not on when cash comes and goes but instead on the total revenues and expenses for the year.

However, this does not mean that the flow of cash in and out of the organization is not also important for its successful management. In order to pay employees and meet other obligations on a timely basis, the organization's managers must know how much cash is expected to be on hand at any given time. The amount and timing of the cash flowing into and out of the organization can impact substantially on the ability of the organization to meet its current cash obligations. Therefore, a distinct, separate, cash budgeting process exists. The fact that the process is separate and conducted primarily by the organization's financial officers should not lead one to believe that the cash budget is not integrally related to the other budgets and decisions of the organization.

At times the cash budget, developed based on the necessity of meeting routine cash requirements for salaries and supplies, will cause the organization to make decisions that seem to make no sense and that impact nurse managers directly. For example, consider a request by nursing to buy new clinic equipment for $200,000. The equipment is expected to have a useful lifetime of 10 years and will generate an extra $40,000 per year in revenues from new patients that the clinic cannot treat without the equipment. The $400,000 of revenues over the 10-year period is enough to make the initial investment of $200,000 profitable. Each year an extra $40,000 of revenue and an extra $20,000 of depreciation expense (one tenth the cost of the equipment would be charged as an expense for each of the 10 years) would be shown. There is a profit of $20,000 per year. (Assume there are no costs for using the equipment.) Yet, the financial officers may say that the organization cannot afford the equipment. How can this decision make any sense?

Even though a profit will be earned each year, it is not clear that the organization can afford to purchase the equipment. The entire price of $200,000 for the equipment will have to be paid in cash this year, even though the revenues are only $40,000 this year. Where will the cash for the initial $200,000 purchase come from?

The potential for profit does not by itself provide the cash needed to make the investment. Certainly, it might be wise to lease the asset rather than pay all the cash up front. Or maybe the organization can borrow the money from a bank. Or perhaps it can raise the money through contributions. While the organization's managers should try to pursue various ways to get the cash for worthwhile investments—whether they are worthwhile because they are profitable or simply because they are good for the patients—there is a responsibility to the well-being of the organization not to spend the money until it is first determined that there will be sufficient cash available to spend.

Financial officers must carefully consider the cash implications of the operating and capital budgets before they are approved. In effect, various departments submit their operating and capital budget requests. A cash budget is developed based on these requests. One reason that departmental budgets may be rejected is that the cash budget may show that the organization would simply run out of cash if it makes all the requested payments. If an organization finds itself without cash to meet its obligations, it may be forced into bankruptcy. Even if the organization is making a profit, without careful management, it may run out of cash and get into financial difficulty.

CASH MANAGEMENT

In a well-run organization, cash is actively managed. This means that an initial projection is made regarding the timing of cash receipts from philanthropy, patients, the government, and insurance companies (including HMOs). An initial projection of the dates payments must be made by the organization is also prepared. The cash excess or shortfall is calculated.

If there is a shortfall, it may be possible to go to a bank and arrange for a line of credit to be available at the projected time cash is needed. Before doing that, however, other approaches must be considered. What if the financial managers take actions to process patient billings more quickly so that payments will be received sooner? Will the extra cost of speedier invoicing be offset by the interest saved by borrowing less money from the bank? What if payments to the organization's suppliers are delayed by 30 days to avoid borrowing money? How angry will this make the organization's suppliers?

Actions taken to speed up the receipt of cash and to slow down the payment of cash are part of the cash management of the organization. Another critical piece of cash management is determining how much cash the organization needs to keep in its bank accounts. Managing cash is much like walking a tightrope. It is important that enough cash be held by the organization to meet its routine needs for payroll and payments to creditors and to provide a cushion of cash to cover any unexpected *contingencies*. On the other hand, the more resources that are kept in cash, the less there is available for capital investment and other organizational needs.

The goal is to have enough cash to meet routine needs and contingencies but not any more than that. If there is no immediate use for excess cash, it can be invested to earn interest, used to repay loans, or used to provide more health care services. Thus, financial managers must be careful to ensure that the organization will always have enough cash to meet obligations, but they should also be careful to assure that the organization is not missing opportunities to provide additional health services because it is keeping too much cash in the bank. Thus, either too little or too much cash leaves the organization in a less than optimal situation.

CASH BUDGET PREPARATION

In health care organizations, the cash budget is generally prepared for the entire coming year on a monthly basis. Some businesses, such as banks, even prepare cash budgets on a daily basis in order to be sure to have cash on hand for particularly busy days of the week or month.

The format of cash budgets is fairly standard. Each month begins with a starting cash balance. The expected cash receipts for the month are added to this. These receipts may be broken down into categories such as inpatient, outpatient, other operating, and nonoperating, or by payer (e.g., Medicare, Medicaid, HMO, other insurers, self-pay patients, donations, and cafeteria sales). The starting cash balance is added to the total receipts to get a subtotal of available cash.

Expected cash payments are subtracted from the available cash. The principal categories of payments include salaries, payments to suppliers, payments for capital acquisitions, and payments on loans. The result of subtracting total payments from the available cash is a tentative cash balance. This balance is considered tentative because the organization will generally have a minimum desired cash balance at the end of each month. This minimum balance is used for cash payments at the beginning of the next month and also serves as a safety net for any required but unexpected cash outlays.

If the tentative balance exceeds the minimum desired balance, the excess can be invested. If the tentative cash balance is less than the minimum desired balance, the organization will borrow funds to meet the minimum level, if their credit is good enough. The final cash balance is the tentative cash balance less any amounts invested or plus any amount borrowed. For organizations in a particularly poor financial condition, banks may be unwilling to lend money. Such a situation will lead to a crisis unless all budgeting is done carefully enough throughout the organization that cash *deficits* are not encountered. Generally, this requires severe service cutbacks.

If a surplus one month is followed by a shortfall the next, it may pay to invest the extra cash in a short-term investment, such as a money market fund. In this way, the excess cash from one month can earn some interest, which can be available to meet the shortage the next month. Borrowing can thus be avoided. In general, the interest rate paid on borrowed money will exceed the rate that can be earned on money invested for a short period. The cash balance at the end of any month will be the starting cash balance for the next month. An example of a cash budget for the first quarter of a year is presented in Table 12–1.

In the example, the beginning cash balance for January is $20,000. Combining the beginning cash balance with the $385,000 expected in receipts during January, there is $405,000 available in cash. Subtracting the expected disbursements of $375,000 leaves a month-end tentative cash balance of $30,000. Assuming that $20,000 is desired as a safety cushion, there is $10,000 available to invest. In February, cash payments have risen by $25,000, but cash receipts have risen even more. The result is that an additional $18,000 is available for short-term investment.

The tables turn in March. Cash receipts are down and cash payments are up. What could logically cause this result? Does it indicate a serious problem? Very possibly not. It is reasonable to assume that during December, substantially fewer

TABLE 12–1. *Cash Budget for One Quarter*

	January	February	March
Starting Cash Balance	$ 20,000	$ 20,000	$ 20,000
Expected Receipts			
Medicare	$120,000	$140,000	$115,000
Medicaid	80,000	90,000	75,000
HMOs	90,000	90,000	90,000
Other Insurers	42,000	40,000	40,000
Self-Pay	40,000	38,000	41,000
Philanthropy	5,000	10,000	8,000
Other	8,000	10,000	9,000
Total receipts	$385,000	$418,000	$378,000
Available Cash	$405,000	$438,000	$398,000
Less Expected Payments			
Labor Costs	$170,000	$180,000	$190,000
Suppliers	25,000	30,000	40,000
Capital Acquisitions	0	10,000	15,000
Payments on Loans	180,000	180,000	180,000
Total payments	$375,000	$400,000	$425,000
Tentative Cash Balance	$ 30,000	$ 38,000	$ (27,000)
Less Amount Invested	(10,000)	(18,000)	28,000
Plus Amount Borrowed			19,000
Final Cash Balance	$ 20,000	$ 20,000	$ 20,000

elective procedures were done because of the Christmas holiday season. The March cash receipts from Medicaid patients are likely to be influenced by what happened in December. On the other hand, because January, February, and March may have colder weather, they are quite possibly busy months with high salary payments for overtime and agency nurses. Thus, it is not surprising to see lower cash receipts in a given month and at the same time see cash payments that are rising during that month. Frequently, health care organizations find that in a given month their payments are greatly influenced by the current month's activity but that their receipts are more influenced by workload in earlier months.

The March tentative balance indicates a cash deficit of $27,000. Additionally, there is a desired $20,000 ending balance. This need can be met in several ways. The organization could simply borrow $47,000. A more likely result is that the $10,000 invested in January and the $18,000 invested in February will be used to reduce the amount needed to $19,000. Then the $19,000 will be borrowed.

Planning for necessary borrowing should take place well in advance. The plan developed should include a projection of when it will be possible to repay the loan. Bankers are much more receptive to an organization's needs if it has specific plans and projections than if it simply tries to borrow money when an immediate cash shortage becomes apparent. From the bank's perspective, an organization that can plan reasonably well is more likely to be able to repay a loan than one that does not even know several months in advance that a cash shortage is likely to occur.

SUMMARY AND IMPLICATIONS FOR NURSE MANAGERS

Cash needs are crucial. As much as nurse managers may like to think of health care services as more than a business, if the organization cannot pay its bills, it will be out of business. The role of cash budgeting is therefore vital to the overall budget process.

Although cash budgets are normally prepared by financial managers, nurse managers should be aware of the crucial role that they play in the overall budget process. Cash sufficiency is essential to making the program, capital, and operating budgets feasible. The cash budget will have a direct bearing on the items that will or will not be approved in operating and capital budgets.

Because of the delays in payments by the government, insurers, and self-pay patients and because of the long-term nature of some investments, cash receipts and payments do not neatly match each other within each month. Some months (or even years) produce cash surpluses and others produce cash deficits. Such surpluses and deficits are not necessarily the results of profits or losses. A profitable year may result in a cash deficit due to the need to make loan repayments or due to major capital acquisitions. Nurse managers must budget their resource needs carefully so that in periods of cash surplus, resources can be wisely invested and cash deficits can be covered by the organization without the need for emergency measures.

SUGGESTED READINGS

Craske, C. (1997, March). Cash control. *Nursing Times.* 93(12), 69–71.

Finkler, S.A., and Ward, D.R. (1999). *Cost Accounting for Health Care Organizations: Concepts and Applications,* Second edition. Gaithersburg, MD: Aspen Publishers.

Gapenski, L.C. (1997). *Financial Analysis and Decision Making for Healthcare Organizations: A Guide for the Healthcare Professional.* Chicago: Irwin Professional Publishers.

Jones, K.R. (1996, September). Cash management in health care organizations. *Seminars for Nurse Managers.* 4(3), 142–143.

McLean, R.A. (1996). *Financial Management in Health Care Organizations.* Albany: Delmar.

Neumann, B.R., Clement, J.P., and Cooper, J.C. (1997). *Financial Management: Concepts and Applications for Health Care Organizations.* Dubuque, Iowa: Kendall Hunt Publishing.

Nowicki, M. (1999). *The Financial Management of Hospitals and Healthcare Organizations.* Chicago: Health Administration Press.

Pelfrey, S. (1990, October). Understanding the tools for managing cash. *Journal of Nursing Administration.* 20(10), 23–27.

Ward, W.J., Jr. (1994). *Health Care Budgeting and Financial Management for Non-Financial Managers: A New England Healthcare Assembly Book.* Westport, CN: Auburn House Publishers.

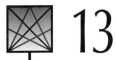

13

Variance Analysis

The goals of this chapter are to:

focus on issues of control, including uses and benefits of control;

define variance analysis;

explain the reasons for doing variance analysis;

distinguish between the concept of an "unfavorable" variance and a bad outcome;

discuss traditional unit or department line-item variances;

outline some possible causes of variances;

explain flexible or variable budgeting;

introduce a flexible budget notation for variance analysis;

define volume, quantity, and price variances;

discuss analysis of revenue variances; and

provide variance analysis tools and examples.

USING BUDGETS FOR CONTROL

Budgets are plans. So far this book has focused on budgets, but the title of the book uses the word budgeting. Budgeting refers not only to making plans; it also refers to using those plans to control operations. If a plan is made and then forgotten, the organization is barely better off than it was without the plan.

Certainly, making plans forces managers to think ahead and anticipate possible future events. Based on such planning, a manager may have made some useful decisions that would not have been made otherwise. Perhaps changes may have been made in the manner in which the organization is operated. For the most part, however, if budgets are not used to control operations, then budgeting is a fruitless process. Health care organizations prepare sophisticated budgets because they recognize a severe need to control their expenses. The government is getting serious about limiting the resources available to the health care sector. Control of costs is vital. In some organizations, such control is critical to survival. In other organizations, cost control is the only way to ensure continuation of all the things the organization is accustomed to—first class equipment and the ability to provide at least adequate and, hopefully, excellent care.

When resources become extremely limited, an organization has a choice. It can reduce the quality of care, or it can become more efficient. True efficiency means providing the same amount of care and quality of care at a lower cost; it requires avoiding waste of resources. Budgeting allows the manager to plan the resources that are needed to do the job. If the budget is not used during the year to control costs, resources may be wasted and quality of care may suffer. Using budgets to control costs will not eliminate all of an institution's financial woes, but without such control, the problems will be far worse.

Using budgets for control can help locate the cause of inefficiency and help avoid waste. In addition, in the hands of a skilled person, budgeting can also help establish a defense for not meeting the budget (if there are valid reasons for spending in excess). Budgeting is a very powerful tool. This chapter and those that follow should be of particular interest to the nurse manager, because they contain important information on methods to defend spending in excess of the budget when that spending is really caused by factors outside the control of the nursing unit or department.

VARIANCE ANALYSIS

Variance analysis is the aspect of budgeting in which actual results are compared to budgeted expectations. The difference between the actual results and the planned results represents a *variance,* that is, the amount by which the results *vary* from the budget. Variances are calculated for three principal reasons. One reason is to aid in preparing the budget for the coming year. By understanding why results were not as expected, the budget process can be improved and become more accurate in future planning. The second reason is to aid in controlling results throughout the current year. By understanding why variances are occurring, actions can be taken to eliminate some of the unfavorable variances over the coming months. The third reason for variance analysis is to evaluate the performance of units or departments and their managers.

In order for variance reports to be an effective tool, managers must be able to understand the causes of the variances. This requires investigating the variances. Such investigation in turn requires the knowledge, judgment, and experience of nurse managers. Variances can be calculated by financial managers. However, those finance personnel do not have the specific knowledge to explain why the variances are occurring. Without such explanation, the reports are not useful managerial aides.

Variance reports are given by finance to nurse managers for *justification.* The word "justification," which is often used, is unduly confrontational. It focuses attention on the evaluation role of variance analysis instead of on the planning and control roles. The goal of the investigation process is to obtain an explanation of why the variances arose. In the majority of cases, the variance report is used to understand what is happening and to control future results to the greatest extent possible. The focus should not be on a defensive justification of what was spent.

If variances arose as a result of inefficiency (e.g., long coffee breaks), then the process of providing cost-effective care is out of control. By discovering this inefficiency, actions can be taken to eliminate it and to bring the process back under control. In this case, future costs will be lower because of the investigation of the variance. The improvement comes, however, not from placing blame on who failed to control past results but on using the information to improve control of future results. It is important to realize that variance analysis provides its greatest benefits when it is used as a tool to improve future outcomes rather than as a way to assign blame for past results.

It would be naive, however, not to realize that in many cases health care organizations do use variances to assign blame for the organization's failures. Therefore, this chapter and the one that follows will provide tools that will aid nurse managers not only in explaining variances but also in deflecting blame for any variances that arise because of factors outside their control.

In many cases, variances are in fact caused by factors outside the control of nursing units or the nursing department. For example, increases in the average level of patient acuity may well cause staffing costs to rise. External price increases may cause more spending on clinical supplies than had been budgeted.

Although these factors are out of the control of nurse managers and should be explained as such, their impact on total costs should not be ignored. Competent nurse managers should be aware of the fact that even uncontrollable variances may require responsive actions to be taken. Uncontrollable spending in excess of the budget in one area may result in a need to restrict spending in another. Adjustments to the entire budget must be considered and either made or rejected in the overall context of the organization and its financial situation.

On the other hand, if uncontrollable spending increases are the result of more patients, then more revenue is likely being received by the organization as well. In that case, there should be less pressure to restrict costs. It therefore becomes critical to understand as much as possible about why variances are occurring. Are they controllable or not? If they are controllable, can actions be taken to reduce or eliminate the variances? If they are not controllable, is their nature such that responsive actions are required or not?

The vast majority of health care organizations carry out at least a minimal amount of traditional variance analysis, in which actual costs are compared to the original budget. If variances are minor, this level of analysis may be adequate. Traditional variance analysis of that type is discussed in the next section. The main weaknesses of that type of analysis are that (1) it ignores changes in the patient workload (volume or acuity) and the likely impact of these changes on cost, and (2) it provides less direction for the investigation of the causes of variances than is possible. Later in this chapter, flexible budgeting will be used as an aid in variance analysis to overcome these limitations of traditional variance analysis.

TRADITIONAL VARIANCE ANALYSIS

At the end of a given time period, the organization will compare its actual results to the budget. Suppose that the organization does this monthly. Several weeks after each month ends, the accountants gather all the cost information and report the actual totals for the month.[1]

The simplest approach is to compare the total costs that the entire organization has incurred with the budgeted costs for the entire organization. For example, suppose that the Wagner Hospital had a total budget for the month of March of $4,800,000. The actual costs were $5,200,000. Wagner spent $400,000 more than they had budgeted. The difference between the amount budgeted and the amount actually incurred is the total hospital variance. This variance will be referred to as an *unfavorable variance,* because the organization spent more than had been budgeted. Accountants use the term *favorable variance* to indicate spending less than expected.

Assuming that the Wagner Hospital begins their year on January 1, their variance could appear in a format somewhat like the following:

This Month

Actual $5,200,000   Budget $4,800,000   Variance $400,000 U

Year-to-Date

Actual $15,150,000   Budget $14,876,000   Variance $274,000 U

In future examples, the *year-to-date* information will be dispensed with, for simplicity. The focus will be on the current month under review. In health organizations, nurse managers are generally provided with information for the year-to-date as well as the current month. The capital U following the variance refers to the fact that the variance is unfavorable. If the variance were favorable, it would be followed by a capital F.

An alternative presentation to using U and F would be to use a negative number for an unfavorable variance and a positive number for a favorable variance. Alternatively, put parentheses around unfavorable variances and no parentheses around favorable variances. Parentheses indicate a negative number. Exercise caution in interpreting variance notation. Any systematic approach can be used to indicate favorable versus unfavorable variances. It would not be wrong to use negative numbers for favorable variances and positive numbers for unfavorable variances, as long as the use is consistent throughout the organiza-

---

[1] One sign of the quality of a finance department is how quickly they provide department and unit managers with variance reports. If finance provides the reports in two weeks or less, they are doing an excellent job. Three weeks is acceptable performance but is not excellent. Longer than three weeks indicates a need for improvement.

tion. There is no consistent approach followed by all organizations in the health care industry.

Why has Wagner had a $400,000 unfavorable variance for the month of March? If variance analysis is to be used to evaluate results, it is necessary to be able to determine not simply that the organization was $400,000 over budget but why that occurred. Given this simple total for the entire organization, the Chief Executive Officer (CEO) has no idea of what caused the variance. The CEO does not even know which managers to ask about the variance, since all that is known is a total for the entire organization.

One solution to this problem would be to have organization-wide *line-item* totals. That is, the total amount budgeted for salaries for the entire organization could be compared to actual total salary costs. The total amount budgeted for surgical supplies could be compared to the actual total amount spent on surgical supplies. The problem with this solution is that there would still be no way to determine what caused the variances. All departments have salaries. A number of departments use surgical supplies. Who should be asked about the variances?

In order to use budgets for control, it must be possible to assign responsibility for variances to individual managers. Those managers can investigate the causes of the variances and attempt to eliminate the variances in the future. The key is that it must be possible to hold individual managers accountable for the variance. This leads to the necessity for determining variances by unit and department. Although the following example uses a hospital, all variance analysis techniques discussed in this book apply equally to all types of health care organizations.

Unit and Department Variances

The overall Wagner variance of $400,000 is an aggregation of variances from a number of departments. Focus on the results for the nursing department.

The Wagner Hospital
Department of Nursing Services
March Variance Report

Actual	Budget	Variance
$2,400,000	$2,200,000	$200,000 U

Apparently, half of the variance for the Wagner Hospital for March occurred in the nursing services area. Now there is more information than there was previously. Previously it was known that there was an excess expenditure of $400,000, but it was not known how that excess came about. Now it is known that half of it occurred in the nursing area. The Chief Nurse Executive (CNE) can be asked to explain why the $200,000 variance occurred.

Unfortunately, at this point the CNE has not been given much to go on. The CNE simply knows that there was $200,000 spent that was not budgeted. Most hospitals would take this total cost for the nursing department and break it down into the various nursing units. Each nursing unit that has a nurse manager who is responsible for running that unit should have both a budget for the unit and a variance report that shows the unit's performance in comparison to the budget.

The variance for one particular nursing unit might appear as follows:

The Wagner Hospital
Department of Nursing Services
Med/Surg 6th Floor West
March Variance Report

Actual	Budget	Variance
$120,000	$110,000	$10,000 U

Line-Item Variances

Even once the total nursing department variance has been divided among the various nursing units, more information is still needed as a guide. Is the variance the result of unexpectedly high costs for nursing salaries? Does it relate to usage of supplies? There is no way to know based on a total variance for the unit or department. More detailed information is needed.

In order to have any real chance to control costs, there must be variance information for individual line items within a unit or department. The CNE must know how much of the nursing total went to salaries and how much to supplies. Nurse managers must have similar information for their own units. For example:

The Wagner Hospital
Department of Nursing Services
Med/Surg 6th Floor West
March Variance Report

	Actual	Budget	Variance
Salary	$108,000	$100,000	$ 8,000 U
Supplies	12,000	10,000	2,000 U
Total	$120,000	$110,000	$10,000 U

This is obviously a great simplification. There should be line items for employee-benefit costs. There should be separate line items for each type of employee. LPNs would be separate from RNs. Each major different type of other than personnel services (OTPS) cost could be a separate line item. For example, see Table 13–1. The more detailed the line items are, the more information that is available. Variance reports with detailed line-item results for each unit and department are generally available in health care organizations today.

TABLE 13–1. Sample Variance Report—March 2001

Cost Center: 6th Floor West Med/Surg

	This Month		Account No./Description	Year-to-Date		
Actual	Budget	Variance		Actual	Budget	Variance
$ 58,951	$ 53,431	$ 5,520	010 Salaries—RN	$164,245	$160,296	$3,949
32,110	31,098	1,012	011 Salaries—LPN	94,930	93,294	1,636
14,124	13,256	868	012 Salaries—Nurses' Aides	41,569	39,768	1,801
4,581	4,088	493	020 FICA	13,742	12,263	1,479
1,081	1,014	67	021 FICA	3,241	3,041	201
351	313	38	022 FICA	1,051	938	113
209	200	9	050 Life Insurance	627	600	27
343	350	(7)	060 Other Fringes	1,029	1,050	(21)
$111,750	$103,750	$ 8,000	(a) Personnel Cost	$320,435	$311,249	$9,185
$ 4,970	$ 3,000	1,970	300 Patient Care Supplies	$ 8,950	$ 9,000	($ 50)
828	800	28	400 Office Supplies/Forms	2,484	2,400	84
650	650	0	500 Seminars/Meetings	1,950	1,950	0
750	750	0	600 Noncapital Equipment	2,250	2,250	0
425	400	25	700 Maintenance/Repair	1,275	1,200	75
45	50	(5)	800 Miscellaneous	135	150	(15)
582	600	(18)	900 Interdepartmental	1,746	1,800	(54)
$ 8,250	$ 6,250	$ 2,000	(b) Other Than Personnel Services (OTPS)	$ 18,790	$ 18,750	$ 40
$120,000	$110,000	$10,000	(c) Total Unit Costs (c = a + b)	$339,225	$329,999	$9,225

Note: In this table, Unfavorable Variances are positive numbers and Favorable Variances are negative numbers.

Understanding Variances

The objective in doing variance analysis is to determine why the variances arose. Nothing can be done with respect to the goal of controlling costs until the nurse manager knows where the unit or department is deviating from the plan and why. The more detailed the line-item information, the easier it will be to identify specific areas where variances are occurring.

Once the variance for each line item for each unit has been calculated, it must be determined whether or not to investigate the variance. Minor variances can be ignored. Variances that are significant in amount must be investigated. (The issue of how to determine if a variance is significant enough to warrant investigation is discussed in the next chapter under the heading of Investigation and Control of Variances.) By dividing variances into nursing units, each unit manager can be assigned the responsibility of determining the causes of the variances for the unit. The manager of 6th Floor West must explain the causes of the $10,000 total unfavorable unit variance.

By dividing the variances into line items, the unit manager can begin the investigation. In the case of the above example, $8,000 of the variance is the result of labor costs, and $2,000 is the result of spending more on supplies than the budget allowed. Note that while the $8,000 labor variance is much larger than the supplies variance in absolute dollar terms, the labor variance is 8% over budget while the supply variance is 20% over budget. Both these variances should be investigated and their causes determined. Where possible, corrective action should then be instituted to avoid similar variances in future months.

Traditional variance analysis requires that the nurse manager proceed to use the unit line-item variance information to attempt to discover the underlying causes of the variances. Consider the $8,000 variance for salaries. Why was $8,000 more than budgeted spent on salaries. No matter how narrowly defined the line items for salaries (e.g., separating RNs from LPNs from Nurses' Aides), the question still arises: Why was $8,000 more than budgeted spent on salaries?

In the absence of supporting evidence, the 6th Floor West unit manager and nurses may be told that they did not do a good job of controlling the use of staff. This is an unwarranted conclusion. Expenditure for staff in excess of the budgeted amount could have a number of possible causes. Investigation may disclose which potential cause was in fact responsible in a given instance.

One potential cause of the $8,000 salary variance is that the unit manager just did not do a good job in controlling the usage of staff. As a result, more hours of nursing care per patient were paid for than had been expected. Another possibility is that the patients were sicker than anticipated, and the higher average acuity level caused more nursing hours to be used per patient. Another possible cause is that the hourly rate for nurses increased. Nurse managers may have no direct control over base salaries. On the other hand, the higher cost could have been due to increased overtime.

Still another possible cause of the variance is that there were more patients, and the additional patients caused more consumption of nursing hours. The most serious problem of traditional variance analysis is that it compares the predicted cost for a predicted workload level (e.g., volume of patient days adjusted for acuity) to the actual cost for the actual workload level.[2] Unless the actual workload is exactly as predicted, there is little chance that a unit will achieve exactly the budgeted expectations.

Essentially, with traditional variance analysis, an attempt is being made to match actual costs to a budget that is relevant for a given workload level. But that workload level is usually not the actual workload that occurs. If a nursing unit has more or fewer patients, the original budget is no longer relevant. If costs fall by 5%, under traditional variance analysis, there is a temptation to praise the manager for coming in under budget. However, if patient volume falls by 20% and costs fall by only 5%, it does not make sense to offer that praise. Such a large patient decline might have warranted a bigger decrease in costs.

Similarly, if patient workload increases by 20% and costs rise by only 5%, it makes little sense to have a variance analysis system that is oriented toward criticizing the unit and manager for having gone over the original budget. The problem with traditional variance analysis is that it is overly focused on the original budget. Many health care organizations are now starting to use a more sophisticated variance approach based on a flexible budget. The main goal of this approach is to allow for changed expectations as workload changes. In such a system, first calculate the portion of the variance caused by changes in workload. Then the remaining portion of the variance can be examined more easily to determine its causes.

FLEXIBLE OR VARIABLE BUDGETS

Flexible or *variable budgeting* takes into consideration the fact that the actual output level often differs from expectations. Managers must have some way of controlling operations, in light of varying levels of activity.

---

[2]The general term "workload" is used here because there is no one, unique measure of workload that will always be relevant for budgeting. Sometimes we will use the technocratic term "output" interchangeably with workload. If we are dealing with a home health agency, then workload is measured by the number of visits. For the radiology department, the workload measure is likely to be the number of x-rays. For a nursing unit, workload would generally be the number of patient days adjusted for acuity. For an operating room, it might be the number of procedures or hours of surgical procedures.

Preparing a budget requires many assumptions and predictions. One of the most prominent of these concerns the workload level. If the volume of services, cost of services, and revenues related to services all rose and fell in equal proportions, this might not create a significant problem. However, that is generally not the case. Revenues may change in a sharply different proportion than costs. Managers need to be able to anticipate such variations. A flexible budget is a tool to aid managers in this area. Flexible budgets are sometimes referred to as variable budgets.

A flexible budget is an operating budget for varying workload levels. For example, suppose that the Best Clinic expects 4,000 visits and had the following operating budget for the coming month:

Best Clinic
Budget for Next Month

Revenues	
Patient Care	$165,000
Expenses	
Salaries	$115,000
Supplies	30,000
Rent	12,000
Other	6,000
Total Expense	$163,000
Surplus	$ 2,000

This budget provides Best Clinic with information that a modest surplus of $2,000 is projected. But what will happen if the number of visits is greater or fewer than expected?

Assume that revenue changes in direct proportion to the number of visits. However, some of the expenses are fixed costs (see Chapter 4 for a discussion of fixed and variable costs). They will not change as the volume of visits changes. For example, rent on the clinic building is a flat monthly amount, regardless of visits. For most organizations, however, some costs are also variable. They vary as the volume of visits goes up or down. Best Clinic will have to buy more supplies if they get very busy. Or they can buy fewer supplies if they have fewer patients.

A flexible budget takes the basic operating budget and adjusts it for the impact of possible workload changes. Assume that revenues and supplies are the only items that vary with the number of visits. For this simple example we will assume that the clinic's staffing is fixed for any likely range of activity. Consider a flexible budget for Best Clinic assuming that 3,600 or 4,400 visits, a 10% decrease or increase, occur next month:

Best Clinic
Flexible Budget for Next Month
Volume of Clinic Visits

	3,600	4,000	4,400
Revenues			
Patient Revenue	$148,500	$165,000	$181,500
Expenses			
Salaries	$115,000	$115,000	$115,000
Supplies	27,000	30,000	33,000
Rent	12,000	12,000	12,000
Other	6,000	6,000	6,000
Total Expense	$160,000	$163,000	$166,000
Surplus/(Deficit)	($ 11,500)	$ 2,000	$ 15,500

This flexible budget shows that if the number of visits increases by just 10%, a surplus or profit of $15,500 will occur. But a 10% fall in visits will result in a loss of $11,500. This information can serve as a warning to the managers in the planning stage. They need to be aware of the potential for losses if volume does not meet expectations, as well as the possible benefits from extra visits.

During the month, if managers see that visits are fewer than expected, they can anticipate the likely financial shortfall without waiting until the end of the month or later to find out. Actions can be taken to increase fund-raising efforts or to find ways to cut costs. Decisions can be made regarding whether the clinic can sustain a financial loss. If it cannot, it may have to find ways to cut costs.

Flexible or variable budgets focus on volume. Nursing units in hospitals have patient days. Home care agencies provide visits. Operating rooms have procedures. In each case, some measure of volume is needed to prepare a flexible budget.

The key to preparing a flexible budget is identification of fixed and variable costs. As volume varies up or down, which numbers in the budget are likely to change and which are likely to remain the same? Will the costs that vary change in direct proportion to volume changes, or will their change be more or less than proportional? Managers must work to understand revenue and cost structures enough to be able to anticipate the changes caused by volume variations.

Flexible budgets not only are useful for planning but also serve a critical role in variance analysis. By understanding flexible budgets the manager is able to interpret more accurately why variances occur and to take any required actions as a result of variances.

FLEXIBLE BUDGET VARIANCE ANALYSIS

Flexible budgeting is a system that requires a little more work than traditional variance analysis but can provide nurse managers with substantially more information. The health care industry has been slow to adopt widely the use of flexible budgeting. This probably reflects a historical lack of emphasis on cost control. As cost control becomes more important to the financial well-being of health care organizations, rapidly increasing adoption of the technique is likely.

It is to the nurse manager's advantage to push administrators and financial officers to adopt the method if they have not already done so. If they will not, then it may be worthwhile for a nursing department to acquire a microcomputer and do the analysis for the department and each unit anyway. The information provided can help managers understand the cause of variances so that they can be controlled. It can also demonstrate that certain unfavorable variances are not the fault of a manager's unit or department but were caused by factors outside of the unit or department's control.

Suppose that the following was the variance report for nursing department salaries:

The Wagner Hospital
Department of Nursing Services
March Variance Report

	Actual	**Budget**	**Variance**
Salary	$1,000,000	$1,000,000	$0

It looks like the department came in right on budget. It is probable that the department's managers would be feeling pretty good about this line item for March. Suppose, however, that the budget of $1,000,000 for nursing salaries was based on an assumption of 25,000 patient days, but there were actually only 20,000 patient days. One would expect that the lower patient-day volume should have allowed for reduction in overtime and elimination of some temporary agency nurse time. The department should have spent less than $1,000,000. The original budget ignores this fact.

When used for variance analysis, the flexible budget is a restatement of the budget based on the volume actually attained. Basically, the flexible budget shows what a line item should have cost, given the workload level that actually occurred.

In variance analysis the flexible budget is prepared after the fact. The actual volume must be known in order to prepare the flexible budget for that specific volume.[3] Keep in mind that because some costs are fixed and some costs are variable, total costs do not change in direct proportion with volume. One would

---

[3]As part of the budget preparation process, some organizations prospectively prepare flexible budgets. This provides the organization with a sense of what costs are likely to be at differing levels of workload.

normally expect that a 10% increase in patient days would be accompanied by less than a 10% increase in costs, since only some costs are variable and increase as census does. On the other hand, a 10% reduction in workload would only be expected to be accompanied by a less than 10% reduction in cost because the fixed costs would not decline.

Using the flexible budget technique allows the variance for any line item to be subdivided to get additional information. Essentially the variance already calculated (i.e., the difference between the budgeted amount and the actual result) is going to be divided into three parts: a *volume variance,* a *price variance,* and a *quantity variance.*

The Volume Variance

The *volume variance* will be defined here as the amount of the variance in any line item that is caused simply by the fact that the workload level has changed. For example, if the budget calls for 25,000 patient days when actually there were 30,000 patient days, then it would be expected that it would be necessary to spend more. Variable costs would undoubtedly rise. The cost of the resources needed for an extra 5,000 patient days constitutes a volume variance.

A substantial number of unfavorable unit line-item variances may result simply from the fact that workload increased above expectations. Such an increase is generally outside of the control of the nurse manager. For many health care organizations, an increase in workload is a good thing. Higher hospital occupancy may mean that there are more patients sharing the fixed overhead of the institution. Similarly, with home health agencies, more visits mean more patients to share the fixed costs of the agency.

Higher volume demands higher cost. If the higher volume was not budgeted for, there will be spending in excess of budget. Note that revenue will likely be higher than budget as well. More often than not, however, nurse managers are held responsible for controlling costs, but they do not receive any benefit from increases in revenues.

The flexible budget approach will allow for specific identification of how much of the variance for any line item is attributable to changes in the workload volume as opposed to other causes. Many health care organizations have adopted use of this portion of flexible budgeting. They recalculate the monthly budget, allowing for the impact on costs of workload changes. Unit managers are then asked to explain the differences between the actual amounts spent, and the amounts that should be spent according to the flexible budget. While this is a major step in the direction of making variance analysis more relevant and useful, it does not yield all the potential benefits of flexible budget variance analysis.

The Price, or Rate, Variance

The *price,* or *rate,* variance is the portion of the total variance for any line item that is caused by spending more per unit of some resource than had been anticipated. For example, if the average wage rate for nurses is more per hour than had been expected, this would give rise to this type of variance. When the variance is used to measure labor resources, it is generally called a *rate variance*, because the average hourly rate has varied from expectations. When considering the price of supplies, such as the cost per package of sutures, it is called a *price variance*, because it is the purchase price that has varied. The terms price and rate are often used interchangeably in practice.

If a unit manager expected to pay $1.00 per roll for bandage tape but actually paid $1.10 per roll, this would give rise to a price variance. Or suppose there is a line item for nurses hired on a temporary basis from an outside agency. If the unit manager expected to pay the agency $45.00 per hour but actually paid an average of $48.00 per hour, this would give rise to a rate variance.

The price, or rate, variance may or may not be under the control of the nurse manager. If the purchasing department predicts all prices used for supplies and then winds up paying a higher price than predicted, it should be possible to measure the price variance so that the responsibility can be placed with the purchasing department. If the nursing department bears the responsibility for price variances on supplies, the purchasing department will have no incentive to find the best prices. On the other hand, if the nurse manager hires temporary nurses directly from the agency, then the responsibility for the rate variance may rest with the nurse manager. Were overqualified people hired? Was an attempt made to seek out an agency that would give the best rate? The manager who can exercise some control over the outcome should be the manager held accountable for the outcome.

The Quantity, or Use, Variance

The third general type of variance under the flexible budgeting scheme is the *quantity, or use,* variance. This is the portion of the overall variance for a particular line item that results from using more of a resource than was expected for a given workload level. For example, if more supplies were used per patient day than expected, this would give rise to a quantity variance because the quantity of supplies that were used per patient day exceeded expectations.

This variance is also frequently referred to as a *use variance* because it focuses on how much of the resource has been used. For example, if one-half roll of bandage tape was used per patient day, while the expected usage was only one-quarter roll, there would be a use variance. The terms "quantity" and "use" are often used interchangeably.

DETERMINATION OF THE CAUSES OF VARIANCES

Before discussing how these different flexible budget variances can be calculated, there is another critical issue to be considered first. The volume, price, and quantity variances are going to be used to find out more information about why the budget differs from the actual results. Using these variances, it will be possible to find out how much of the variance was caused simply by a change in the workload volume, how much by a change in prices, and how much by changes in the amount of each resource consumed for a given level of workload.

What the nurse manager will not get from this analysis is the ultimate explanation of causes of the variances. The nurse manager will still have to investigate to find out *why* these variances have occurred. The analysis provides significant new information by pointing a finger in a specific direction instead of waving a hand in a vague direction.

For instance, if twice as many surgical supplies were used per patient day as expected, the nurse manager knows exactly what to investigate. The analysis does not tell why there was a variance, but it does tell where. Rather than simply saying that the operating room is over budget, it is known that the line item for surgical supplies is over budget. Furthermore, rather than simply noting that too much was spent on surgical supplies, it has been determined that the problem was not caused because there were extra procedures. Nor was it caused because the price of surgical supplies went up. It is specifically known that the problem lay in using more surgical supplies per procedure than had been budgeted. Managers must take over at this point and investigate why this occurred. Why were more surgical supplies used per procedure than expected? Was it sloppy use? Clear-cut waste? Was it pilferage? Was there a major disaster that did not increase the number of procedures considerably but did bring in patients requiring a great amount of surgical supplies? Is the budget wrong and it is not really possible to get by with the budgeted amount of surgical supplies per procedure?

If answers to these questions were not needed, the variance process could get by with a lot more accountants and computers and a lot fewer nurse managers. Accountants and computers, however, cannot answer these questions. Ultimately, the nurse manager must find out the actual underlying cause of the variance.

THE MECHANICS OF FLEXIBLE BUDGET VARIANCE ANALYSIS

The first step in flexible budgeting is to establish the flexible budget for the actual workload level. Given the actual cost for a particular line item and the original budgeted amount, it must be determined what it should have cost for that line item given the workload level that actually occurred.

For example, consider the supplies budgeted for and used by the Med/Surg 6th Floor West nursing unit at the Wagner Hospital in March:

The Wagner Hospital
Department of Nursing Services
Med/Surg 6th Floor West
March Variance Report

	Actual	Budget	Variance
Supplies	$12,000	$10,000	$2,000 U

The actual consumption was $12,000. The budgeted consumption was $10,000. Suppose that the budget assumed that there would be 500 patient days for this unit for March, but there actually turned out to be 600 patient days. (For the time being, ignore the acuity level of the patients. Using acuity in the variance model is explicitly addressed in Chapter 14.) Assuming that the consumption of supplies would normally be expected to vary in direct proportion to patient days, the planned consumption was $20 per patient day. This is calculated by dividing the $10,000 budget by the 500 expected patient days.

For 600 patient days at $20 per patient day, $12,000 would have been budgeted for supplies. This is the flexible budget. It is the amount the department would have expected to spend had the actual number of patient days been known. Notice that in this case the flexible budget and the actual amount spent are identical:

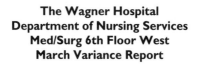

**The Wagner Hospital
Department of Nursing Services
Med/Surg 6th Floor West
March Variance Report**

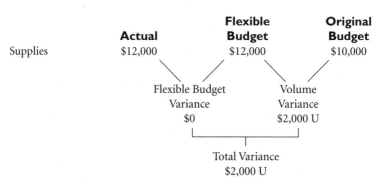

The difference between the original budget and the actual amount spent is the total variance. This is still $2,000 U. The difference between the original budget and the new flexible budget is the volume variance. In this case, the difference is $2,000 U. Note that this volume variance is considered to be unfavorable because the flexible budget requires more spending than was expected. The increased workload may well have been a favorable event for the organization, but the accountant always refers to cost in excess of the original budget as being an unfavorable variance.

The difference between the flexible budget and the actual amount spent can be referred to as a flexible budget variance. Here the flexible budget variance is zero. The entire variance in supplies has been explained by the fact that there was a different volume of patients than had been anticipated.

What about the nursing salaries for the unit? Recall the variance report for nursing salaries:

The Wagner Hospital
Department of Nursing Services
Med/Surg 6th Floor West
March Variance Report

	Actual	**Budget**	**Variance**
Salary	$108,000	$100,000	$8,000 U

To keep the discussion relatively simple at this point, assume that nursing salary costs should vary in direct proportion to the number of patient days. In other words, assume that nursing salary costs are variable. A more realistic example is discussed in Chapter 14, once flexible budget mechanics have been fully developed.

Nursing salaries had been budgeted at $100,000, with an expectation of 500 patient days. This is a cost of $200 per patient day. Assuming nursing salary costs are variable, had it been known that there would be 600 patient days, $120,000 would have been budgeted. The variance report can be restated as follows:

The Wagner Hospital
Department of Nursing Services
Med/Surg 6th Floor West
March Variance Report

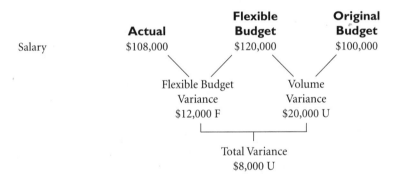

	Actual	**Flexible Budget**	**Original Budget**
Salary	$108,000	$120,000	$100,000

Flexible Budget Variance $12,000 F   Volume Variance $20,000 U

Total Variance $8,000 U

Subtracting the original budget from the flexible budget, the volume variance is found to be $20,000 U. When the flexible budget is subtracted from the actual cost, it turns out that the flexible budget variance is $12,000 F. Note that the volume variance is unfavorable because the extra patients require more spending. However, the actual amount spent was less than the flexible budget, resulting in a favorable flexible budget variance.

If the volume and flexible budget variances for salaries are combined, there is an unfavorable total variance of $8,000. Note that if both variances were favorable they could be added together and the result would be $32,000 F. If they were both unfavorable, they could be added and the result would be $32,000 U. Since one of the variances is favorable and one is unfavorable, the smaller one must be subtracted from the larger one to get a combined total variance. The total variance will have the same label (i.e., favorable or unfavorable) as the larger of the two variances. Hence, $20,000 U − $12,000 F = $8,000 U.

At this point in the analysis, there is not yet sufficient information to determine the causes of the flexible budget variance. Suppose that the CNE of the organizations had come to the unit manager in the middle of April and complained about a total lack of cost control on the unit. The unit had a $2,000 unfavorable supplies variance and an $8,000 unfavorable salary variance. Based on traditional variances (without using a flexible budget), there would be no way the CNE could determine the exact cause of the problem.

Certainly, the unit manager is aware of increased patient volume and would argue that extra patient days were a major factor. But how major? By using a flexible budget, it is possible to find out exactly what dollar impact the extra patient days should have had. In the example, flexible budgeting has shown that the entire variance in supplies is attributable to the extra patient days. The volume variance for supplies was $2,000 U, the same as the amount of the total supply variance. Furthermore, the volume variance was $20,000 U for salaries. The department manager should have expected to spend $20,000 more on nursing salaries than was in the original budget, given the 100 extra patient days. In fact, only $8,000 was spent above the original salary budget. Rather than being blamed for having gone over budget, the unit manager can now show that given the actual number of patient days, the unit actually spent $12,000 less than should have been expected!

Flexible Budget Notation

The next step in the process is to try to determine what caused the flexible budget variance. In order to do this it is necessary to formalize the flexible budgeting process by introducing some notation. The letter A will be used to refer to an actual amount. The letter B will be used to refer to a budgeted amount. The letter P will stand for a price or rate, and the letter Q will stand for a quantity. The letter i will be used to stand for an input, and the letter o to stand for an output or workload.

Inputs are resources used for each line item. If one is considering how much was spent on nursing salaries, then the input is nursing time. If one is considering the cost of bandage tape, then the input is rolls of bandage tape. *Outputs* are a measure of what is being produced. Since improved health cannot readily be measured, proxies will be used to measure how much output is produced. Frequently used output measures include patients, patient days, visits, treatments, and procedures.

The notation is combined to form six key variables. Pi stands for the *price* of the *input,* such as $1 per roll of bandage tape or $25 per hour for nursing salary. Qo stands for the total *quantity* of *output.* Qi stands for the *quantity* of *input* needed to produce one unit of output. The letter B in front of other letters indicates a *budgeted* amount. The letter A in front of other letters indicates an *actual* result. The definitions of the notation can be formalized as follows:

BPi: *budgeted price per unit of input*
BQi: *budgeted quantity of input for each unit of output*
BQo: *budgeted quantity of output*
APi: *actual price paid per unit of input*
AQi: *actual quantity of input for each unit of output produced*
AQo: *actual quantity of output*

The notation can best be understood in an example.

An Example of Volume, Price, and Quantity Variances

Suppose that Wagner Hospital had the following line item in their variance report for a nursing unit for the prior month:

	Actual	**Budget**	**Variance**
Nursing Labor	$34,038	$28,800	$5,238 U

The unit manager wants to find out what caused the variance, so the following information is gathered:

BPi: $24.00 per hour budgeted nursing rate
BQi: 3.0 hours of budgeted nursing time per patient day
BQo: 400 budgeted patient days
APi: $24.40 actual average nursing rate per hour
AQi: 3.1 hours of actual nursing time per patient day
AQo: 450 actual patient days

Before proceeding to use these data, consider what is involved in obtaining the information. Information is worthwhile only if it is more valuable than the cost to collect it. All three of the budgeted items are already known. It would not have been possible to prepare an operating budget without a forecast of patient days, the average rate for nurses, and the budgeted hours per patient day (or at least the total budgeted time, which can be divided by the expected patient days to get the budgeted time per patient day). What about the actual information? The actual number of patient days is readily available. The actual wage rate and the amount of actual paid nursing time is available from the payroll department. Given the nursing time and the actual number of patient days, one can divide to get the nursing time per patient day. Therefore, all the data needed for flexible budget variance analysis is readily available.

The first step in utilizing this data is calculating the original budget in terms of the notation. The original budget is simply the expected cost per patient day multiplied by the expected number of patient days. In this case, the expectation is that nurses will be paid $24.00 per hour; the department will pay for an average of

3.0 hours per patient day. Therefore, the expected cost is $72 per patient day. For the month, 400 patient days are expected, so the budget is $28,800 ($24.00 × 3.0 hours × 400 patient days). In terms of the notation, this can be shown as follows:

Original Budget

$BQi \times BPi \times BQo$

$3.0 \times \$24.00 \times 400$

$\$28,800$

That is, BQi, the budgeted quantity of input per patient day, is 3.0 hours; BPi, the budgeted price per hour of nursing time, is $24.00; and BQo, the budgeted quantity of patient days, is 400. If these three numbers are multiplied together, the result is the originally budgeted amount for nursing labor.

The next step is to find the flexible budget. Keep in mind that the flexible budget is the amount that one would have expected to spend if the actual number of patient days had been known in advance. Therefore, leave the BQi at the budgeted 3.0 hours per patient day, and leave the BPi at the budgeted $24.00 per hour. The only change is from a BQo of 400 patient days to a new AQo of 450 patient days. The flexible budget can then be calculated as follows:

Flexible Budget

$BQi \times BPi \times AQo$

$3.0 \times \$24.00 \times 450$

$\$32,400$

Note that the difference between the original budget and the flexible budget is caused by a difference in the number of patient days. Other than that, the calculations are the same. The originally budgeted amount of $28,800 can be compared with the flexible budget amount of $32,400 to determine the volume variance of $3,600 U. Since patient days are higher than expected, cost will be higher than expected. This will give rise to an unfavorable variance. The comparison between the original budget and the flexible budget can be shown as follows:

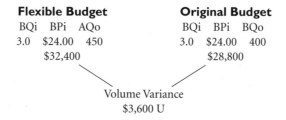

Flexible Budget			**Original Budget**		
BQi	BPi	AQo	BQi	BPi	BQo
3.0	$24.00	450	3.0	$24.00	400
	$32,400			$28,800	

Volume Variance
$3,600 U

At this point, the flexible budget can be compared to the actual results in order to find the flexible budget variance. First, restate the actual costs in terms of the notation:

Actual

$$AQi \times APi \times AQo$$
$$3.1 \times \$24.40 \times 450$$
$$\$34,038$$

Note that for the actual cost, the actual paid time per patient day, the actual price paid per hour, and the actual number of patient days are used. If desired, the flexible budget can be compared to the actual results to determine a *flexible budget variance:*

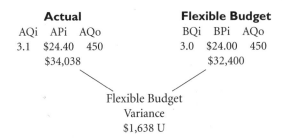

Actual			**Flexible Budget**		
AQi	APi	AQo	BQi	BPi	AQo
3.1	$24.40	450	3.0	$24.00	450
	$34,038			$32,400	

Flexible Budget
Variance
$1,638 U

The flexible budget variance is $1,638 U. If it is true, as has been asserted, that the total variance is simply being broken into its component parts, then it should be possible to combine the volume variance and the flexible budget variance and come out with the total variance. The difference between the original budget and the actual result is $5,238 (i.e., $34,038 − $28,800). Consider all the information available so far in notation form:

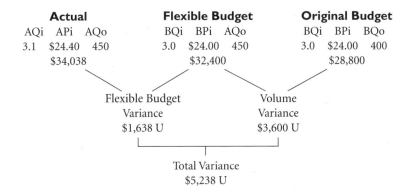

Actual			**Flexible Budget**			**Original Budget**		
AQi	APi	AQo	BQi	BPi	AQo	BQi	BPi	BQo
3.1	$24.40	450	3.0	$24.00	450	3.0	$24.00	400
	$34,038			$32,400			$28,800	

Flexible Budget　　　　　　Volume
Variance　　　　　　　　　Variance
$1,638 U　　　　　　　　　$3,600 U

Total Variance
$5,238 U

As can be seen, the total variance still is $5,238, but it has now been separated into a flexible budget variance and a volume variance. If the $1,638 U flexible budget variance is added to the $3,600 U volume variance, the result is the $5,238 total variance. The flexible budget variance is of greater concern to the nurse manager than is the volume variance. The volume variance results from changes in the workload. This is usually outside of the nurse manager's control. The flexible budget variance is caused by the difference between the budgeted and actual price per hour for nursing services and because of differences in the amount of nursing time per patient day. If possible, more should be found out about what makes up this variance.

In order to find out this extra information, it is necessary to derive something called a *subcategory.* This subcategory is simply a device to allow for separation of the flexible budget variance into two pieces: the price variance and the quantity variance. The subcategory is defined as the actual quantity of input per unit of output, multiplied by the budgeted price of the input, times the actual output level. In terms of the notation, the subcategory can be calculated as follows:

Subcategory

$$AQi \times BPi \times AQo$$
$$3.1 \times \$24.00 \times 450$$
$$\$33,480$$

If the subcategory calculation is compared to the actual costs, the price variance can be determined. First, consider the following:

Actual	**Subcategory**
$AQi \times APi \times AQo$	$AQi \times BQi \times AQo$

What is the difference between the actual and the subcategory calculations? The Qi, quantity of input per unit of output, is exactly the same for both; it is the actual value. The Qo, quantity of patient days, is exactly the same for both; it is the actual value. The price is different, however. The actual uses the actual price, while the subcategory uses the budgeted price. This is the only difference between the two. Therefore, if the actual amount spent does not equal the subcategory, it must be due to a difference between the price paid for the resource and the price budgeted.

Now insert numbers and see what that variance is:

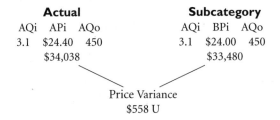

Actual			**Subcategory**		
AQi	APi	AQo	AQi	BPi	AQo
3.1	$24.40	450	3.1	$24.00	450
	$34,038			$33,480	

Price Variance
$558 U

The price variance of $558 U results from the fact that on average $24.40 was paid per hour for nursing time instead of the budgeted $24.00. It is possible that this occurs because of poor scheduling, which results in unnecessary overtime. On the other hand, perhaps it results from a larger raise for nursing personnel than the nurse manager had been told to put into the budget by the personnel department. Then again, look at the volume variance. Whenever there is a large unfavorable volume variance, it means that the workload was much greater than expected. Such unanticipated increases in workload put a great strain on nursing time, frequently requiring added overtime or the addition of high-priced agency nurses. All these possibilities should be investigated by the nurse manager.

What effect will added patient load have on the quantity of nursing time per patient? It is possible that busy nurses will tire and start to work slower. It is also possible that as patient volume increases, the nurses on staff will work harder to cover all of the patients. There may be a favorable variance or an unfavorable variance. Look at the quantity variance, first examining the relationship between the subcategory and the flexible budget:

Subcategory	**Flexible Budget**
$AQi \times BPi \times AQo$	$BQi \times BPi \times AQo$

What differences are observed between the subcategory and the flexible budget? The Pi, price per hour of nursing time, is the budgeted amount in both cases. The Qo, quantity of patient days, is the actual amount for both. The only difference between the two is in the Qi, quantity of nursing time per patient day. The flexible budget uses the budgeted time per patient day; the subcategory uses the actual paid nursing time per patient day. Any difference between the subcategory and the flexible budget must be related to the quantity of nursing time per patient. It is possible to insert values and calculate that variance:

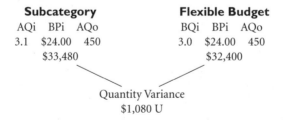

Subcategory			**Flexible Budget**		
AQi	BPi	AQo	BQi	BPi	AQo
3.1	$24.00	450	3.0	$24.00	450
	$33,480			$32,400	

Quantity Variance
$1,080 U

The quantity variance of $1,080 U can be explained in a number of ways. It is possible that because of the substantial increase in patient days above expectations, many part-time nurses were hired. These nurses were unfamiliar with the institution and therefore were not as efficient as the regular nurses. Another possibility is that the population was sicker than anticipated and required more care. Of course, there is also the possibility that supervision was lax and that time was simply being wasted. Again, variance information can only point out the direction; the manager must make the final determination regarding why the variance occurred and how to avoid it in the future.

In order to use flexible budgeting, one should have an idea of how the pieces fit together. Review the price and quantity variances, looking at how they together comprise the flexible budget variance:

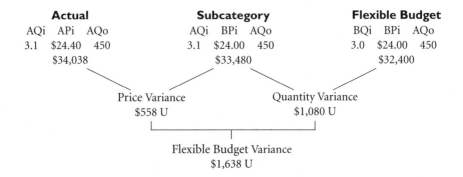

Notice that combining the price variance of $558 U and the quantity variance of $1,080 U results in the flexible budget variance. Recall that the flexible budget variance and volume variance add up to the total variance. Figure 13–1 shows that the three individual variances—price, quantity, and volume—add up to the total variance for the line item.

Recall that without flexible budgets, the total variance for the line item would be the only piece of information available for analysis. There was an unfavorable variance of $5,238. Using Figure 13–1, it is possible to determine at the outset that of this total variance, $3,600 was caused by the increase in patient days. It is now also known that $558 of the variance was caused by having paid a higher average rate to the nurses than was anticipated and that $1,080 of the variance was caused by a longer average amount of nursing time per patient day than had been anticipated. Why these specific variances occurred is not known, but there is a much better focus on where the problem areas are.

A generic model for flexible budgeting variances is presented in Figure 13–2. In looking at this model, several things should be kept in mind. First of all, recall that basically all the necessary data is generally readily available. Second, the accounting and information systems departments can calculate all these variances when they do monthly variance reports. If they are not willing to do so, then it is possible to either calculate these variances by hand or on a computer.

It sometimes is not obvious whether a variance is favorable or unfavorable. Looking at Figure 13–2, an easy rule of thumb is that as one moves from the right side toward the left, larger numbers on the left indicate unfavorable variance. For example, if the flexible budget amount is larger than the originally budgeted amount, the volume variance is unfavorable. If the subcategory is greater than the flexible budget, the quantity variance is unfavorable. This is true because as one

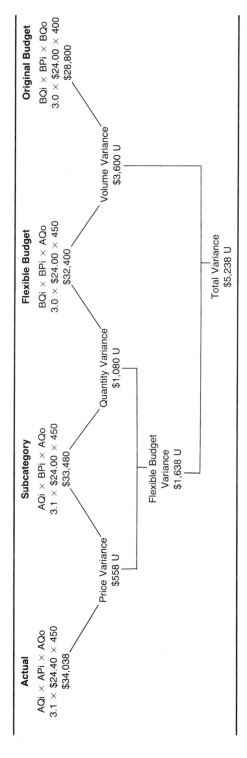

FIGURE 13–1. Price, quantity, and volume variances for 6th Floor West.

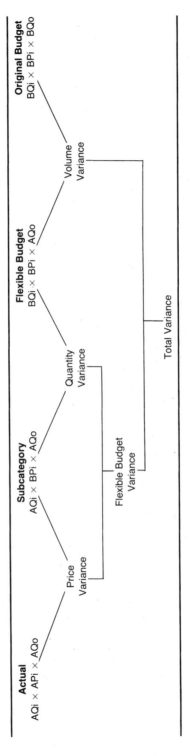

FIGURE 13–2. Price, quantity, and volume variances for a generic model.

moves from the original budget toward the left, movement is toward the actual result. If the actual result is larger than the original budget, then more was spent than budgeted. The result is an unfavorable variance. Given the way this model is set up, this also holds true for each of the individual variances making up the total variance.

REVENUE VARIANCES

The nurse manager's primary variance analysis effort focuses on expenses. This is predominantly because managers of health care organizations have a greater degree of control over expenses than they do over revenues. However, the information that can be yielded from revenue variance analysis is also important. For example, changes in revenue that result from changes in patient volume may be outside the control of the organization and its managers. Such changes, however, may require management actions or reactions to protect the organization's financial position.

Revenue variance methodology follows the same pattern as expense methodology. There is a traditional variance that tends to focus on the total revenue expected and actually achieved for a unit or department. There is also a flexible budget methodology that helps to identify the various underlying causes of variances. The total revenue variance for a unit, department, or organization can be broken down into a volume variance, a mix variance, and a price variance.

Consider an outpatient surgery department that has budgeted revenues of $1 million for the month just ended. Actual revenues were $850,000. Traditional variance analysis identifies a $150,000 unfavorable revenue variance. What caused the $150,000 shortfall?

The first step for flexible budget revenue variance analysis would be to identify the revenue per patient. Unlike costs, which may be fixed or variable, revenues are often all variable. Therefore the total $1 million budget could be divided by the number of patients budgeted to get an average revenue per patient. This allows calculation of a volume variance. Suppose that 800 patients were expected for the month. In that case the average revenue per patient was expected to be $1,250 (i.e., the $1 million total revenue divided by 800 patients = $1,250 of revenue per patient). See Figure 13–3.

If there were actually only 750 patients, then a flexible budget for revenue of $937,500 (i.e., 750 patients × $1,250 price) would be calculated. The revenue flexible budget indicates the amount of revenue that would have been budgeted if the number of patients had been forecast exactly correctly. The difference between the original budget for 800 patients and the flexible budget for 750 actual patients is an unfavorable volume variance of $62,500. Less revenue than expected is considered unfavorable.

The next calculation concerns the mix of patients. Not all patients would be expected to be charged $1,250. That figure represents an average. Assume that half the patients were expected to be type A patients charged $1,000 and half were

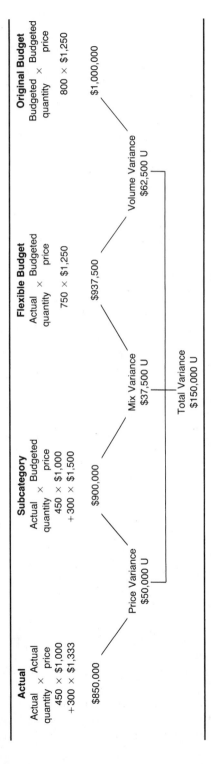

FIGURE 13–3. Revenue variances.

expected to be type B patients charged $1,500. Any number of different types of patients with different prices is possible, but for this discussion we will limit it to just types A and B.

Suppose that of the 750 actual patients, 450 were type A and 300 were type B. Not only are there fewer patients than expected, but the mix of patients has changed as well. Less than half the patients are the more highly priced type B patients. Based on the actual number of patients and the actual mix, revenues would be expected to be $900,000 (i.e., 450 patients @ $1,000 + 300 patients @ $1,500). If we compare the flexible budget of $937,500 (what revenue would have been expected to be for 750 patients) to this new "subcategory" value based on the actual mix, the difference is $37,500. This is the mix variance, which is unfavorable. The variance is unfavorable because there is a greater proportion of lower-revenue patients.

This still leaves an unexplained variance of $50,000. This is a price variance. It is a result of charging a different price than expected. Although the outpatient surgery intended to charge $1,500 for type B patients, it is possible that because of government regulation or negotiated rates with insurance companies, the average price for type B patients was only $1,333.33. In that case actual revenue would be $850,000 (i.e., 450 patients @ $1,000 + 300 patients @ $1,333.33). The $50,000 difference between the $900,000 from the mix calculation is an unfavorable price variance. It is unfavorable because the price was less than budgeted.

The calculations for these variances can be seen in Figure 13–3. Note that in each case the number of patients is multiplied by the price per patient. For the budget and flexible budget the total number of patients and the budgeted average price per patient are used. For the subcategory, the mix of patients is used, splitting the total into the number of actual patients of each type. For the subcategory the budgeted price for each type of patient is used. For the actual costs the actual number of each type of patient and the actual prices for each type of patient are used.

Often revenue variances are calculated based on the contribution margin rather than the revenue. (See Chapter 4 for a discussion of contribution margin.) Revenue places too great a focus on the total charge for different types of patients rather than on the profit implications of each type patient. A patient with high revenue could have even greater expenses and cause losses. Another patient with only modest revenues could be quite profitable. Managers do not just need information about changes in revenues. They need to know whether the revenue changes are in profitable areas or unprofitable ones.

It is possible therefore to use the budgeted contribution margin rather than the revenue in all the calculations just discussed. There still would be a volume variance. Fewer patients would imply less overall contribution margin. There still would be a mix variance. However, whether the mix variance is favorable or unfavorable would depend on whether there is a greater or lesser proportion of the types of patients with higher contribution margins. The price variance would still depend on the actual price charged for each type of patient.

Knowing whether variances are caused by changes in prices, the mix of patients, or the volume of patients is important information that managers can use in taking actions to respond to increases or decreases in revenues. If the number of patients is falling, then steps should be taken to find out why and to make sure that there are corresponding reductions in organizational expenses. If the mix of patients is changing, it may be necessary to shift resources within the organization. If prices differed from budget, an effort must be made to understand why it occurred and its overall implications for the organization's finances.

SUMMARY AND IMPLICATIONS
FOR NURSE MANAGERS

Budgeting is a process of planning and controlling. If a budget is prepared but is not used to control results, a substantial part of the potential benefit of budgeting is lost. The key issue to remember, however, is that organizations do not control costs, people do.

The difference between the budget and what actually occurs is called a variance. Comparing actual results to budgeted expectations and analyzing the resulting variances should be done monthly. This can allow for midstream corrections that will improve the year-end results. It also provides information for preparing the coming year's budget, and for evaluating units, departments, and managers' performance.

Many health care organizations prepare variance reports by comparing the information in the original budget to the actual results. There are several problems with that type of comparison. First, it does not tell as much about the cause of the variance as one would like to know; for instance, traditional variance analysis does not indicate whether a variance is caused by more resource use per patient or by higher prices for resources used. Second, traditional variance analysis ignores the fact that resource consumption would be expected to vary with workload volume. One can compare the budgeted cost for an expected patient volume to the actual cost for the actual patient volume. Part of the variance, therefore, will just be the result of changes in workload levels, rather than being related to efficiency.

This has caused many health care organizations to start using a method called flexible budgeting. Flexible budgeting establishes an after-the-fact budget; that is, what it would have been expected to cost had the actual workload been known in advance. Using flexible budgets, it is possible to break a unit or department's line-item expense variances down into components caused by (1) changes in prices or salary rates from those expected; (2) changes in the amount of input used per unit of workload or output, such as the amount of nursing time per patient day; and (3) changes in the workload volume itself. It is also possible to divide revenue variances into the portion caused by volume, mix, or price changes.

Managerial expertise and judgment are still needed to investigate and evaluate the variances that are determined by using flexible budgeting. Ultimately, this technique can make the manager's job easier by segregating the variance into its component parts. This allows the manager to spend more time understanding and explaining why the variance occurred.

SUGGESTED READINGS

Bautista, C.L. (1994). Meeting the challenge of cost containment: A case study using variance analysis. *Hospital Cost Management & Accounting.* 6(2), 1–8.

Cavouras, C.A., and McKinley, J. (1997, May). Variable budgeting for staffing analysis and evaluation. *Nursing Management.* 28(5), 34–36, 39.

Douglas, D.A., and Mayewske, J. (1996, February). Census variation staffing. *Nursing Management.* 27(2), 32–33, 36.

Felteau, A. (1992, February). Budget variance analysis and justification. *Nursing Management.* 23(2), 40–41.

Finkler, S.A. (1996). Flexible budgeting allows for better management of resources as needs change. *Hospital Cost Management & Accounting.* 8(3), 1–5.

Finkler, S.A. (1991). Variance analysis. Part I: Extending flexible budget variance analysis to acuity. *Journal of Nursing Administration.* 21(7/8), 19–25.

Finkler, S.A. (1991). Variance analysis. Part II: The use of computers. *Journal of Nursing Administration.* 21(9), 9–15.

Finkler, S.A., and Ward, D.R. (1999). *Cost Accounting for Health Care Organizations: Concepts and Applications,* Second edition. Gaithersburg, MD: Aspen Publishers.

Horngren, C.T., Foster, G., and Datar, S.M. (1999). *Cost Accounting: A Managerial Emphasis,* Tenth edition. Englewood Cliffs, NJ: Prentice-Hall.

Maitland, D. (1993). Flexible budgeting and variance analysis: Why leave staff nurses in the dark? *Hospital Cost Management Accounting.* 5(9), 1–8.

Swansburg, R.C. (1997). *Budgeting and Financial Management for Nurse Managers.* Boston: Jones & Bartlett Publishers.

Wilburn, D. (1992, February). Budget response to volume variability. *Nursing Management.* 23(2), 42–45.

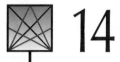

14

Variance Analysis

EXAMPLES, EXTENSIONS, AND CAVEATS

The goals of this chapter are to:

provide additional variance analysis examples;

provide insight into the problems encountered when variance information is aggregated;

introduce the concept of exception reports and explain their benefits;

explore further the interpretation of variances;

explain how flexible budgeting can be used even if staffing patterns are rigid;

provide a tool for determining the variance due to changes in patient acuity;

reiterate the dependence of flexible budget variance analysis on variable costs;

discuss causes of variances;

discuss when a variance is large enough to warrant managerial attention and investigation; and

discuss variance analysis as related to performance budgeting.

INTRODUCTION

Chapter 13 presented the basic mechanics of flexible budgeting. Although the topic has tremendous potential value, it may be new to even those readers with substantial experience as managers. This chapter provides several exercises to help the reader become more familiar with the notation and process of flexible budget variance analysis. Flexible budgets differ from original budgets because some costs are variable. Those costs should be expected to change as workload levels change. Therefore, one may have questions regarding how to integrate flexible budgets with fairly rigid staffing patterns. Integration of acuity measures into flexible budgeting will be of interest to many as well. These extensions are discussed in this chapter. Finally, issues concerning fixed versus variable costs, the causes of variances, and variance investigation and control, and variance analysis of performance budgets are addressed in the last part of this chapter.

AGGREGATION PROBLEMS

The Nearby Hospital had the following results for labor costs for the last month:

Salary	Actual	Original Budget	Variance
All departments	$499,700	$500,000	$300F

Should the hospital administrator investigate this variance? Is more information about the variance required? Your immediate reaction is probably to leave well enough alone. The total amount of the variance is small—and favorable at that. Why worry about a $300 variance?

The problem with these results is that when variances are combined, there is a tendency to lose information. Some of the favorable and unfavorable variances may offset each other. The net result is small, and the two variances cannot be observed. For example, assume that the departmental breakdown of the $300 variance was as follows:

Salary	Actual	Original Budget	Variance
Operating Room	$150,000	$125,000	$25,000 U
Dietary	100,000	125,000	25,000 F
Nursing	124,900	125,000	100 F
Lab	124,800	125,000	200 F
Totals	$499,700	$500,000	$ 300 F

Given this extra information, it becomes apparent that it would be a mistake not to investigate further. In this case, which departments need to be investigated? It is fairly obvious that one should be especially concerned with the operating room. And, even though the dietary variance is favorable, it would probably be wise to find out what is happening in that department as well.

However, focus attention on the nursing department. Suppose that the following information for the nursing department is available[1]:

---

[1]Recall that our notation from Chapter 13 was as follows:
BPi: *budgeted price* per unit of *input*
BQi: *budgeted quantity* of *input* for each unit of output
BQo: *budgeted quantity* of *output*
APi: *actual price* paid per unit of *input*
AQi: *actual quantity* of *input* for each unit of output produced
AQo: *actual quantity* of *output*

BPi:	Budgeted nursing rate is $20.00 per hour
BQi:	2.5 hours of budgeted nursing time per patient day
BQo:	2,500 budgeted patient days
AQo:	2,000 actual patient days
Budgeted Total Cost:	$125,000
Actual Total Cost:	$124,900

Although the variance for the nursing department is only $100 and is favorable, the number of patient days is down substantially from expectations.

What variances can be calculated? Is all the desired information available? What is meant by a favorable variance in this context? The original budgeted cost was $125,000, and the actual cost was $124,900. It would appear that everything is fine, since there is a $100 favorable variance. However, it would be nice to calculate the price, quantity, and volume variances to see if everything is in fact okay.

To calculate a volume variance, it is first necessary to determine the flexible budget (i.e., the amount that would have been budgeted if the actual workload level had been predicted accurately). The flexible budget is the budgeted quantity of input, multiplied by the budgeted price of inputs, multiplied by the actual quantity of output. Information about all those variables is available, and the volume variance can be calculated as follows:

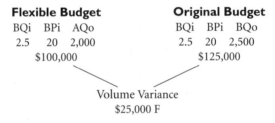

Flexible Budget

BQi	BPi	AQo
2.5	20	2,000

$100,000

Original Budget

BQi	BPi	BQo
2.5	20	2,500

$125,000

Volume Variance
$25,000 F

The volume variance is a favorable $25,000. This means that the workload was down substantially. If it is assumed that nursing staff costs are variable (this assumption will be relaxed later in the chapter), then a volume variance should be accompanied by reduced spending. For most hospitals, a reduction in patient days from the expected level would often be an *unfavorable* event. It probably means that admissions and revenues are down substantially. It is called a *favorable* variance because treating fewer patients implies that less would be spent. However, that does not mean that something *good* has happened. It is important for managers to be aware of favorable volume variances as quickly as possible, so that adjustments can be made to staffing if necessary.

In order to calculate price and quantity variances, it is necessary to be able to calculate the subcategory value. This requires multiplying the actual quantity of input by the budgeted price by the actual quantity of output. Information on the actual quantity of input was not given, so it is not possible to calculate the subcategory value. However, the actual spending can be compared to the flexible budget to determine a flexible budget variance.

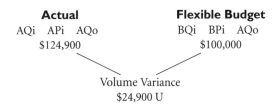

Actual

AQi APi AQo
$124,900

Flexible Budget

BQi BPi AQo
$100,000

Volume Variance
$24,900 U

This variance is unfavorable. It is not known why it has occurred, and there is not enough information here to break this variance into its price and quantity components. It is possible, however, that the reduced patient load was not accompanied by reduced staffing. If staffing was kept virtually the same, the amount of nursing time available per patient day would rise and an unfavorable quantity variance would occur. This means that workload and possibly revenue is falling but that costs are not decreasing. This would mean financial losses would occur.

The point of this example is not to be able to determine what really happened at Nearby Hospital but to get a good understanding of the problems that get buried when variances are aggregated and evaluated in total. When the overall variance for the hospital was examined, the offsetting variances in the operating room and dietary departments were not apparent. Variance information for each department separately is needed. One would certainly want to investigate the large unfavorable variance in the operating room and, even though it is favorable, would probably want to determine what caused the large favorable variance in the dietary department as well.

However, looking at department variances did not point out the problem within the nursing department. It is possible that different units in the nursing department might have variances that would offset each other. So it is really necessary to look at variances for each unit. Within a nursing unit, it is possible that an unfavorable salary variance could be offset by a favorable supply variance. Managers must look at each line item of each unit. Traditional variance analysis would allow that.

In this example, however, falling patient volume was offset by a flexible budget variance. A manager who simply examined the line-item variance for nursing salaries in a particular nursing unit would not be aware of that problem. Only by using flexible budget variance analysis can the manager get more information about what is going on within a line item. Once managers have such information, they can investigate the variances. In this example, the flexible budget variance might have been the result of a failure to reduce staffing as workload decreased. It might have been the result of a salary rate increase. It might have been the result of a change in patient mix. The expertise of the manager is needed to make the final determination. However, the ability of managers to use their knowledge and expertise is substantially enhanced if price, quantity, and volume variances are calculated for each line item for each unit.

EXCEPTION REPORTING

Aggregation problems create substantial difficulty. The only way to be sure that one variance is not being offset by another variance is by examining every single price, quantity, and volume variance, of every single line item of every single unit of every single department of the hospital. This creates a potentially unmanageable burden. Should the Chief Executive Officer (CEO) of the hospital have to examine every individual variance for the entire organization? Should the Chief Nurse Executive (CNE) have to examine every individual variance for all units of the nursing department? The time required would be enormous. A solution to this problem is the use of *exception reports*.

Assuming a computer prepares all the variances for each cost element, it is a simple process to have the computer prepare a list for the CEO of only those individual variances that exceed a certain limit. This is called an exception report. It only lists the variances that are large. How large depends on the desires of the individual CEO. When tight, centralized control is desired, smaller variances are of interest. For example, while some CEOs might be interested only in monthly or year-to-date variances that are greater than 20% of the budget or $50,000, a CEO running a more centralized operation might be interested in variances greater than 10% or $10,000.

This does not mean that variances less than $10,000 must go unnoticed. Each department head, such as the CNE, would get a report for their department at a more detailed level, perhaps 5% or $1,000. Continuing the process, nurse managers would receive detailed exception reports for the variances in units under their supervision. Ultimately, the nurse manager who has direct control over a unit would want to review all variances for that unit. In all cases, if a nurse manager feels that a particular variance indicates a problem that is likely to grow worse in future months, the higher levels of nursing administration should be alerted to the problem rather than waiting until the variance is great enough to appear on the CNE's exception report.

INTERPRETATION OF VARIANCES

Assume that you are the nursing administrator for a medical group. This may be either a fee-for-service organization or a prepaid-group practice. Suppose that the organization is expecting a severe outbreak of the Hoboken flu this winter, so it has hired extra agency nurses to treat the patients and administer shots. The budgeted expectation was that 1,000 hours of part-time services would be needed at $40.00 per hour, for a total cost of $40,000. It was also expected that the part-time nurses would average a half hour for each of 2,000 patients. The results at the end of the flu season are as follows:

Salary	Actual	Original Budget	Variance
Part-time nurses	$50,000	$40,000	$10,000

Would this be considered to be a favorable or unfavorable variance? On the surface, more was spent than was expected; therefore, it would be recorded as an unfavorable variance from an accounting viewpoint. The physician director of the medical group may well be complaining about the total lack of budget control exhibited by the unexpected $10,000 excess cost. At this stage, however, there is more to the variance than simply what was expected to be spent and what was actually spent. Consider how much work was done for the $50,000 actually spent.

Suppose that 2,600 patients were actually treated by the part-time nurses, who worked a total of 1,200 hours. What are the variances that can be computed from this information? The original budget is $40,000 and the actual cost was $50,000. The number of patients actually treated was 2,600, the budgeted time per patient was one-half hour, and the budgeted hourly rate was $40.00. Therefore, the flexible budget would be $52,000 ($\frac{1}{2} \times \$40 \times 2,600$). The subcategory would compare the actual quantity of hours to treat the actual number of patients at the budgeted hourly rate of $40.00. The actual time taken to treat the actual number of patients has been given as 1,200 hours. For 2,600 patients to be treated in 1,200 hours, an average of 0.461 hours must have been used per patient (1,200 hours divided by 2,600 patients = 0.461 hours per patient). Therefore, the subcategory is $48,000 (0.461 hours per patient $\times$ $40 per hour $\times$ 2,600 patients).

The resulting variances are shown in Figure 14–1. Although the actual wage rate is not known, it is known that the actual costs were $50,000. The rate variance is $2,000 U, the quantity variance is $4,000 F, and the volume variance is $12,000 U. Let's discuss the volume variance first, since it is the largest. That variance is attributable to the fact that there were 2,600 patients instead of the expected 2,000 patients.

Is this result good or bad for the organization? What is the likely effect of these extra patients on revenues? If the medical group is a *prepaid-group plan*, such as an HMO, the volume variance is bad news. It means that the number of patients treated has gone up substantially without any increase in revenue. On the other hand, if it is a *fee-for-service* organization, the extra cost will be associated with

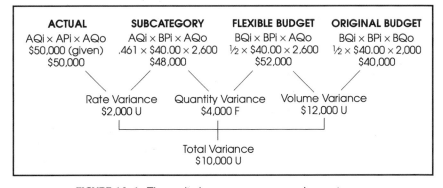

FIGURE 14–1. The medical group agency nurse salary variances.

increased billings. The number of patients treated is 30% greater than expected. Therefore, even if the actual costs were $12,000 more than the budgeted $40,000, the organization would be better off, if it makes a profit on each patient.

In any case, a clear argument can be made that the portion of the unfavorable variance caused by increased patient flow is beyond the control and therefore beyond the responsibility of the nursing administrator.

What about the two remaining variances—the $2,000 unfavorable rate variance and the $4,000 favorable quantity variance? Certainly, one can come up with several possible scenarios. For instance, because more part-time hours were needed than had been expected, some experienced RNs were hired rather than just new graduates (i.e., there were not enough new graduates available to fill the need). The experienced RNs, however, were so skillful that their higher wage rate (resulting in the unfavorable rate variance) was more than offset by the speedy efficiency with which they worked (resulting in the favorable quantity variance). If this was in fact the case, the organization should learn for the future that it may be more cost-effective to use experienced RNs.

An alternative scenario would be that the rate variance was simply the result of overtime wages. Once the patients started coming, there was not enough time to hire anyone else, so the organization just worked the agency nurses it had for longer hours, resulting in an overtime premium. However, the overtime premium that caused the rate variance was more than offset by the fact that there were so many patients that the nurses never had idle time. Because some idle time had been built into the budget, the favorable quantity variance resulted.

This can also tell something about the future. Perhaps the nurses were thrilled that they did not have to sit around bored. In this case, next time fewer nurses should be hired and they should be kept relatively busy. On the other hand, one possible implication of a favorable quantity variance is a reduced level of quality of care, with each patient receiving less time and attention. Reduced quality of care will normally show up as a favorable quantity variance. If quality of care suffered, one would want to avoid that situation in the future. Another possibility is that the nurses worked hard and fast (the patients were lined up right out into the hall, so it was continuous work), but they are so mad at being overworked that they will never work for the organization again. A "favorable" quantity variance does not always mean favorable things for the organization.

Nothing can be concluded for certain about the rate and quantity variances for the medical group because the reader was not actually there and knows little about the organization. A really useful variance report can only be developed by someone with knowledge of the specific situation. The value of flexible budgeting, however, should be reasonably clear.

The methodology does help to separate out the elements that are totally beyond the unit or manager's control, such as the number of patients. It is then possible to see clearly the magnitude of the rate and quantity variances. If they are substantial, the manager can turn attention to finding out why they occurred. This information is needed for two reasons: first, so that the organization can be managed more efficiently in the future, and second, so that the manager can reasonably defend the way the department or unit was run.

RIGID STAFFING PATTERNS

The medical group example presents an extreme in that nurses were hired by the hour. Flexible budgeting makes the assumption that if one more patient is treated, it is possible to consume just one more tongue depressor, one-quarter roll more of bandage tape, or one-half hour more of nursing time. This may be true in the case of tongue depressors and bandage tape, but it implies a lot more flexibility of nurse staffing than most organizations have.

Health care organizations often have some flexibility to transfer nurses from one shift to another or from a unit with a temporarily low occupancy to one with a higher occupancy. In some cases, however, such flexibility may be limited. This is particularly the case at unionized organizations with strong work rules. The key to flexible budgeting is that if the workload (such as patient days) increases or decreases, costs should increase or decrease as well. But nursing costs cannot be reduced if patient days are just one or two fewer than expected. Nurse staffing tends to be variable only if there are more substantial workload changes.

Suppose that a department has rigid work rules. No nurses can be shifted into or out of the department. Either new nurses are hired or nurses are let go if the patient volume changes significantly. Obviously, for small changes in workload, a manager will not change staffing levels. However, flexible budget variance analysis can still be used.

For simplicity's sake, this example examines variances for an entire year, using annual FTEs and annual salaries. (In practice, one would want to find the variances on a monthly basis.) Suppose that the staffing pattern is as follows:

Staffing Guide	
FTEs (RNs)	**Patient Days**
4	0– 6,000
5	6,001– 7,000
6	7,001– 8,000
7	8,001– 9,000
8	9,001–10,000

Further assume that for the year just past:

	Actual	**Original Budget**	**Variance**
Nurses salaries	$286,000	$320,000	$34,000 F

Also assume for that year, that:

Expected patient days   = 10,000
Expected salary per FTE = $40,000
Actual patient days   = 7,750
Actual salary   = $44,000
Actual FTEs   = 6.5

Although the variance is listed as $34,000 F, one can readily see from the Staffing Guide that for the actual workload of 7,750 patient days, staffing should have been 6 FTEs. The so-called favorable variance may largely stem from a volume variance, and there may be underlying price and quantity variances that would warrant investigation.

With a rigid staffing guide, there is no need to find both the quantity of input per unit of output (Q_i) and the quantity of output (Q_o) and then multiply these to find the total quantity of input. The staffing guide can be used to simplify this process.

The original budget is concerned solely with budgeted amounts. At the BQ_o of 10,000 patient days, the staffing guide calls for 8 FTEs. This can be referred to as the TBQ (total budgeted quantity of input). If the TBQ is multiplied times the budgeted price per FTE, the result is the original budget (see Fig. 14–2).

Both the actual results and the subcategory are based on the actual quantity amounts. In this example, the actual total quantity consumed is 6.5 FTEs. Refer to that as the TAQ (total actual quantity of input). If the TAQ is multiplied times the actual price per FTE, the result is the actual; if TAQ is multiplied by the budgeted price per FTE, the result is the subcategory value.

The flexible budget is what would have been budgeted had the actual workload level been known. In this case, patient days were actually 7,750. According to the staffing guide, 6 FTEs should have been used for that number of patient days. Refer to that as the TBAQ (total budgeted quantity of input for the actual quantity of output). If TBAQ is multiplied by the budgeted price per FTE, the result is the flexible budget.

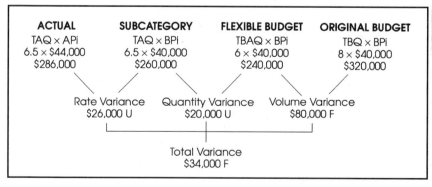

FIGURE 14–2. Rate, quantity, and volume variances with rigid staffing.

Looking at Figure 14–2, the variances can now be found. Notice that the Pi shown in each case is the cost per FTE, not per hour of nursing time. This is necessary because of the rigid nature of the staffing patterns, where quantity measures are given as the number of FTEs rather than in hours.

Figure 14–2 indicates that the actual cost of $286,000 came about because 6.5 FTEs were used at an actual rate of $44,000 each. The same quantity of nursing labor (6.5 FTEs) at the budgeted salary of $40,000 per FTE would have cost $260,000. There is a $26,000 rate variance due to the fact that the average salary paid exceeded expectations by $4,000 per FTE. The flexible budget next compares the actual amount of labor used with the amount of labor that would have been budgeted had the actual number of patient days been known in advance. Thus it is seen that there was a $20,000 unfavorable variance as a result of having used 0.5 FTE more than would have been budgeted for 7,750 patient days.

The largest variance is the volume variance. This is a favorable variance only in the sense that the unit expected to need 8 FTEs for 10,000 patient days. In fact, the unit should have needed only 6 FTEs for 7,750 patient days. If the manager had reacted immediately, $80,000 less would have been spent. Spending less implies a favorable variance even if the workload decline is bad for the organization.

Now the results can be evaluated in the same way as if nurses could be moved around by the hour, but one must be cognizant of the implications of the staffing pattern. The volume variance is not of much interest, assuming that it is outside the manager's control. This may not always be the case. There are situations in which poor management can keep beds empty when there are patients waiting to fill them. In such cases, the volume variance may be at least partly a nursing responsibility.

The quantity variance is of some concern. Did the nurse manager of this unit do a good or bad job in controlling staffing costs? Despite the large unfavorable variance, there is strong reason to believe that the manager did a reasonably good job. In order to come down to 6 FTEs, a full 25% of the unit's staffing had to be either laid off or permanently reassigned elsewhere. Given the high costs associated with attracting, training, and retaining qualified nurses, a manager must be most reluctant to let a nurse go unless there is evidence that a downturn in patient days is not merely a passing aberration but rather a permanent trend. Finishing the year with additional consumption of only 0.5 FTE would appear to indicate that the manager sized up the situation and acted reasonably quickly.

What about the price variance? Certainly, if it is the result of overtime or unexpected shift-differential increases, that might indicate poor scheduling control, in light of the decrease in patient days. A much more plausible explanation is that the two nurses who were released had the least seniority and the lowest pay rate. The six nurses who were retained are likely to have been earning a higher rate. This would raise the average rate and therefore cause the price variance.

Thus, even in the case where staffing patterns are relatively rigid, managers can still benefit from flexible budget variance analysis.

FLEXIBLE BUDGETING AND ACUITY

Acuity measures can lead to substantial improvements in budgeting and reimbursement. The budgeting improvements stem from the recognition of the fact that different patients require different amounts of nursing care. If patient acuity can be measured and predicted, then the amount of staffing budgeted can be adjusted, based not simply on the number of patients or patient days but also on the degree of illness of the patients and their likely requirement for nursing inputs.

If acuity is used in preparing the operating budget, then acuity should be included when that budget is used as a tool for control. If average acuity is different from the expected level, then it is logical that resource consumption in terms of nursing requirements will also differ from the budgeted amount.

Acuity can be built into variance analysis through the flexible budget model (Fig. 14–3). Begin on the right-hand side of the figure with the original budget. The budgeted quantity of input per unit of output, BQi, has been replaced by BQiBA, which is the budgeted quantity of input per unit of output at the *budgeted acuity level.* In other words, BQiBA is the amount of nursing time budgeted per patient day, assuming a particular expected acuity level. The BPi and BQo are the same as in the earlier model.

Moving to the left is the flexible budget. The only change between the original budget and the flexible budget is that the budgeted quantity of output has been replaced with the actual quantity of output. Thus, the flexible budget indicates what the cost would have been expected to be had the actual output level (e.g., number of patient days) been known when the budget was being prepared. This assumes that the model is using the actual output level but the expected acuity level. The difference between the original and flexible budgets is the volume variance.

The next category is a new one—the acuity subcategory. The price of inputs

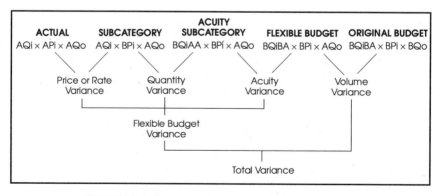

FIGURE 14–3. Rate, quantity, acuity, and volume variances.

and the quantity of outputs are the same for the flexible budget and the acuity subcategory. However, the flexible budget uses the budgeted quantity of input per unit of output for the budgeted acuity level, BQiBA. The acuity subcategory uses the budgeted quantity of input per unit of output for the actual acuity level, BQiAA. The difference between the flexible budget and the acuity subcategory is called the acuity variance.

The acuity subcategory represents what would have been budgeted for the actual output and acuity. The flexible budget represents what would have been budgeted for the actual output level, using a budgeted acuity level. Because the quantity of output in both cases is the actual and the price of inputs in both cases is the budgeted, the difference between these two categories must be attributable to the fact that the actual and budgeted acuity levels do not agree. If the acuity subcategory is larger than the flexible budget, the actual acuity was greater than expected. The logical outcome of greater acuity is that there would be a need to consume more resources. The result is an unfavorable acuity variance.

Moving to the left, next is the subcategory, which is the same as the subcategory that has been used up until now. The AQi (actual quantity of input per unit of output), inherently represents the actual quantity of input per unit of output for the actual acuity level. The resulting quantity variance tells whether more or less input per unit of output was used than expected, given the actual acuity level. The price variance is unchanged.

It is important to note that if the price, quantity, acuity, and volume variances are totaled, the result is the same total variance as it would have been without using acuity in the model. Additional amounts of variance have not been added. Rather, the variance is subdivided so that the causes of the overall variance can be more easily determined. Where did the acuity variance come from? Until this discussion, the acuity variance was buried in the quantity variance. What has been done here is to separate the quantity variance into the part caused by a change in acuity and the remainder, resulting from other causes.

This is a significant separation if in fact nursing resources are supposed to be added as acuity increases. Suppose that the department has an unfavorable overall variance. How did that variance arise? The part of it caused simply by increased patient days (the volume variance) or by a larger than anticipated hourly raise (the rate variance) can be identified. But what if most of the unfavorable variance resides in the quantity variance? Was that unfavorable variance the result of factors beyond the control of the nurse manager?

With Figure 14–3, it is possible to separate the portion caused by an unexpected change in the acuity level. Thus, it is a little easier to determine if the remaining quantity variance is the result of *controllable* or *uncontrollable* events. The reader should keep in mind that the quantity and acuity variances combined in Figure 14–3 would equal the quantity variance if the acuity component was not being segregated.

FIXED VERSUS VARIABLE COSTS

The basic approach surrounding flexible budgeting is that the original budget assumes a specific level of workload, such as a fixed number of patient days. If the actual level differs from that expected, the amount of resources consumed would change. The starting point for a flexible budget analysis, therefore, is that it is expected that resources will be consumed in some direct relationship to output. However, with respect to fixed costs, this is not the case.

By definition, a fixed cost is one that does not vary with the level of output. Examples include the depreciation on a hospital building or the salary paid to a nurse manager. These costs do not change in proportion to the number of patients or patient days. This does not mean that they will not have any variances. They may well have variances. However, no part of the variance can be related specifically to any workload volume measure. As a result, there cannot be a volume variance.

Furthermore, in the case of fixed costs, it may be difficult to determine what portion of the variance represents a price variance and what portion a quantity variance. In some cases, price and quantity variances can be calculated for fixed costs. The cost of heating a clinic can be evaluated in terms of the price of fuel and the quantity of fuel. In many cases, however, there will be only one variance for fixed cost items. Although flexible budgeting can be very helpful in the case of costs that vary with output levels, the reader should be aware of this limitation with respect to fixed costs.

CAUSES OF VARIANCES

Throughout the last several chapters, there have been numerous examples of variances and suppositions as to what might have caused them. It is important to be aware of the fact that variance analysis is only a tool to point the right direction. The nurse manager must make the investigation and final determination of what caused a variance to arise.

Common internal causes of variances include shifts in quality of care provided, changes in technology being used, changes in the efficiency of the nurses, changes in organization policy, or simply incorrect standards. Variance analysis can highlight a quantity variance, but it cannot indicate whether quality of care is improving or if coffee breaks are getting longer. Both might show up as an unfavorable quantity variance. Poor staff scheduling may be resulting in undue overtime, or pay raises may have increased labor costs. Both would show up as an unfavorable rate variance.

External causes of variances commonly include price changes for supplies, volume changes in workload, and unexpected shifts in the availability of staff. Flexible budgeting is somewhat more helpful in these cases than with the internally caused variances. Shifts in workload can be isolated in the volume variance. Going over budget on supplies can be isolated in the price variance, if the problem is in the purchasing department as opposed to lax nursing control over the quantity of supplies used.

In any event, flexible budget variance analysis can greatly ease the problem of determining the cause of a department's overall variance. It can even simplify the problem of determining the cause of the variance in any one specific line item. However, the final responsibility for determining the cause of the variance ultimately rests on the shoulders of the nurse manager.

INVESTIGATION AND CONTROL OF VARIANCES

Probably the most difficult aspect of variance analysis is determining when a variance is large enough to warrant investigation. As has been shown in this chapter, even a small variance can be hiding significant problems when variances are aggregated. But suppose that variances have not been aggregated and information is available on each individual price, quantity, and volume variance for each cost element. Should a manager investigate $5, $50, $100, or $1,000 variances? How big a variance is too big to tolerate without investigation?

It must be kept in mind that budgets are "guesstimates" of the future. They cannot be expected to come out exactly on target. Small variances can generally be ignored. Hopefully, over the course of a year, the small unfavorable variances will be balanced out by small favorable variances.

This still does not tell when to investigate a variance. Unfortunately, there is no set answer. The solution favored by this author is as follows: when a manager looks at a variance, it should be assumed that it will occur in the same amount month after month until the end of the year. For instance, suppose that a $500 unfavorable variance was found for January for nurses' aides salaries. If that variance occurred every month, it would total $6,000 for the year. If $6,000 is an unreasonably high variance, investigate the $500 January variance as soon as possible.

Suppose that the January variance was only $100 and that $1,200 is a variance that would be acceptable for the year. No immediate investigation would take place. In February, the variance might be $200, but perhaps the unit can live with a $2,400 variance as well. If the variance is $300 in March, the manager must be concerned even if $3,600 would be an acceptable level. The monthly increase in the variance indicates a growing problem. At this point, the manager would probably investigate the variance to make sure that it does not continue to grow even further out of control.

The key to controlling variances is to be timely, to correct behavior if necessary, and to use the information from variances to correct rates promptly.

If variances are not investigated promptly after each month's variance report is received, then the budget will only serve as a planning tool and not a tool to help the organization control its operation. Information about last month's performance should be used to improve the performance for the remaining months of the year.

Such improvement will likely depend on taking actions to correct behavior when necessary. This may mean meeting to discuss areas of waste, tightening rules on coffee breaks or on personal use of supplies, and so forth. For the most part, the key to improvement is simply a heightened awareness of the budget throughout the year. Everyone is enthusiastic about meeting the budget for the first month or two, but then they gradually slip back into old, sometimes wasteful, habits. By bringing budget variances to the attention of relevant employees whenever the variances start to get out of line, the manager can reinforce the beneficial motivating aspects of the budget that were prominent right after the budget was adopted. If necessary, more forceful means should be used to modify behavior when budget variances are the result of employees not doing their jobs properly.

Finally, in some cases, it will be found that the variances are simply out of the unit or manager's control. A shortage of a key raw material may drive the price of supplies up. If there appears to be a protracted change that is outside the control of the manager and that will result in continuing unfavorable variances, it is important to bring this to the attention of the organization's rate-setting personnel. The sooner this is known and the rates are corrected upward, the better it is for the financial stability of the organization.

PERFORMANCE BUDGETS AND VARIANCE ANALYSIS

Performance budgeting was the topic of Chapter 11 of this book. In a sense, most of this chapter on variance analysis revolves around performance budgeting. Flexible budgets are an attempt to match actual costs incurred with the costs that should have been incurred based on the actual workload. By looking at the actual workload rather than the original budgeted expectations, variances are being calculated with at least some measure of performance being taken into account. However, in developing performance budgets, Chapter 11 went beyond the flexible budget. Performance budgets were established based on a variety of key performance areas.

In the example in Chapter 11, it was suggested that a percentage of the cost of each line item could be allocated to each key performance area. For example, 15% of the nurse manager's time might be devoted to quality improvement (see Table 11–1). Based on these percentage allocations, a cost could be budgeted for each key performance area. For example, $51,500 might be budgeted for quality improvement (see Table 11–2). A budgeted cost could then be determined for each unit of output in each key performance area. For example, the budgeted cost might be $5,150 per 1% drop in the rate of failure to comply with patient care plans (see Table 11–3). How can these performance budget calculations be compared to actual results, and variances between budget and actual determined?

The first step is to assess how much output was actually accomplished in each key performance area. In establishing the performance budget, output measures are chosen that are quantifiable. For example, at the end of the month or year, the percent reduction in failures to comply with patient care plan procedures can be determined and compared with the budgeted reduction. Similar measures are used for the other key performance areas. For example, the number of patient complaints can be compared with the budgeted number of complaints; the nurse turnover rate can be compared with the budgeted turnover rate. Thus, getting a variance in terms of volume of output achieved is readily possible.

The next step would be to compare the actual cost per unit of work accomplished to the budgeted cost. For instance, suppose $51,500 was budgeted for reducing patient care plan errors, with a budgeted goal of a 10% reduction in the rate of failures to comply (a budgeted cost of $5,150 per 1% drop in the failure rate). Suppose that the actual results were that the failure rate fell by 12%. If the total actual cost for this quality improvement is divided by 12, the actual cost per 1% drop can be determined and compared to the budgeted cost of $5,150.

Unfortunately, it is difficult to calculate the actual amount that was spent on quality improvement. This amount consists of a percentage of the cost of each line item. The actual costs for each line item will be known. This cost information is used in the traditional and flexible budget variance analyses discussed earlier. However, there is no ready mechanism for determining the exact percentage of each line item that actually was devoted to each key performance area.

Consider the following information, abstracted from the tables in Chapter 11. It includes the budgeted percent effort (just for the quality improvement key performance area) for each line item (Table 11–1), the budgeted cost for each line item, and the budgeted cost for quality improvement (Table 11–2). A total of $51,500 was included in the performance budget for quality improvement.

Line Item	Line Item Total Cost		Percent Effort Devoted to Quality Improvement		Cost Budgeted for Quality Improvement
Nurse Manager	$ 50,000	×	15%	=	$ 7,500
Staff	800,000	×	5	=	40,000
Education	20,000	×	20	=	4,000
Supplies	40,000	×	0	=	0
Overhead	90,000	×	0	=	0
Total					$51,500
Divided by budgeted outcome (% reduction in failure to comply with patient care plan)					÷ 10
Budgeted cost per percent reduction in failures					$ 5,150

In the example, the nurse manager was budgeted to devote 15% of her total effort to quality improvement. Did she in fact devote 20%; perhaps only 10%? In most organizations (if not all), the data collection systems will not be nearly sophisticated enough to capture such information. Therefore, it will generally be necessary to estimate the actual percentage allocations.

Suppose that the nurse manager was budgeted to cost $50,000 but that, because of a change in fringe benefit rates, the actual manager cost was $51,000. Also suppose that the manager makes an ex post allocation of her total time and estimates that 16% of her effort was devoted to quality improvement. In that case, instead of the budgeted $7,500 of manager cost for quality improvement, the actual manager cost for quality improvement was $8,160 (total nurse manager cost of $51,000 multiplied by 16% effort on the quality area).

Assume that the actual results for each line item in the quality improvement area were as follows:

Line Item	Line Item Total Cost		Percent Effort Devoted to Quality Improvement		Cost Budgeted for Quality Improvement
Nurse Manager	$ 51,000	×	16%	=	$ 8,160
Staff	823,000	×	6	=	49,380
Education	19,000	×	15	=	2,850
Supplies	38,000	×	0	=	0
Overhead	94,000	×	0	=	0
Total					$60,390
Divided by budgeted outcome (% reduction in failure to comply with patient care plan)					÷ 12
Budgeted cost per percent reduction in failures					$ 5,033

The actual cost information would come from the unit's regular variance reports. The percentages of actual effort would be based on estimates by the unit manager and the unit's staff. The budgeted cost for quality improvement was $51,500, while the actual cost was $60,390. The difference between these two numbers represents an $8,890 unfavorable variance. However, this variance does not consider actual work accomplished.

Just as with the flexible variance analysis discussed earlier, it is necessary to consider more than simply the absolute amount of money spent. In terms of accomplishing the goal of reducing the rate of failures to comply with patient care plans, the budgeted cost was $5,150 per 1% reduction in the failure rate. The actual result was a cost of $5,033 per percent reduction in the failure rate.

Had one anticipated the 12% reduction, the budgeted cost would have been $61,800 ($5,150 multiplied by 12). Although there is a total variance of $8,890 unfavorable, the volume variance was $10,300 unfavorable ($51,500 budgeted minus $61,800 flexible budget for a 12% reduction). The cost for the actual volume was less than would have been expected for that volume.

In analyzing performance budget results, it is also interesting to look at each line item. In this case, staff salaries of $49,380 were devoted to quality improvement. In the original budget, the amount was $40,000. This greater effort has apparently led to a greater reduction in the failure rate. Even though the cost per percent reduction was less than budgeted, this result would require careful scrutiny by the nurse manager. If greater efforts were being made in this area, where were efforts less than budgeted? Perhaps this represents more attention to charting, and less direct patient care. In that case, this may not be considered to be a favorable use of time. A unit could have perfect, failure-free patient care plans but poor quality care because of insufficient direct care time. On the other hand, if the reduction in effort elsewhere was in the area of other indirect time, this may represent a favorable outcome.

As with all areas of variance analysis, the calculations provide raw information about what has occurred. The judgment and experience of competent managers is needed to interpret the variances and determine both their underlying causes, as well as whether they represent favorable or unfavorable events for the unit and organization.

SUMMARY AND IMPLICATIONS FOR NURSE MANAGERS

Flexible budget variance analysis is a useful but complex tool. Care must be taken to make sure the analysis helps the manager. For example, aggregation of variances can hide serious problems. Offsetting variances are quite common. If variances are aggregated, offsetting variances may go undetected. Exception reports are particularly useful to keep large variances from going unnoticed.

Flexible budgeting assumes that costs are variable. With fixed costs, there will be no volume variance, since fixed costs by definition do not vary with volume. However, nursing labor costs, even with rigid staffing patterns, can be evaluated in a flexible budget analysis. Varying levels of acuity can also be readily built into the model.

Variances are generally caused by internal changes in efficiency, technology, or quality of care, or by externally caused changes in workload volume or prices. Whatever the cause, efficient management requires investigation and evaluation of variances on a timely basis, followed by actions to correct variances whenever possible.

SUGGESTED READINGS

Dove, H.G., and Forthman, T. (1995). Helping financial analysts communicate variance analysis. *Healthcare Financial Management.* 49(4), 52–54.

Felteau, A. (1992, February). Budget variance analysis and justification. *Nursing Management.* 23(2), 40–41.

Finkler, S.A. (1991). Variance analysis. Part I: Extending flexible budget variance analysis to acuity. *Journal of Nursing Administration.* 21(7/8), 19–25.

Finkler, S.A. (1991). Variance analysis. Part II: The use of computers. *Journal of Nursing Administration.* 21(9), 9–15.

Finkler, S.A., and Ward, D.R. (1999). *Cost Accounting for Health Care Organizations: Concepts and Applications,* Second edition. Gaithersburg, MD: Aspen Publishers.

Horngren, C.T., Foster, G., and Datar, S.M. (1999). *Cost Accounting: A Managerial Emphasis,* Tenth edition. Englewood Cliffs, NJ: Prentice-Hall.

Mailhot, C.B., Binger, J.L., and Slezak, L.G. (1990, May). Managing operating room budget variances. *Journal of Nursing Administration.* 20(5), 19–26.

Voss, G.B., Van Ooij, A., Brans-Brabant, L.J., and Limpens, P.G. (1997, February). Cost-variance analysis by DRGs: Technique for clinical budget analysis. *Health Policy.* 39(2), 153–166.

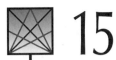

15

Benchmarking, Productivity, and Cost-Benefit and Cost-Effectiveness Analysis

The goals of this chapter are to:

define benchmarking;

explain the benchmarking technique and the critical steps in the benchmarking process;

define productivity and productivity measurement;

provide tools for productivity analysis;

discuss productivity standards;

introduce the concept of unit costing;

explain the relationship between productivity standards and unit-costing;

explore the notion of productivity improvement;

define the concepts of cost-benefit analysis and cost-effectiveness analysis; and

explain the principles of cost-benefit analysis and cost-effectiveness analysis.

INTRODUCTION

Budgeting is not simply about preparing a plan for the organization to do what it has always done, the way it has always done it. Rather, budgeting should help the organization constantly get better—be more effective and efficient in providing its services. Benchmarking, productivity measurement, and cost-benefit/cost-effectiveness analysis are approaches that organizations use to become better at what they do.

Benchmarking is a technique aimed at finding the best practices of other organizations and incorporating them into an organization. Benchmarking will be the first major topic covered in this chapter.

Many health care organizations today are also concerned with *productivity*. As financial resources become more constrained, improvements in productivity represent one way of cutting fat rather than lean. The area of productivity measurement, however, remains somewhat of a mystery in many industries, not just health care. In health care, the difficulties are compounded by problems related to quality and outcomes measurement.

As an organization works to improve productivity in health care, one must always guard against the motivation to sacrifice mission to achieve productivity increases. It is possible to reduce the number of hours of care per patient day. Many health care providers consider such a reduction to be a sign of increased productivity. However, if the reduction is accompanied by a decrease in the quality of patient care, then productivity has not really improved. True productivity improvements are those that enable the organization to use less resources for each unit of service provided, without decreasing the quality of the services provided.

In recent years there has been a trend to reorient the focus of nursing productivity measurement from hours per patient day or FTEs per adjusted occupied bed[1] toward the cost per unit of service provided. The essence of this *unit-costing* is that if we can lower the dollar cost of providing a unit of a specific service, we do not need to worry about things such as the number of care hours used to provide the service. Unit-costing will be discussed in the productivity section of the chapter.

The chapter concludes with a discussion of cost-benefit and cost-effectiveness analysis. These are two techniques that are frequently used by managers as they attempt to improve the productivity of their departments. The techniques are defined and their basic principles are discussed.

BENCHMARKING

One of the roles of budgeting is to help the organization continuously improve over time. The budget should incorporate changes that will allow it to provide services more efficiently. Ultimately such constant improvement helps the organization to accomplish its mission better, while at the same time providing it with an edge over its competitors. Benchmarking is a technique that many organizations employ to help set the direction for change. Simply stated, *benchmarking* is a technique that organizations use to find best practices and to incorporate those practices within the organization.

Benchmarking is linked closely with a variety of process improvement techniques such as Total Quality Management and Continuous Quality Improvement. However, those techniques may be employed using a totally internal focus on an

---

[1]*Adjusted occupied beds* is a measure that combines both inpatient days and outpatient care by using a formula for the number of outpatient visits considered to be the equivalent of one inpatient day.

organization's processes. The essence of benchmarking is examination of what others are doing. By forcing the organization to look beyond itself, many useful approaches developed elsewhere can be used to benefit the organization. This means that an organization may benefit from rare insights or the costly trials and errors of others. It allows the organization to avoid spending substantial resources to reinvent the wheel every time it needs to improve in some area.

Benefits of Benchmarking

There are a number of different ways that benchmarking leads to improved organizational results. Some of the most prominent focuses of benchmarking studies are in the areas of meeting customer requirements, developing accurate measures of productivity, and improving competitiveness.

As health care becomes increasingly competitive, it becomes more important than ever to concentrate on the customer. The knowledge of the services that other organizations are providing to customers is incredibly valuable. To remain competitive, organizations must be aware of what the competition is doing. If it can be determined that elsewhere in the country a service is provided that is not offered by any local competitors, then the organization can gain insights on how to provide its customers with even more than they expect. The most successful organizations are those that are proactive rather than reactive. The organization that introduces new services first has an edge over those that follow. Since the health care industry is largely localized, one does not have to invent all new services. Rather, organizations should strive to keep abreast of innovations around the country and to have the flexibility to be "the first ones on the block" to offer those services.

One of the greatest difficulties in assessing productivity is trying to determine the right level of productivity. How long should it take to do a certain procedure? We can measure productivity in terms of improvement over time. However, some would argue that the organization cannot be productive unless it has some optimum standard for comparison. Benchmarking evaluates the level of productivity of other organizations. This allows the organization to compare itself to the best organizations, creating productivity targets that are challenging, yet attainable. Productivity will be discussed later in this chapter.

Rates of change within organizations are highly variable. Some organizations change rapidly. Others tend to maintain what they believe is a good way of providing care. It is surprising that, despite the rapid change in clinical techniques, health care management techniques often tend to be stagnant. It is difficult to spend a great deal of time being innovative while at the same time trying to complete the day's work that has to be done. Benchmarking helps by allowing organizations to change, without having to invent all the changes. This not only reduces the amount of effort required to find changes that truly results in improvements but also allows the organization to leapfrog over competing organizations.

Benchmarking Approaches

There are three primary approaches to benchmarking. These three approaches are competitive benchmarking, cooperative benchmarking, and collaborative benchmarking.[2] Competitive benchmarking refers to finding specific information about individual organizations providing the same services as yours. Cooperative benchmarking refers to seeking information from organizations in other industries. Collaborative benchmarking refers to finding information within your industry but based on industry-wide statistics.

When people think of benchmarking, they often focus their thoughts on competitive benchmarking. Hospital managers may desire to determine how a specific function is done at the hospital that does that function the best. A visiting nurse agency may want to know the best practices related to supplies inventory at other home care agencies. This is the hardest type of benchmarking data to obtain. Naturally, organizations are reluctant to share their secrets with the direct competition. For this reason, it is often easier to fly across the country and observe several organizations that are not in direct competition with the organization than to observe practices of direct competitors in the same area as the organization. It is not unusual for exchanges to be worked out in which organizations that are similar but in different markets allow visitors to examine their procedures.

Sometimes competitive benchmarking is done without direct permission. This can occur through informal observation or by using a variety of publicly available information. Health care providers generally issue many reports to the public and government that can be useful in assessing their approaches. Consultants have access to many organizations and are often willing to share the best practices that they have observed. As Pavlock notes, "The goal is to find out what the competitors are doing, how, and how well in order to compare their practices with the benchmarker's operations."[3] Agency nurses often work for many different providers. They can be an invaluable source of information on how other organizations do things.

Cooperative benchmarking takes a substantially different approach. Rather than focusing on specific competitors, it looks at organizations in totally different industries. While this might seem odd at first, it actually has great merit. Suppose that a health care provider finds that it consistently ranks low in customer satisfaction. A cooperative benchmarking approach would be to select an organization that is known for its great customer service. For example, Nordstrom's department store over the years has had such a reputation. Spending some time visiting Nordstrom's, learning their philosophy and how they operationalize that

---

[2]Info-Line, *Understanding Benchmarking: The Search for Best Practice,* Alexandria, VA, American Society for Training and Development, Issue 9207, July 1992, pp. 5–6.

[3]Ernest J. Pavlock, *Financial Management for Medical Groups,* Center for Research in Ambulatory Health Care Administration, Englewood, Colo, 1994, p. 588.

philosophy and maintain high customer satisfaction might be enlightening. Why should Nordstrom's agree to let you do this? For several reasons. First, everyone loves flattery. And seeking to learn from any organization certainly flatters that organization. Second, many organizations will view helping health care providers to be an act of public service. Finally, the time may come when you will have some information that might benefit Nordstrom's.

It is important to bear in mind that as long as benchmarking is limited to the benchmarker's industry, you never really become a leader. You are always following someone in your industry. By going outside of the industry, you gain the possibility of becoming the industry leader yourself.

Some organizations actually make a business of allowing themselves to be used for benchmarking purposes. Disney now offers a formal program called "The Disney Approach to Quality Service for Healthcare Professionals." In a three and a half day program costing about $3,000 per participant, Disney offers "A Unique Benchmarking Opportunity." In the program Disney provides not only information about how Disney does things but also linkages to how their approaches can be employed in the health care industry.

Collaborative benchmarking is a process whereby a number of organizations in the same industry pool data so that all members of the pool can determine where they stand relative to the best members of the pool. Generally there is confidentiality, with members of the pool being anonymous. Each organization sees its own data and where it stands relative to everyone else but does not know who has better or worse ratings.

This collaborative approach is more of a *how much* approach rather than a *how* approach. With competitive or cooperative benchmarking the benchmarker tries to learn as much about the best practice process, to make it easy to adopt that practice. Collaborative benchmarking doesn't allow for an understanding of process. On the other hand, if collaborative benchmarking is used, it can help highlight weaknesses. The organization can then move aggressively into one of the other approaches of benchmarking to find ways to convert that weakness into an area of competitive strength.

The Benchmarking Process

The process for benchmarking has been summarized by Camp as having ten steps[4]:

1. Decide what to benchmark
2. Identify organizations with best practices
3. Collect data for comparison
4. Assess gap between best practice and your performance

---

[4]Robert C. Camp, *Benchmarking: The Search for Industry Best Practices That Lead to Superior Performance*, American Society for Quality Control, Milwaukee, 1989, pp. 9–12.

5. Project likely improvement in best practices over the next three to five years
6. Communicate findings
7. Establish goals
8. Create specific plans for improvement
9. Implement plans
10. Reestablish benchmarks as they change over time

Every organization does too many things to be able to benchmark fruitfully all processes. Benchmarking usually focuses on problem areas. The organization must first decide where it is most in need of outside comparison (step 1). The focus should start with areas for which a difference in performance will lead to a difference in achievement of mission. In other words, one must select areas where change might result in a meaningful impact. There is a difficult chicken and egg problem. How do you know where you fall short until you benchmark? How do you know what you want to benchmark until you know where you fall short? Collaborative benchmarking can highlight where some problems are likely to exist. However, ultimately managers must thoroughly understand their own processes. It can be especially beneficial to focus efforts on those areas that are costly (because they have the most potential for cost-savings) and those areas that are creating morale problems.

Second, the benchmarker must select organizations with best practices (step 2). This requires a fair amount of investigation. Reading publications, asking around, talking to consultants, and general networking is essential to this step. Pavlock suggests that you "talk with industry experts, the firm's employees, customers, suppliers and others knowledgeable about the areas or business practices being targeted. Ask whose products, services or business practices are similar in some way to the benchmarking firm. A benchmarking consultant may be helpful."[5] The more you have to offer in return to a benchmarking partner, the more likely they are to allow you to review their organization. So part of the selection process must include consideration of what you have to offer in exchange and who would be likely to want it.

Step 3 concerns data collection. The data collection process involves not only data but also people. In collecting data about your own organization and the comparison organization it is critical to involve the right people. That includes the managers most familiar with the existing processes at both organizations, as well as the person responsible for implementing any changes. To the extent possible, the staff members who will ultimately have to make any changes succeed should be involved in the process. If they do not view the changes as their changes, they will not have a vested interest in having them succeed. The data to be collected must be usable. So, before collecting the data one should question

---

[5]Pavlock, ibid., p. 589.

what types of changes might be needed. Although this cannot be answered fully before the data is collected, it will help formulate the measurement instruments so that the data is collected in a usable form.

Change is difficult and costly. If the gap between best practice and your performance is not great, it may not be worthwhile trying to implement change. So it is important to assess the gap between current and best practices (step 4). If the measurement tools are well designed and a sizable gap is evident, the benchmarker will be able to see where change is needed.

Knowledge of the gap allows the organization to set targets for improvement. However, the targets should not necessarily be set at the level that exists in the best practices organization now. That organization is likely to make improvements during the period the benchmarker is implementing changes. Therefore, the benchmark established needs to be set at the level that will likely exist at the best practices organization several years in the future (step 5).

It is critical that the findings of the benchmarking process be widely communicated (step 6). There will undoubtedly be ripple effects resulting from any change. The more support developed for changes, the more likely they are to succeed. But support is not possible without clear communication of what was found and why the findings dictate that changes would be beneficial.

Step 7 is the establishment of goals. These goals should be those that the study team believes are appropriate in order to maximize the benefit gained from adopting the best practices. These goals should be developed with a careful eye toward both the existing gap as well as the estimation of where the best practices organization will be in several years, as discussed above.

The goals must be translated into objectives that form the basis for specific plans for improvement (step 8). To the extent possible, all persons who will be involved in the implementation of the changes should be involved in designing the plans for change.

Next comes the actual implementation of the plans (step 9). Assuming that the new benchmarks are well communicated and the action plans well designed, the organization should start to make progress fairly quickly. If progress is not visible in a short time, staff may become discouraged and fall into old patterns of behavior. Although the process of gathering the benchmarking data can be challenging and time-consuming, one cannot relax once the data has been collected. Unless the actual implementation is supervised carefully, all the preceding efforts may turn out to have been wasted.

The final step is to reestablish benchmarks as they change over time (step 10). One of the fundamental principles on which benchmarking is based is that change is essential. There is no one correct way to do things. It is not as simple as getting all aspects of the organization to reach that correct plateau. Rather, processes need to be improved continuously. Even if the organization achieves the status of an industry leader that everyone wants to evaluate for its benchmarking efforts, continued improvement is essential.

Requirements for Successful Benchmarking

One thing that should be clear from the above discussion is that benchmarking is a big deal. It is not a brief activity undertaken at little cost. It involves the time of many managers over substantial periods of time. Benchmarking is unlikely to work unless there is a strong management commitment to the process. Managers in the organization must study their current processes. It is difficult to change to something else, unless you first know where you are now. And there must be a willingness to change. Such willingness is much harder to obtain than we often think. Someone once described change as being similar to heaven. Everyone is ready to extol its virtues, but no one is actually in much of a rush to get there.

PRODUCTIVITY

Contrary to rumor, productivity is not focused primarily on getting people to work harder. The concern, rather, is to have employees' efforts be more productive. What is meant by productivity? The most common productivity measure is the amount of output produced by each unit of input. This can be calculated as follows:

$$\text{Productivity} = \frac{\text{Total Outputs}}{\text{Total Inputs}}$$

For example, suppose that a nurse practitioner can see 250 patients during a month when 100 hours are devoted to seeing patients. The productivity measure would be:

$$= \frac{250 \text{ Patients}}{100 \text{ Hours}} = 2.5 \text{ Patients per Hour}$$

If the practice can be cleared to allow the nurse to see more patients per hour, productivity would improve, assuming that the care provided remains the same. For example, suppose that the nurse practitioner currently records everything manually in the patient chart after the visit. However, a computer program is available with a touch screen function that allows for faster data entry and chart updating. Since less time is spent charting, more patients can be scheduled. Suppose that after the implementation of the computer system the nurse can now see 270 patients in the same 100 hours. Productivity has improved to:

$$= \frac{270 \text{ Patients}}{100 \text{ Hours}} = 2.7 \text{ Patients per Hour}$$

If the cost of each hour is the same and visits per hour rise from 2.5 to 2.7, the practice is more productive. Assuming that the extra visits per hour generate more revenue, it is more profitable as well. (Note that we have not yet considered the cost of the computer. That will be addressed later in this chapter.)

Productivity Standards

In the above example it was hypothesized that a nurse practitioner used computers to improve productivity from 2.5 patients per hour to 2.7 patients per hour. One problem with such a measure of productivity is that the only comparison is over time. Often managers would prefer to also have a benchmark or standard for comparison. Standards can be based on broad industry average experience, best industry practice, or simply on the organization's budget.

For example, suppose that the nurse practitioner believes that an ideally functioning practice would see 3 patients per hour. The nurse practitioner has determined this based on reading many articles about similar practices and also talking to peers around the country. Productivity can be measured by comparing actual results of this practice to that standard. For example, originally the practice productivity was 2.5 patients an hour. Compared to the standard, this represents an 83% productivity rate calculated as follows:

$$\frac{\text{Actual Productivity}}{\text{Standard Productivity}} \times 100 = \text{Productivity Percent}$$

$$\frac{2.5 \text{ Patients per Hour}}{3.0 \text{ Patients per Hour}} \times 100 = 83\%$$

After the innovation with the computer charting, the practice productivity rose to 90%.

$$\frac{2.7 \text{ Patients per Hour}}{3.0 \text{ Patients per Hour}} \times 100 = 90\%$$

If an industry standard cannot be found, the productivity percent can be calculated as a percent of the budget or of some perceived ideal. It should be noted, however, that the resulting percentage must be interpreted differently based on the type of standard used. If the budget is used as the denominator of the fraction, then the goal should be to attain 100% productivity or better. That would imply that the organization is achieving or exceeding its budget. In contrast, what if the denominator of the fraction is based on a perceived ideal? It is highly unlikely that an ideal result can ever be attained. Therefore, the manager must bear in mind that we would always expect productivity to be less than 100%, and performance should be assessed based on how close we come to 100%.

Unit-Costing

In the above example, productivity rose from 83% to 90% after the computer charting was introduced. However, we must still question whether that productivity change is an improvement. In recent years there has been a movement to stop looking at productivity simply in terms of inputs and outputs and to make sure that the cost per unit of service is considered in the calculation. This approach is called unit-costing.

For example, hospitals have long used hours per patient day (HPPD) as a productivity measure. This is actually an inversion of the typical productivity measure. Consider a nursing department that consumed 10,000 hours of nurses' time in a month when it provided 2,500 patient days of care. The standard productivity measure would be outputs divided by inputs to find the amount of output per unit of input. For the nursing department the calculation would be:

$$= \frac{2,500 \text{ Patient Days}}{10,000 \text{ Hours}} = 0.25 \text{ Patient Day per Hour}$$

The result here is cumbersome because each unit of output (i.e., a patient day) requires more than one unit of input (an hour of care). One-quarter of a patient day of care is generated by each hour of nursing care. By inverting the fraction, we can measure the HPPD:

$$= \frac{10,000 \text{ Hours}}{2,500 \text{ Patient Days}} = 4 \text{ HPPD}$$

This is a common hospital productivity measure. However, in today's environment of tight financial resources, this measure fails to indicate the cost of care, which is critical. If we replaced all LPNs with RNs, it is possible that we could reduce the HPPD. But would that make the organization more productive? That is a complicated question. An RN can do activities that an LPN cannot do. But the cost per hour for an RN is also higher than it is for an LPN. Consider the following example. Suppose that an RN earns $35 per hour including benefits and an LPN earns $25 per hour including benefits. Suppose further that an LPN requires 20% more time to accomplish activities than an RN would require for the same activities. (Some activities can only be performed by an RN.) Assume that currently we have 100 hours of RN time and 120 hours of LPN time and we have an output of 50 patient days. The HPPD under the current staffing would be:

$$\frac{100 \text{ RN Hours} + 120 \text{ LPN Hours}}{50 \text{ Patient Days}} = 4.4 \text{ HPPD}$$

and the cost per unit of service would be:

100 RN Hours × $35	=	$3,500
120 LPN Hours × $25	=	3,000
Total Cost	=	$6,500
		÷ 50 Patient Days
Cost per Patient Day		$ 130

If we shifted to an all RN staff, we could replace the 120 LPN hours with 100 RN hours. The HPPD would then be:

$$\frac{100 \text{ RN Hours} + 100 \text{ RN Hours}}{50 \text{ Patient Days}} = 4.0 \text{ HPPD}$$

The HPPD have fallen from 4.4 to 4.0. But is the unit more productive? What has happened to the cost of care provided:

$$200 \text{ RN Hours} \times \$35 = \$7,000$$
$$\div 50 \text{ Patient Days}$$

Cost per Patient Day $ 140

Productivity is difficult to assess in absolute terms. Shifting from a staff with RNs and LPNs to an all RN staff resulted in fewer required hours of care for each patient day in the above example. But the cost per patient day rose from $130 to $140. Clearly, simply measuring productivity based on HPPD does not make sense. HPPD can fall while cost per patient rises. We cannot say this makes us more productive. On the other hand, productivity measures should take quality of care into consideration. Shifting to the all RN staff did raise the cost per unit of service, but it may also have raised the level of quality of care. So we cannot say clearly that the increased cost per patient day reduced productivity.

On the other hand, we could identify an acceptable level of quality of care. As long as that level of quality is maintained, reductions in the cost per unit of service would be considered to be productivity increases. In the above example, if the care being provided by 100 RN hours and 120 LPN hours was of acceptable quality, then the shift to an all RN staff would reduce productivity because it increases the cost per patient day. We cannot let traditional productivity measures such as the reduction in HPPD from 4.4 to 4.0 lead us to believe productivity is improving when the cost per patient day is increasing. Financial resources are too limited for us to focus solely on measures such as HPPD. The productivity measure provided by cost per unit of service is much more meaningful to managers who are trying to make the best use of their limited financial resources.

Therefore, at least one author has called on health care organizations to shift their measures of productivity toward the cost per unit of service, or unit-costing. This calls for replacing measures of input with measures of cost.[6] Rather than thinking about the hours per patient day, we could consider the cost per patient day. Similarly, in various situations we could measure productivity in terms of the cost per patient, cost per procedure, or cost per visit.

For example, consider the case of the nurse practitioner and the rise in productivity percent from 83% to 90% after purchase of a computer. Did productivity really rise or fall? Maybe the cost of the computer was greater than

---

[6]Janet Barron, "Productivity and Cost Per Unit of Service," in *Nursing Management Desk Reference,* edited by Roxane Spitzer-Lehmann, W.B. Saunders, 1994, Philadelphia, pp. 260–277.

the benefit. Suppose that the total costs of the practice for the month (including the salary of the nurse practitioner) without the computer system were $8,000. The computer system is leased for $300 per month (for all hardware and software). The cost of the practice rose from $8,000 to $8,300. What happened to the cost per unit of service? Originally it was:

$$\frac{\$8,000 \text{ Cost}}{250 \text{ Patients}} = \$32.00$$

After the computer implementation the cost per unit of service was:

$$\frac{\$8,300 \text{ Cost}}{270 \text{ Patients}} = \$30.74$$

It turns out that productivity has indeed improved as a result of the computer, since the cost per visit, even including the cost of the computer, fell from $32.00 to $30.74.

Notice also that the cost per unit of service approach does not require us to measure the amount of different resources used. In the example as initially stated, it was assumed that the nurse practitioner worked 100 hours in both situations. Most likely, the number of hours spent seeing patients would vary from month to month. However, we can calculate productivity of the practice from month to month without having to track the number of hours worked or the amount of other resources used. All that is needed is the total cost for the services provided each month and the number of units of service provided.

On the other hand, the measurement of costs can be complicated. The last chapter in this book looks at costing out nursing services in some detail. If one wants, the methodologies of that chapter can be used to measure costs in a fairly sophisticated manner. However, in many instances, simple measures of cost can be used. For example, an operating room department or outpatient surgery unit can simply divide its total costs by the number of hours of surgery to get a cost per hour or cost per minute. If the cost per hour of surgery falls from month to month, then productivity is improving, assuming that case mix is constant. Similarly, a home care agency could calculate the cost per home care visit by dividing total costs by the total number of visits. Such measures can be tracked either over time or compared to some budget or standard, as discussed above.

The problem with this approach is that you must be willing to accept some averaging. For instance, if a home care agency provides visits by aides, LPNs, and RNs, the average cost per visit may be misleading. What if the number of visits by RNs is falling and the number of visits by aides is rising? It is likely that the cost per visit will fall. But that may not be indicative of true productivity improvement. This is especially so if the profit of RN visits is greater than the profit on visits by aides.

One way to handle such a situation is to divide the costs of the health care unit or organization into separate categories and measure productivity for each category. We could measure the costs of RN visits, costs of LPN visits, and costs of aide visits, and then divide those costs by the number of visits of each type to assess productivity. For example, suppose that the costs for the agency for the month were $100,000 and there were 4,000 visits. One productivity measure would be:

$$\frac{\$100,000 \text{ Cost}}{4,000 \text{ Visits}} = \$25 \text{ Cost per Visit}$$

but a more sophisticated approach would be to determine the volume and cost by type of visit and calculate productivity as:

$$\frac{\$50,000 \text{ Cost of RN Visits}}{1,000 \text{ RN Visits}} = \$50 \text{ Cost per RN Visit}$$

$$\frac{\$30,000 \text{ Cost of LPN Visits}}{1,000 \text{ LPN Visits}} = \$30 \text{ Cost per LPN Visit}$$

$$\frac{\$20,000 \text{ Cost of Aide Visits}}{2,000 \text{ Aide Visits}} = \$10 \text{ Cost per Aide Visit}$$

Over time we could track changing productivity for each type of visit.

The difficulty of such productivity measurement is assigning costs to each group. Clearly, the cost of RN visits would include the cost of RNs, the supplies they use, and their travel and charting costs. The problem is determining what share of rent, supervision, billing, and other costs to assign to one group versus the other groups. There is no simple rule for such allocations. Overhead costs can be allocated based on the number of visits (if half the visits are by aides, assign half the overhead to aides) or based on the revenue from visits (if half the revenue comes from RN visits assign half the overhead to them) or based on a number of other approaches. No one approach is more valid or correct than any other.

Although many organizations use arbitrary ways to allocate overhead or indirect costs, an alternative approach is to ignore overhead costs. Productivity could be measured based on just the direct costs per unit of service. This approach will help assess productivity improvement or declines related to direct costs. Unfortunately it does not provide information about changes in productivity in overhead areas of the organization, such as the billing department. This is especially important if changes in RN productivity are associated with changes in overhead departments. However, we could separately measure productivity for overhead by measuring things such as the cost per bill issued.

As you can see, productivity measurement is complex. Managers cannot simply apply productivity formulas blindly. Thought must go into deciding how to measure productivity and also how to interpret productivity measures. Nevertheless, unit-costing is feasible. We must define the unit (such as patient day, RN visit, or nurse practitioner treatment) and divide the number of units of service into the cost of providing that service. We can have broad average costs or more specifically measured costs based on approaches discussed in Chapter 16.

Barron nicely summarizes the issue related to productivity measurement as follows:

> Managers cannot be held to both dollar and hour limits. Either they manage the hours and watch what happens to the dollars, as is the common practice, or they manage the dollars and watch what happens to the hours. Past practice has led to tightly controlled hours and escalating dollars. A dollars per unit of service system tightly controls dollars while allowing flexible hours.[7]

Barron's point is important because it focuses on the fact that productivity is unlikely to improve in health care organizations until management changes its thinking. If there is a goal to control costs, then finance should not persist in holding managers accountable for measures such as HPPD. That thinking stiffles innovation instead of encouraging it. Executives who say that they support innovation and creativity but then evaluate employees based on adherence to a measure such as HPPD clearly are not putting their money where their mouth is. They are forgetting that people respond well to the incentives that the organization provides. If the goal is to control spending per visit, per treatment, or per patient, then the productivity measurement and evaluation must be based on those units of service as well.

Unit-Costing and Productivity Standards

If unit-costing is used to assess productivity we can still employ productivity benchmarks or standards. For instance, in the home care agency example above, we could assess the cost of each visit versus a benchmark. If we believe the ideal cost per RN visit is $44, then we could divide the actual $50 cost (see calculation above) into the ideal $44 cost as follows:

$$\frac{\$44 \text{ Ideal Cost}}{\$50 \text{ Actual Cost}} \times 100 = 88\% \text{ Productivity}$$

As the actual cost per visit declines, we would get closer to 100% productivity. Such measures require careful thought about what should go in the numerator and denominator to get a meaningful indicator.

Productivity Improvement

For most health care organizations, the focus on productivity does not exist simply for the purpose of measuring the level of productivity. Rather, we are concerned with improving productivity. Such improvements can be accomplished by forcing staff to work harder. Generally, however, such efforts are self-defeating. They result in declining morale. Although short-term improve-

---

[7]Barron, op. cit., p. 271.

ments may be possible as a result of such strategies, in the longer term declines in productivity may occur as a result of the pressures placed on employees. Further, the quality of care provided may decline as a result of the pressure on employees.

Working smarter, not harder, is the key to improving productivity. Productivity measurement should be used to generate information to follow the progress of serious process improvement efforts. Learning how to do things more efficiently is likely to result in permanent productivity gains and should not require increased and often unsustainable individual efforts by employees.

The key to working smarter, not harder, lies in changing processes. Benchmarking, discussed earlier in this chapter, is one approach to improving productivity. Adopting the best practices of others is likely to change processes in a way that increases productivity. Reengineering, total quality management (TQM), continuous quality improvement (CQI), and value-added approaches similarly are aimed at improving underlying processes. The essence, however, does not lie in the use of a specific technique such as TQM or CQI but rather in a review of the way the organization provides its services.

Managers must be given the time and support necessary to promote change. Productivity improvement is unlikely to occur without change. The organization must foster an environment that encourages change. Managers must know that innovation is expected from them. If the message given to managers is that they are overseers of an existing operation, then they will simply oversee that static provision of care. Improvement is likely to occur only when innovation is actively supported, encouraged, and rewarded.

Productivity improvements also require an understanding of why resources are consumed. We must know first why an organizational unit exists. What is the mission of the unit or department? Next, the unit must be examined to determine if all the resources it consumes are really necessary to accomplish that mission. This is not to say that some resources are simply wasted. Rather, one must take a cost/benefit perspective. Are the benefits of each of the unit's activities great enough to justify the cost of those activities? Some long-standing practices may need to be eliminated because their costs have risen so high over the years that they can no longer be justified.

For example, for each activity of the organizational unit one might ask:

- When is it performed?
- How often is it performed?
- Where is it performed?
- Who is performing it?
- Is it necessary to perform it at all?[8]

The answer to these questions may provide the information needed to make changes that will result in productivity increases without substantial reduction in

---

[8]Pavlock, op. cit., p. 595.

services provided. We might find that a function always handled by one department has been superceded by an activity now done with new technology for a lower cost in another department. The old activity not only may be duplicative but also may be providing inferior information to that already available in the other department.

Over time, space needs change as well. Productivity relates to all resources consumed, not just to labor. If the organization is not using space wisely, then it is possible that money is being wasted. Organizations often grow haphazardly. Space is allocated based on immediate necessity rather than careful planning. It may be worth an organization's time to have a space planner examine operations and reallocate space. It is possible that space savings will occur that might allow the organization to rent less outside space, thus saving money.

For example, the last decade has seen substantial movement in hospitals from inpatient care to outpatient care. While new outpatient facilities have been built, what has happened to the excess space formerly needed for inpatients? It is possible that much of that space is being used in suboptimal fashion. Spending some money for redesign and even remodeling could result in substantial reductions in the cost of space and could even make provision of care more efficient, resulting in reduced labor costs as well.

At this point we have questioned the need for the organization to exist and have evaluated its activities to see if they could be eliminated or performed differently. The facilities used by the organization have also been considered. Finally, productivity improvement requires careful evaluation of the staff and supplies used. It is often difficult to assess whether staffing patterns are appropriate. Collaborative benchmarking, as discussed earlier, can be helpful. By considering issues such as the number of visits per home care worker at other home care agencies, one can get a sense of the organization's productivity in the use of staff. This information can be a starting point in at least getting a sense of where an organization is on a continuum of resource consumption.

However, it is critical to keep in mind that collaborative benchmarking results in "how much" type information rather than "how" information. Many consulting firms tell health care providers that they can provide their services with fewer staff because others do so, but they don't provide the "how" piece of information. It may be that there are unique factors relating to the organization's physical structure, patient mix, or even culture that make such productivity standards impossible.

For example, suppose that abortions are relatively inexpensive compared to other obstetrical procedures. Hospitals that do more abortions in its labor and delivery department will need fewer RNs per 1,000 patients than hospitals that perform fewer abortions. Suppose that a hospital with many abortions has a ratio of 2 RNs per 1,000 obstetrical procedures. Suppose further that the average hospital that does some abortions uses 2.5 RNs per 1,000. A consultant tells a Catholic hospital that does no abortions that best practice for obstetrics calls for the use of 2 RNs per 1,000. The Catholic hospital currently has a ratio of 2.7 RNs per 1,000. How useful is that information? Not very. And it may be destructive if top management blindly calls for departments to use benchmarked data without an understanding of how the numbers were achieved. Productivity improvement requires careful analysis, rather than simplistic pursuit of targets that are not well understood.

Finally, supplies and equipment should also be considered when an organization is trying to assess productivity improvement. For example, a thorough review of the process related to supplies may find that the hospital does not get the best buy on supplies. Or it may show that it did get a good price but purchased too much and then had to dispose of some supplies that reach their expiration date. Or it may show that the hospital buys the correct amount but has trouble distributing the supplies to where they are needed, when they are needed, creating bottlenecks that delay patient treatment. Often productivity improvement requires nothing more than a careful examination of how the organization does things, a determination of where problems are occurring, and then development and implementation of solutions to avoid the problems in the future.

Where do we often find room for productivity improvement? Pavlock notes that, "Scheduling modifications for patients, staff and physicians are probably the most important way to improve the overall productivity."[9] This requires a delicate balance. Patients do not like to wait for care. However, if caregivers have to wait for patients to arrive, they are being paid for time when they are not productive. This problem is exacerbated by the fact that it takes different amounts of time to treat different patients, and the time needed for any one specific patient cannot accurately be anticipated in advance.

All productivity improvement efforts should include a component to assure that quality is not negatively impacted. Productivity measures implicitly assume that quality is held constant. If a car maker shifts from producing luxury sedans to economy models, the cost per car made will decline. However, that doesn't represent a productivity gain. The company is simply making a different, less expensive product. In health care, it is incorrect to consider a reduction in hours or cost per treatment to be a productivity gain if it was accomplished by reducing quality.

COST-BENEFIT AND COST-EFFECTIVENESS ANALYSIS

Cost-benefit analysis (CBA) and cost-effectiveness analysis (CEA) are methods that are used to consider the advantages and disadvantages of decisions. These techniques are often used in assessing the implementation of best practices based on a benchmarking study or other changes designed to improve productivity. They are employed in a variety of other situations as well.

---

[9]Ibid., p. 597.

CBA is a method that compares the benefits related to a decision to the costs of that decision. The method holds that the decision makes sense if the benefits related to the decision will exceed the costs. In terms of numbers, if

$$\frac{\text{Benefits}}{\text{Costs}} > 1$$

then the project has a positive benefit/cost ratio and adds value. In order to determine the ratio, it is necessary to assign values to both the costs and the benefits in monetary terms. In practice, it is difficult to assign monetary values to health care outcomes. We have trouble measuring the value of a life and even more difficulty in measuring the difference in health outcomes that do not involve life or death.

CEA is not as ambitious as CBA in that it does not require a measurement of the value of the benefits. Rather, it relies on using comparisons. One considers whether a project is cost-effective in comparison with some alternative approach. An approach that achieves a specific desired outcome for the least possible cost is considered to be cost-effective.

Cost-Benefit Analysis

Cost-benefit analysis, as its name implies, compares the costs and benefits of an action or program. The method is used primarily by the government, since it can take into account not only private costs and benefits but public ones as well. However, many health care organizations use the method. Cost-benefit analysis has been defined as being an

> analytical technique that compares the social costs and benefits of proposed programs or policy actions. All losses and gains experienced by society are included and measured in dollar terms. The net benefits created by an action are calculated by subtracting the losses incurred by some sectors of society from the gains that accrue to others. Alternative actions are compared, so as to choose one or more that yield the greatest net benefits, or ratio of benefits to costs. The inclusion of all gains and losses to society in cost-benefit analysis distinguishes it from cost-effectiveness analysis, which is a more limited view of costs and benefits.[10]

In the minds of many people, cost-benefit analysis is associated with large-scale public projects, such as the building of a dam. However, the technique can be extremely useful even for evaluating small purchases such as a personal computer. Health care policy makers will be likely to include the impact on society in their cost-benefit analyses. Health care managers are more likely to focus specifically on the impact of a decision on their organization.

---

[10]J.L. Mikesell, *Fiscal Administration—Analysis and Application for the Public Sector.* Fourth edition. Harcourt Brace College Publishers, Fort Worth, 1995, pp. 559–560.

All organizations attempt to determine if the benefits from spending money will exceed the cost. If the benefits do outweigh the costs, it makes sense to spend the money; otherwise it does not. Careful measurement of costs and benefits provides the information needed to support a spending decision.

There are several key elements in performing a cost-benefit analysis:

- Determine project goals
- Estimate project benefits
- Estimate project costs
- Discount cost and benefit flows at an appropriate rate, and
- Complete the decision analysis.

Determine Project Goals

In order to determine the benefits, it is first necessary to understand what the organization hopes the project will accomplish. So identification of goals and objectives is essential. Suppose that a home care agency is trying to decide if it should acquire a van that would drop off nurses and aides at patient homes. The first question is why it believes that it would be better off with a van. The goals may be few or numerous, depending on the specific situation. Perhaps staff currently have difficulty parking. They spend a lot of time searching for parking and often incur parking tickets for illegal parking because there are no legal spaces available. The agency may wish to reduce the cost for parking lots and parking tickets, and to save the time staff spend searching for parking.

Estimate Project Benefits

Once the goals have been identified, the specific amount of the benefits must be estimated. The benefits should include only the incremental benefits that result from the project. For instance, the manager would not include the benefit of providing existing services to existing customers, since the services are already provided. However, if freeing up staff time allows for more patients to be cared for, then the revenue from that extra service should be included in the analysis. Benefits may also arise from cost reductions. All additional benefits should be considered, estimated, and included in the cost-benefit calculation.

In the home care agency example, it is likely that the manager will be able to calculate the benefits fairly directly. For example, the agency may have logs showing travel time separately from visit time. It can use that information to calculate the labor cost of time spent by staff searching for parking. It certainly knows the amount it currently pays for parking lots and parking tickets. Measurement of other benefits is more complicated. If we are able to see more patients, the benefit would really be the profit from those additional patients, rather than their entire revenue.

Estimate Project Costs

Projects have costs as well as benefits, and those costs must also be estimated as part of the cost-benefit analysis. In the case of the van, the primary costs relate to the acquisition of the van and the labor cost for the driver. However, care should be exercised to include all costs, such as the cost of gasoline and maintaining the vehicle. Some consideration is also needed for coverage when the driver is sick or on vacation. In cost-benefit analysis it is also critical to consider *opportunity costs.* Opportunity cost refers to the fact that when a decision is made to do something, other alternatives are sacrificed. In the case of buying a van, the agency buys the van with cash that might have been used to pay rent on a new office location in an adjoining community. Perhaps the money in that alternative use would generate many more patients and great amounts of additional revenues and profits.

Discount Cost and Benefit Flows

Often project benefits and costs occur over a period of years. This creates a calculation problem because money has a different value at different times. Money is more valuable today than the same amount of money in the future. If one pays $40,000 for a van today and receives $15,000 of net benefits per year over the four-year life of the van, one cannot compare the $40,000 to the sum of $15,000 for four years. At a minimum, the agency could have invested the $40,000 and earned interest each year.

This creates a problem in comparing benefits and costs. They cannot simply be totaled for the life of the project and then compared to see if the benefits exceed the costs. The timing is critical. This is especially true because projects often have higher costs in early years and higher benefits in later years. Simple addition of total benefits and total costs could lead to improper decisions. The approach to deal with the problem is referred to as discounting cash flows. This approach uses an interest rate, referred to as the discount rate, to convert all costs and benefits to their value at the present time. See the Time Value of Money discussion in the Appendix to Chapter 10 for additional discussion related to discounting of future cash flows.

Complete the Decision Analysis

Once all the relevant costs and benefits of a project have been estimated and adjusted in a discounting process, they can be compared to each other in the form of a ratio. Generally benefits are divided by costs. If the result is greater than 1, it means that the benefits exceed the costs and the project is desirable. The greater the benefit to cost ratio, the more desirable the project.

Cost-Effectiveness Analysis

As noted earlier, an approach that achieves a specific desired outcome for the least possible cost is considered to be cost-effective. If we do not have a comparison, we run into difficulties. Consider, for example, a project that will save lives. If we know that we can save lives at a cost of $50 per life, would we consider that to be cost-effective? Certainly. However, in drawing such a conclusion, we are implicitly placing at least a minimum value on a human life by implying it is worth more than $50. This creates a difficulty in trying to establish a cutoff point. Is a project that saves lives at a cost of $10,000 per life cost-effective? How about $1 million? How about $1 billion?

Some might argue that there are many alternative options that could save lives for less than $1 billion per life saved. Therefore, the project that costs $1 billion per life is not cost-effective. In comparison with other alternatives, the billion dollar per life project costs more to accomplish the outcome of saving lives than alternatives cost. The problem with assuming that $50 per life saved is cost-effective is that it puts a value on the benefit, rather than simply holding the benefit constant. A more CEA-oriented approach would consider different approaches to save a life and find out which one costs least. That would be the cost-effective alternative.

Therefore, to operationalize CEA, one must compare alternatives that generate similar outcomes. For example, suppose that a hospital has been treating a certain type of patient using a particular approach. Now an alternative approach is suggested. Is the new approach cost-effective? We must first establish that the clinical outcomes are equal. Then we must show that the new approach costs less money than the old approach. If a new approach generates the exact same outcome for less money, then it is cost-effective.

Note how this avoids the problem of measuring the value of the benefits. Because we hold the benefits constant, any approach that costs less must inherently be superior to other approaches. In reality, however, it is difficult to find different techniques that yield the exact same health care outcomes.

As a result, researchers have developed a variety of techniques to enable the comparison of outcomes across interventions, conditions, and diseases. Researchers have been able to model the long-term effects of clinical treatments on patients. With this ability, CEA can now go beyond simple comparisons of the cost per life saved to more precise comparisons of cost per life-years saved (LYS), cost per quality adjusted life years (QALYS), and cost per disability adjusted life years (DALYS). The latter two outcome measures (QALYS and DALYS) assume that a life year in a fully functional state is different (more valuable) than a life year in an impaired state.

Will this approach work in all cases? No. It is possible for an alternative to yield an improved health benefit but to cost more. Will that approach be deemed cost-effective? No, even though the improved health may be worth the extra cost, it is not considered cost-effective because it costs more. CEA is limited to evaluating less costly alternatives with at least the same outcome. It cannot comment on the advisability of more costly alternatives that provide better outcomes.

Finally, many managed care programs are looking at cost-effectiveness analysis as a guide for deciding what treatments will be covered. CEA provides information to assist in decision making. It does not provide the answer. Although strictly allocating resources based on the results of CEAs may be problematic politically or ethically, CEA at least brings information to the table to inform the decision-making process. If an alternative is shown to be cost-effective, then we know that it is a superior alternative because we get at least as good a result for a lower cost.

SUMMARY AND IMPLICATIONS FOR NURSE MANAGERS

Budgeting in the twenty-first century requires a lot more than simply "minding the store." Nurse managers must find ways to improve the performance of their units proactively. To do this managers can benefit by understanding productivity and productivity measurement and by using the techniques of benchmarking and cost-benefit and cost-effectiveness analysis.

How does an organization get to be outstanding? It must foster and facilitate innovation and improvement. Unless there is an environment that is supportive and even encouraging of change, progress is likely to be hampered severely. Many organizations like to say that they believe in innovation, but the culture they create stifles change rather than rewarding it. Suggestions for change are viewed as criticism of the way top management is doing its job. Often, such criticism is not welcomed. Staff quickly learn that it is wiser to be quiet and allow the waste and inefficiency they observe to continue. It should not be surprising that the most significant changes in organizations occur only after the top management has been replaced. At those times the new top management can admit openly to problems and the need for change. After all, the existing problems can be attributed to those who have just left.

For change to occur, it is critically important for managers to assess their current situation. The better existing processes are understood, the easier it is to be willing to take the risk of replacing some of them. Benchmarking is an invaluable aid, especially for organizations that are looking to make quick, significant improvement. The task of undertaking a benchmarking study is involved and can be costly. Most organizations are well advised to use bench-marking (at least competitive and cooperative benchmarking) only when they feel there is potentially room for significant improvement.

The true benefit of benchmarking does not come from knowing *how much* the benchmarking organization differs from the best practices organization that it studies. The benefit comes from an understanding of *how* it differs. Knowing that another organization has a lower cost does not really motivate managers to match that cost. It frustrates them, since they have no idea of how to match the cost. Clear efforts must be made to assure that benchmarking is not just a tool for leverage to try to make staff work harder. Benchmarking should be used to show the way to true improvements in productivity.

Productivity assesses the amounts of inputs needed to produce an organization's outputs. Health care organizations need to work constantly on reducing the resources needed to provide high-quality patient care. Such improvements may come about from implementation of technological change or from low-tech changes in procedures. Nurse managers must develop an approach to measuring productivity so that changes in productivity can be monitored. And the measure should be meaningful. As discussed in the chapter, measures such as hours per patient day may be inadequate. If the real goal of improved productivity is to decrease the cost per patient, that goal must be incorporated into the measurement. One approach is to focus on unit-costing. Ultimately, however, it is not measurement but improvement in productivity that is essential for healthy organizations.

Two techniques that are sometimes used by managers to help assess whether changes are likely to improve productivity are cost-benefit and cost-effectiveness analysis. Cost-benefit analysis is a technique that compares the benefits of a change to its costs. If the benefits are greater than the costs, the change is worthwhile. Often, however, managers will not be able to measure benefits. Benefits are particularly hard to value when human life is involved. What is a life really worth?

Cost-effectiveness analysis has an appeal because it only requires that the manager estimate costs. In the cost-effectiveness approach, an alternative is evaluated to see if it produces at least as good a benefit as another alternative but for a lower cost. Nurse managers may frequently find themselves faced with whether or not to make a change in the way a unit or organization does something. CEA is helpful because if the change will at least keep results as good as they currently are, the analysis only needs to focus on whether the change will cost less.

SUGGESTED READINGS

Allred, C.A., Arford, P.H., Mauldin, P.D., and Goodwin, L.K. (1998). Cost-effectiveness analysis in the nursing literature, 1992–1996. *Image—the Journal of Nursing Scholarship.* 30(3), 235–242.

Anonymous. (1998, November). Benchmark data, improved productivity help team save $6.9 million in labor costs. *Data Strategies & Benchmarks.* 2(11), 161, 168–170.

Anonymous. (1998, March). For best results, critically examine process behind benchmarking data. *Healthcare Benchmarks.* 5(3), 29–32.

Anonymous. (1989, July). Productivity standards can help forecast cuts in staffing. *Hospital Materials Management.* 14(7), 10.

Bolster, C.J., and Binion, R. (1987). Linkages between cost management and productivity. *Topics in Health Care Financing.* 13(4), 67–75.

Buerhaus, P.I. (1998). Milton Weinstein's insights on the development, use, and methodologic problems in cost-effectiveness analysis. *Image—the Journal of Nursing Scholarship.* 30(3), 223–227.

Camp, R.C. (1989). *Benchmarking: The Search for Industry Best Practices That Lead to Superior Performance.* Milwaukee: American Society for Quality Control.

Chizever, S.D., editor. (1989). Hospital productivity. *Topics in Health Care Financing.* 15(3).

Choich, R., Jr. (1988, May). Relationship of productivity analysis to departmental cost-accounting systems. *American Journal of Hospital Pharmacy.* 45(5), 103–110.

Finkler, S.A. (1986). Productivity measurement. *Hospital Cost Accounting Advisor.* 1(8), 1–4.

Fitzgerald, K. (1998, June). Clinical benchmarking: Implications for perinatal nursing. *Journal of Perinatal & Neonatal Nursing.* 12(1), 23–30.

Gelinas, M.V., and James, R.G. (1999, June). Is your benchmarking missing the mark? *Healthcare Benchmarks.* 6(6), 68–70.

Hellman, E.A. (1991, December). Analysis of a home health agency's productivity system. *Public Health Nursing.* 8(4), 251–257.

Horngren, C.T., Foster, G., and Datar, S.M. (1999). *Cost Accounting: A Managerial Emphasis,* Tenth edition. Englewood Cliffs, NJ: Prentice-Hall.

Info-Line. (1992, July). Understanding Benchmarking: The Search for Best Practice. *American Society for Training and Development,* 92(7), 5–6.

Jeffries, E., and Timms, L. (1998, September). Sharing good practice: Developing network forums. *Nursing Standard.* 12(50), 33–34.

Kobs, A.E. (1998, January–March). Getting started on benchmarking. *Outcomes Management for Nursing Practice.* 2(1), 45–48.

McIntosh, E., Donaldson, C., and Ryan, M. (1999, April). Recent advances in the methods of cost-benefit analysis in healthcare. Matching the art to the science. *Pharmacoeconomics.* 15(4), 357–367.

Mikesell, J.L. (1995). *Fiscal Administration—Analysis and Applications for the Public Sector.* Fourth edition. Fort Worth: Harcourt Brace College Publishers.

Patterson, P. (1986, February). Mastering the fundamentals of OR productivity monitoring. *OR-Manager.* 2(2), 1, 6–7.

Ried, W. (1998, October). QALYs versus HYEs—what's right and what's wrong. A review of the controversy. *Journal of Health Economics.* 17(5), 607–625.

Serway, G.D., et al. (1987). Alternative indicators for measuring hospital productivity. *Hospital & Health Services Administration.* 32, 379–398.

Siegel, J.E. (1998). Cost-effectiveness analysis and nursing research—is there a fit? *Image—the Journal of Nursing Scholarship.* 30(3), 221–222.

Stone, P.W. (1998). Methods for conducting and reporting cost-effectiveness analysis in nursing. *Image—the Journal of Nursing Scholarship.* 30(3), 229–234.

Williams, M. (1998, May). Benchmarking: Simply the best. *British Journal of Theatre Nursing.* 8(2), 19–24.

Wilson, C.K. (1998, February). Implementing best practices. *Aspen's Advisor for Nurse Executives.* 13(5), 2.

16

Costing Out Nursing Services

The goals of this chapter are to:

discuss the various reasons for costing out nursing;

explain why costing nursing was not always done;

consider the potential role of computers in costing out nursing;

identify patient classification systems as one basis for costing out nursing;

discuss the use of DRGs in costing nursing;

provide a specific RVU approach and example for costing out nursing services;

discuss the limitations of an RVU approach; and

introduce product-line costing and budgeting.

INTRODUCTION

As financial pressures faced by health care organizations continue to grow, the focus on costing out nursing services has increased. Ideally, by costing out nursing, one would like to find the dollar value of the resources consumed to provide nursing care. However, this is a complex problem—one in which even the goals are unclear.

Does a health care organization want to know what it costs them to employ a nurse? Is this costing out nursing? No. The focus of costing is on the cost of providing nursing care to patients. However, this does not solve the problem. Is it desirable to find the nursing cost per patient or per patient day or per patient care hour? Should the costing focus on the cost per acuity adjusted patient day? Per DRG? Per visit?

The cost per patient (or visit or treatment) is the simplest approach. It merely requires dividing total nursing costs by the number of patients (or visits or treatments). This method provides little information to aid management in decision making. Knowing the cost per patient tells the manager little about which types of patients are particularly costly to care for.

Acuity-adjusted measures attempt to separate patients into homogeneous groups. This information is more sophisticated. For example, the cost for a day at patient classification level 1 can be distinguished from a day at level 2 or 3. However, one must consider whether the organization makes decisions about groups of patients in a particular patient classification level. Hospitals, for example, are more likely to make decisions on the basis of DRGs for two reasons. First, DRGs are groupings used for setting prices or charges. Second, decisions can be made about whether or not to provide care for particular DRGs. A hospital could decide it is losing a lot of money on open-heart surgery and so stop offering the associated DRGs. It would not be feasible for a hospital to decide that it loses money on patients when they are at patient classification level 3 and to decide only to treat patients when they are classified as 1, 2, and 4.

The problem is even more complex. Costs, whether based on an acuity-adjusted patient day approach or a DRG-type approach, can be either resource-based or based on direct care hours. If resource-based costing is done, then resource consumption data must be collected for each patient or patient group. An hourly approach would charge a certain standard amount per nursing hour to each patient or patient group, for each hour of nursing care consumed. This hourly charge would include all nursing costs. In this case, only hours would have to be collected, instead of resources consumed. The hourly approach is the one that lawyers and accountants commonly use in their practices.

If nurse managers want to budget the appropriate amount of staff and other resources for the patients they expect to encounter, they must know the cost of providing nursing care to various types of patients. The characteristics of patients that make a difference in the cost of providing nursing is crucial. What are the key determinants of how much nursing care a patient needs? Can patients be grouped by nursing resource requirements? What costing approaches exist and how technically and financially feasible are they? These issues are the subject of this chapter.

WHY STUDY THE COST OF NURSING SERVICES?

The original impetus for developing advanced methods for costing nursing services was a desire to "take nursing out of the room and board side of the ledger and put us on the revenue-producing side."[1] Historically, nursing has not been treated as a revenue center in health care. Instead, it has been included in the per diem charge in hospitals, along with hotel-type costs for room and meals or in the overall fee for most other types of health care organizations. This has created many misconceptions. Some administrators view nursing costs as a burden—a substantial outlay not generating any revenue inflows.

Such a perspective is clearly incorrect. The presence of the nursing staff and the quality of nursing care offered are critical factors in attracting patients to the

---

[1]Franklin A. Shaffer, *Costing Out Nursing: Pricing Our Product,* National League for Nursing, 1985 p. 5.

institution. Without quality nursing care there would be no revenue. Nevertheless, without some costing mechanism superior to the one historically used, nursing cannot be treated as a revenue center. This causes the "burden" view to persist.[2] To address this problem, many researchers started trying to develop costing methods that would allow nursing to become a revenue center.

The more that nurse managers understand about the nursing services that are provided to patients and what it costs to provide those services, the better position they are in to control those costs. Many health care organizations are in a critical financial position. To survive, they must know which patients generate profits and which generate losses. Even if they feel morally bound not to turn away patients that generate losses, added knowledge can allow them to focus marketing attention on those patients that are profitable. The profits made from those patients can then support the care for the remaining patients. Therefore, efficient management requires that nurse managers understand costs by type of patient.

CURRENT COSTING APPROACHES

The essence of the costing problem is that often nursing costs are charged to patients as part of a general charge, rather than being charged separately on the patient's bill. As a result, different patients all receive the same charge for nursing care services. In terms of providing management with an understanding of the cost implications of different patients, this provides extremely poor information. It implicitly assumes that all patients consume exactly the same amount of nursing care, even though different patients have different nursing care requirements.

Why has costing for nursing care taken this direction to begin with? In order to charge different amounts to different patients, it must be possible to determine different amounts of resource consumption for different patients. In some areas it would be virtually impossible to measure differential consumption. For example, how much of the Chief Financial Officer's time is consumed by each patient? One would be hard pressed to show that different patients receive different amounts of benefit from the CFO. Even if they did, it would be impossible to measure.

In the case of nursing, however, different patients do consume different amounts of nursing resources. This is particularly true for hospitalized patients whose nursing requirements vary considerably. Nevertheless, until the decade of the 1980s, measuring differential consumption was, if not impossible, at least too costly to consider. Hospitals are faced with two extreme alternatives. One choice is to take the total annual costs of nursing care and divide that by the number of patients treated for the year, to come out with an average cost per patient. At the other extreme, the hospital could hire a data collector to follow each nurse and determine exactly how much of that nurse's time was used by each patient. Figure

---

[2]There are political and power issues related to this "burden" view. However, they are beyond the scope of this book.

16–1 reflects this extreme choice. Alternative A is a simple and inexpensive approach at one extreme. Alternative Z is an extremely detailed and expensive approach at the other extreme.

What hospital could afford to assign a data collector to each nurse to observe how much of the nurse's time was being devoted to each patient? The value of information should always justify its cost. Alternative Z in Figure 16–1 was just too costly to undertake. Figure 16–2 adds a compromise. In most cases, a patient with a 3-day length of stay would consume less nursing care than a patient with a 15-day length of stay. If total nursing care costs are divided by total patient days, patients who are in the hospital for more days can be assigned more nursing cost than patients in the hospital for fewer days. This is Alternative B. It is still not nearly as precise and accurate an approach as Alternative Z. However, it is not much more expensive than Alternative A, and it gives a much better approximation of the nursing care cost for different patients.

However, under Alternative B, the approach most hospitals use, the nursing cost is assumed to be the same for all patient days. More days imply more cost, but for the same number of patient days, all patients are assumed to use the same amount of nursing care. While this is much better than Alternative A, it is still a poor measure of nursing cost. Differing acuity of different patients results in a need for more or less nursing care per patient day.

SOLUTIONS TO THE COSTING PROBLEM

Computerization of the Costing Process

How can the cost of each individual patient be better measured, without having an accountant follow every nurse? One solution that many hospitals are beginning to examine is computerization. The addition of computers, not only at nursing stations but also by each bedside, is seen by many nurses to be the future for all hospitals. Many hospitals have already installed bedside computer terminals.

There will be a variety of uses for such computers. Nursing documentation may improve dramatically. Immediate access to information, such as lab test results, also has the potential for great improvement. Quality of care is improved by using computers for functions such as checking medications before they are administered, for correct dose, timing, and medication. Another use of bedside computer systems is to better track nursing costs.

In Figure 16–3, computers have been added to the continuum from low-accuracy, low-cost information to high-accuracy, high-cost information. This alternative has been labeled as Y. With computers, nurses record not only when they are with each patient but also what they are doing for each patient. The specific cost of the nurse giving care can be associated with the patient by having the computer multiply the time spent by the salary of the particular nurse providing the care. When nurses are doing some indirect activities, such as

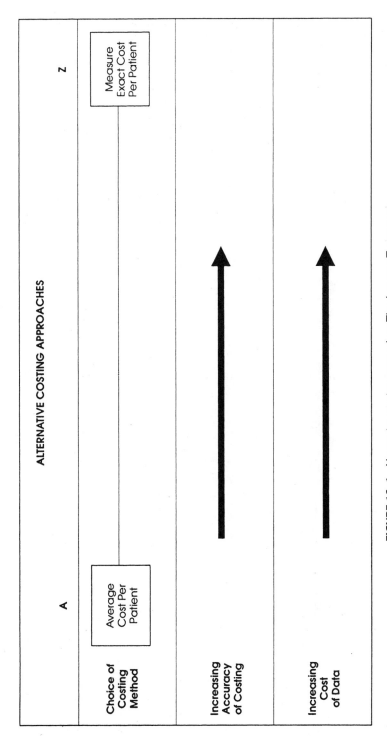

FIGURE 16–1. Alternative costing approaches: The A versus Z extremes.

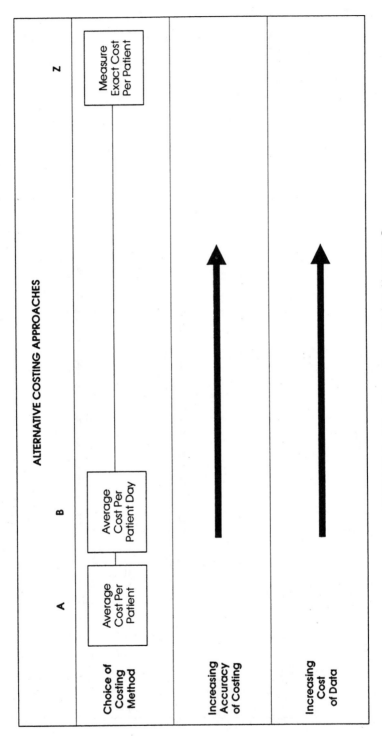

FIGURE 16–2. Alternative costing approaches: Alternative B.

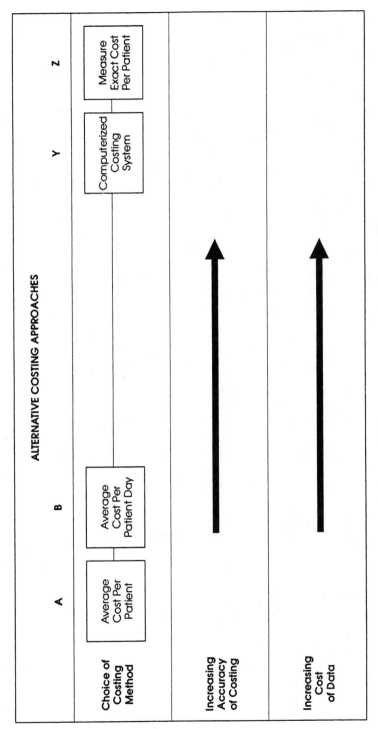

FIGURE 16–3. Alternative costing approaches: Alternative Y.

371

documenting a patient's record, the computer can also assign that cost to the appropriate patient, since the documentation is being done on the computer.

Substantial progress is currently being made in a variety of areas to ease the input of data into the computer. Uniform price codes (bar coding) are becoming more widely used on a variety of supplies consumed by health care organizations. Employee identification cards are being issued by most health care organizations, with magnetic strips containing the employee number in computer readable form. This allows nurses to slide their card into the computer to identify themselves. Light pens have been replaced with touch sensitive screens. Such screens allow the user to simply touch a particular item on the screen to select menu choices and enter data. The result of progress in the computer area is that bedside terminals can accurately capture most of the costs (both the direct and many indirect costs) of providing nursing care to specific patients.

Note that Alternative Y is close to Alternative Z in several respects. The data to be gained is potentially accurate and clearly can be patient-specific. For patients that require the presence of a nurse at the bedside for substantial amounts of time, that cost will be captured. It would be able to assign different patients costs (and ultimately charges) based on their differing consumption of nursing resources.

Current Solutions

Another approach to estimating the cost of nursing care is a *patient classification system.* Patient classification systems require rating patients based on the likely nursing resource requirements resulting from their acuity. Sicker patients requiring more nursing care are assigned higher acuity or higher classification levels. Many hospitals have developed their own systems, while several commercial systems are widely used in hospitals throughout the United States. Patients are rated on scales, such as 1 to 5. Patient classification systems were discussed in Chapter 8.

Nonhospital health care organizations also have a variety of approaches for classifying patients by resource consumption. However, these often focus on physician time or total resources. Work is needed on improving the ability to assess nursing resource consumption by different types of patients in various types of health care organizations.

Patient classifications will not generally be perfectly accurate measures of the resources needed for each patient. Some patients that are classified as a level 2 patient will require more care than level 2 calls for, and some level 2 patients will require less care than would be expected based on that classification. However, if the system is functioning reasonably well, on average patient resource consumption will match that which is expected, based on the classification system. And certainly it would generally be expected that a level 2 patient will consume resources closer to the level 2 average than to the level 1 average or the level 3 average.

If a mechanism to cost out patients based on their patient classification can be established, it will not provide the precise accuracy of Alternative Z. It will not even provide the Alternative Y accuracy that a computer system can generate. However, it can create a new alternative, called X (see Fig. 16–4). Alternative X is inaccurate in that all patients are assigned the same nursing cost for a day at the same classification level. If two patients are both level 2 on a given day, their cost is assumed to be the same, even though it is known that they will probably not consume exactly the same nursing resources. However, Alternative X is much more accurate than Alternatives A and B. Alternative B assumes that the cost is the same per patient day for all patients, regardless of acuity.

Alternative X is an improvement because the cost is considered to be the same per patient day only for patients in the same acuity level. Different costs are assigned to patient days at different acuity levels. Users of Alternative X must recognize that the information has some degree of inaccuracy. However, the system may be accurate enough, given the current high costs of using either Alternative Y or Z. Therefore, patient classification systems can be the basis for a system that allows more accurate estimates of the cost a hospital incurs for nursing care for different types of patients.

Somewhere between X and Y on the scale from A to Z, one could place workload measurement tools. These are variants of patient classification. Workload measurement tools attempt to determine the nursing care time required for each individual patient each day. The approach of these tools is to identify the time required for each of the types of nursing interventions that take up most of the nurses' time. Each patient is evaluated each day to determine which interventions will be needed. Thus, such tools can track required care hours specific to each patient. This is contrasted with patient classification systems that use an average hour figure for all patients within a broad category or level of care.

Such an approach is not as sophisticated as Alternative Y, where the actual care hours are entered into the computer as the patient receives the care. It is likely that some interventions will take longer than typical for some patients and less time for others. Therefore, the cost ultimately assigned to the patient will be based on average times, not actual times. However, the workload measurement approach is more sophisticated than Alternative X, which uses average nursing care hours for all patients in a given patient classification category.

WHY CHANGE THE COSTING APPROACH?

The mere fact that the ability to improve costing now exists does not in itself explain why a nurse manager would want to improve costing. What is to be gained from having a more accurate measure of the different costs for nursing care for different types of patients?

One argument that is sometimes offered is that separate costing for different types of patients will allow for *variable billing*. Variable billing refers to the fact that the amount billed to each patient per patient day or per treatment varies.

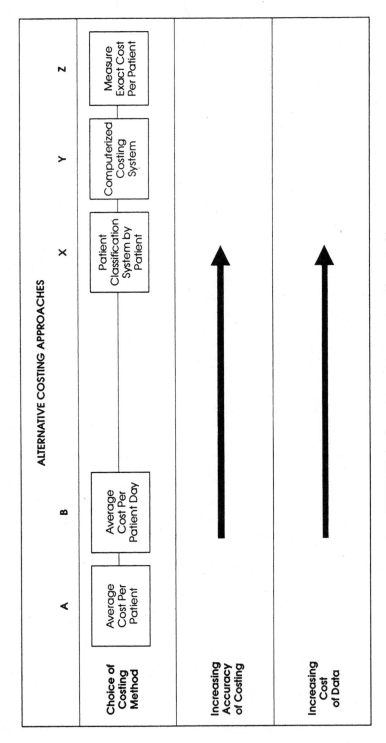

FIGURE 16–4. Alternative costing approaches: Alternative X.

Instead of simply charging all patients the same amount per day for their nursing care, different patients will be charged different amounts, based on their differing resource consumption. Once the different costs of caring for different patients are known, they can be charged accordingly.

To the extent that all patients are paid on a *prospective payment* basis, such as capitation or DRGs, variable billing holds little appeal. On the other hand, in most states at least some patients are charged for their services on a fee-for-service basis. In these cases, variable billing may be a way to better justify bills and, in some cases, increase overall revenues. Variable billing may be beneficial to nursing because it shows in a dramatic way the specific contribution that nursing makes to the overall revenue structure of the organization.

Variable billing is not the only advantage of better costing. A critical benefit from improved costing of nursing services is that the organization can generate information for better management decisions. Is a particular service too costly? What price can be bid for an HMO or PPO contract? Health care costing has long been based on averages and cross-subsidizations. In the current environment, errors in the calculations of costs become more serious, as negotiations for discounted prices becomes more intense. Thus, if the organization's managers are mistaken about the resources that a particular class of patient consumes, the ramifications can be serious. Less averaging of costs is acceptable today than was acceptable in the past. This means that managers are being pushed along the increasing accuracy of the costing line in Figure 16–4, even though this also moves in the direction of increased cost of data.

In addition, as costing becomes more specific and more accurate, not only is it possible to deal better with pricing problems, but managers can be more efficient in managing costs as well. Controlling budgets improves as another measure of expected cost becomes available. Flexible budget systems can provide better analysis and control of costs, and productivity can be monitored better if more is known about costs. It is possible to assess how costs should change based on changing numbers of patient days. It is also possible for information about the cost per patient for a given DRG to be used to assess the change in total costs as the number of patients in each DRG changes.

SHOULD COSTING BE LINKED TO DRGs?

If health care organizations are going to move in the direction of more accurate costing of nursing services, one of the critical questions is to determine how to categorize the cost. Should there be one nursing cost for medical patients and another for surgical patients? Should the cost for men as opposed to women be determined or for young people as opposed to old people? Should there be one nursing cost for each type of patient based on ICD or CPT code? Should the cost be found by DRG or based on Medicare outpatient ambulatory groupings?

The problem managers are faced with is the definition of the product of nursing care. What is it that nursing produces? If a nurse changes a dressing or gives a patient a medication, are those the products of nursing care? Probably, most people would consider those activities to represent only intermediate products. The ultimate product is care of the patient, not any one part of that care.

However, health care organizations treat many different kinds of patients. They do not have only one final product: care of a patient. They have many final products represented by the different patients that nurses give care to. Yet currently all patients are costed for nursing care as if they were the same. This needs to be changed. Final products need to be defined so that nurse managers can assess the cost of each. Patients could be divided into categories called *Nursing Resource Groupings* (NRGs). Ideally, the patients should be divided into homogeneous NRGs based on nursing care consumed. Any patient in one NRG would consume a similar set of nursing resources as any other patient in that grouping.

What should be the basis for costing nursing services in the interim until a NRG-type system is in use? One approach is to fall back on Alternative X. A patient classification system can be used to determine how many days a given patient is at each classification level. If the cost of each day at each classification level (discussed later in this chapter) can be determined, the manager can add up the costs to determine the patient's total nursing care cost.

However, this requires determining the patient classification for every patient for every day. Some hospitals will feel that the advantages of being at Alternative X on the costing accuracy scale are sufficient to warrant this investment in data collection. Doing this not only will improve costing but also will collect information that can be used for calculating acuity variances (see Chapter 14).

However, many health care providers will not want to spend the resources needed to classify every patient every day or to classify every treatment or visit. The alternative is to take a sample of patients from each DRG or other categorization and determine the average nursing cost for patients in each DRG or category, based on a sampling approach. All patients within a specific DRG will not consume the exact same nursing resources for each day at a specific patient classification level. Nor will all patients in one DRG have the same number of patient days at each classification level, nor even have the same total number of patient days. The same is true regardless of the patient categorization system used. This approach is based on an *average* length of stay and an *average* number of days at each patient classification level, as well as *average* nurse resource consumption within each patient classification level. As a result, the *average* amount of nursing resources for each type of DRG can be found.

For example, if a hospital uses a nursing patient classification system that has a scale from 1 to 5, a group of patients from each DRG can be sampled to find out, on average, how many days of the patients' stay was at level 1, how many at level 2, and so on. The averaging of all patients in a given DRG at a given hospital will not give a measurement alternative accurate enough to be labeled W on the scale from A to Z. Such an estimate of cost would probably be considered to be R on such a scale. It would not be nearly as accurate as X, but it would be substantially more accurate than Alternatives A and B. This new alternative R (see Fig. 16–5) would be substantially less expensive than Alternatives X, Y, or Z.

Thus, it seems that DRGs or similar groupings or categorizations, although perhaps not ideal for the purpose of costing nursing care, are an adequate categorization for the assignment of average differential nursing costs. Many hospital decisions are based on particular DRGs or clusters of DRGs, so the DRG-based cost information generated will be of considerable management value. Organizations caring for ambulatory patients similarly will have to find a workable system for grouping patients that improves the accuracy of costing while being relevant for decision making.

A SPECIFIC APPROACH TO COSTING NURSING SERVICES

Nursing care costs consist of the staff costs of direct patient care, the staff costs of indirect patient care (supervisors, secretaries, etc.), patient care related costs (e.g., patient and unit supplies), and overhead (allocated from other departments). Note that the cost of nursing care is more than just the hourly salary and benefits of the nurse giving care at the bedside. Nursing management, assessment, planning, evaluating, teaching, and discharge planning are also critical elements of nursing care. Additionally, supplies, secretaries, and overhead are elements of overall nursing care cost. A manager could try to determine the costs of each of these elements separately for each category of patient or could do the costing in a more aggregate fashion. Start with the assumption that all nursing department costs are aggregated.

The key element that allows for improved costing of nursing services for hospitals is the fact that nursing patient classification systems are currently in place in almost every hospital. Without such systems, different patients consume different amounts of resources, but the manager has no way to measure the differential consumption. With a classification system, once a patient has been classified, the manager has some idea about the nursing resources they consume.

For example, suppose that a nursing unit has the following hypothetical patient classification resource guidelines:

Acuity Level	Hours of Care
1	3.0
2	4.0
3	4.8
4	6.6
5	9.0

In developing the patient classification system, various clinical indicators are used to determine if a patient should be classified as a 1, 2, 3, 4, or 5. Once the

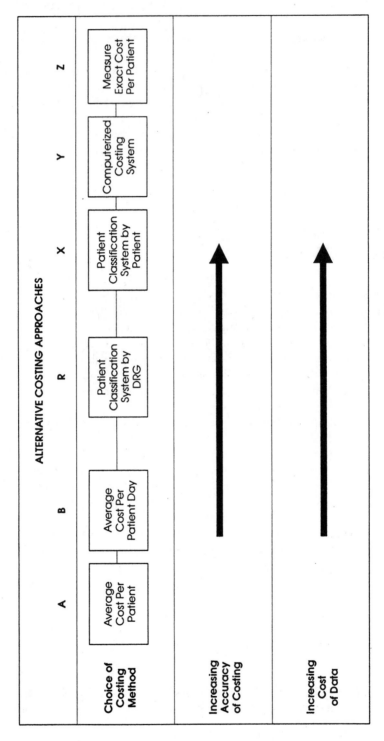

FIGURE 16–5. Alternative costing approaches: Alternative R.

patient has been classified, the classification system tells how many hours of nursing care should be required to treat that patient in your hospital. In the above example, a patient classified as a 4 would typically require on average 6.6 hours of care.

Note that the scale is not proportional. A patient classified as a 2 does not require exactly twice as many hours as a 1. While a level 1 needs 3 hours of care, a level 2 patient needs 4 hours. Rather than double, this is only 33% more care. A level 3 patient needs 4.8 hours. This is 20% more than a level 2. A level 4 patient requires 38% more care than a level 3. As one moves from level to level, the amount of additional care does not change in proportion. It changes based on the specific classification system and the clinical needs of a patient at each level in that system.

This complicates the cost calculation. If the scale were strictly linear, one could add up all the patient days at each level and divide into total nursing cost to get a cost per unit of patient classification. For example, suppose the unit had one patient day that was a level 1, one patient day that was a 3, and one patient day that was a 4. The total of $1 + 3 + 4$ is 8. If total nursing costs were $1,000, then the cost per patient classification unit would be $125 (i.e., $1,000/8). The cost for a patient day classified as a 4 would be $500 ($4 \times \$125$).

However, since the scale is not linear, it is necessary to create a relative value unit (RVU) scale. This scale will allow determination of how much care each level requires relative to the care needed for a typical level 1 patient. A patient classified as a 1 will be given a value of 1 on the *relative value scale*. Each other classification level would then be calculated in relative proportion. This can be accomplished by dividing the required hours of care for each level by the number of hours required for level 1. For example,

$$\frac{\text{Level 2}}{\text{Level 1}} \frac{4.0 \text{ hours}}{3.0 \text{ hours}} = 1.33$$

Therefore, the relative value assigned to classification level 2 is 1.33. This value of 1.33 represents the fact that a level 2 patient consumes .33 more nursing care hours than a level 1 patient. Continuing for all classification (acuity) levels:

Acuity Level	Hours of Care	RVU
1	3.0	1.00
2	4.0	1.33
3	4.8	1.60
4	6.6	2.20
5	9.0	3.00

Assuming the following information, the reader will be able to see how the RVU system can be used to develop cost information:

Total nursing costs:		$250,000
Number of patient days at each acuity level:	Level	1: 100 days
		2: 220 days
		3: 350 days
		4: 110 days
		5: 40 days

The first step is to determine the total amount of work performed by the nursing department. This is done by multiplying the RVUs for each acuity classification level by the number of days at that level. Using the number of patient days given above and the RVUs calculated above, the total RVUs would be:

Acuity Level	Patient Days	3	RVU	5	Total RVUs
1	100	×	1.00	=	100.00
2	220	×	1.33	=	292.60
3	350	×	1.60	=	560.00
4	110	×	2.20	=	242.00
5	40	×	3.00	=	120.00
	820				1,314.60

There were 1,314.6 units of nursing work performed. We can divide this into the total nursing cost to find the cost for each RVU of nursing work.

$$\frac{\text{Total Nursing Costs}}{\text{Total RVUs}} = \text{Cost per RVU}$$

$$\frac{\$250,000}{1,314.60} = \$190.17 \text{ per RVU}$$

Here one can see that the nursing cost for a patient for one day with classification 1 would be $190.17. The cost for a patient with classification 4 would be $190.17 multiplied by 2.20 (the RVU for classification level 4).

How would a manager calculate the nursing cost for a patient from admission to discharge? Suppose that the average DRG 128 patient had a length of stay of seven days, with two days classed as a 1, four days classed as a 2, and one day classed as a 4. The nursing cost for DRG 128 would then be:

Acuity Level	Patient Days	3	RVU	3	Cost per RVU	5	Total Cost
1	2	×	1.00	×	$190.17	=	$ 380.34
2	4	×	1.33	×	190.17	=	1,011.70
3	0	×	1.60	×	190.17	=	0.00
4	1	×	2.20	×	190.17	=	418.37
5	0	×	3.00	×	190.17	=	0.00
	7						$1,810.41

Would all patients in a given DRG be expected to consume the same resources? Not really, but the manager can still be confident that an approach such as this, on average for any given DRG, will give a much more accurate assignment of cost than simply assigning to every patient in a nursing unit the same daily cost for nursing care.

LIMITATIONS OF THE RVU APPROACH

Patient Classification vs. Other Workload Measurement

The purpose of the RVU–Patient Classification approach is to provide a workable costing approach accessible to the majority of health care organizations in the country. However, it does not generate perfectly accurate measures of cost and is subject to a variety of limitations.

For example, the idea of an alternative to patient classification was discussed earlier. If a workload measurement tool is in place in a hospital and is being used on an ongoing basis to categorize resource needs of each patient each day, then it can be used to provide cost information that is potentially more accurate. Rather than being limited to perhaps 5 patient classification levels for a given Med/Surg unit, such an approach collects indicators of hours of resource consumption for each patient. It is more patient-specific than the RVU approach. Putting such an approach in place and following through with it on a continuous basis may be a considerable undertaking. However, if it is used, costing is made potentially easier.

Under such an approach, the required interventions for each patient are translated into required hours of care. Total nursing care costs for direct and indirect expenses must be calculated as with the RVU system. Dividing total nursing costs by total hours of care generates a cost per hour of care. This cost per hour can be multiplied by the required hours of care for each patient for each day as determined by the system. This will give the cost per patient for each day in the hospital. If aggregate information is desired by DRG, it can be obtained by averaging the costs of each patient in that DRG. However, the majority of hospitals do not have patient-specific work measurement systems in place. Many ambulatory settings do not have an adequate classification system to use to improve costing accuracy. They may have to leapfrog directly to a computerized system to achieve accurate costing.

Indirect Nursing Costs

A problem with both the RVU and more detailed work measurement systems, as described so far is that this chapter has been assuming implicitly that all nursing costs vary in proportion to the hours of nursing care. Does that make sense for indirect costs? For example, will a sicker patient who requires more direct nursing care also require more indirect nursing care? More charting time?

More supplies? More overhead? The answers to these questions depend on the specific situation of your institution.

Is it true that secretarial costs will be greater for patients that are more acutely ill? It may well be that a simple per diem allocation is a more appropriate way to allocate such costs. Costing could therefore be improved by dividing total nursing costs between those costs that vary with nursing care hours (such as RN staff and LPN staff, and perhaps clinical supplies) and those costs that do not vary with nursing care hours (such as office supplies, nurse manager time, and secretarial time). The costs that vary with nursing care hours would be allocated by the RVU or work measurement approaches described above. The other costs could be divided by total patient days and assigned to patients based on their number of patient days.

Staffing Mix

A significant problem is the fact that most nursing classification systems provide required hours of care but do not specify the mix of care. If 30% of all nursing care hours are provided by LPNs, then it is assumed that 30% of the care for each patient is provided by LPNs.

It is possible that one patient at level 2 might require 4 hours of RN care while another might require 3 hours of LPN care and only 1 hour of RN care. Obviously, both patients do not consume the same amount of nursing care resources, even if they consume the same number of hours of care. Therefore, there will be some distortion of costs unless the hospital uses a system that not only indicates how many hours of care are needed but also how many hours of care by staff type.

This problem is not unique to costing, however. It represents a weakness of patient classification systems. If the organization does not know the required mix of care providers, the classification system is not going to be useful for staffing decisions. Part of this problem stems from the fact that different organizations have different views on which functions can be done by different types of staff. However, over time one can expect that classification systems will improve. As they do, this mix problem should become less serious.

In the meantime, managers could attempt to separate the cost of RNs from LPNs and aides and assign those costs separately to patients. Special studies could be undertaken for each DRG to determine whether their care was biased toward more than an average amount of RN care or toward more than an average amount of LPN care. Then the cost of nursing care for that DRG could be adjusted accordingly.

How complex are managers willing to make the costing system? Health care organizations must decide how much refinement they are willing to make to their costing system, realizing that generally the more accurate the costing system is, the more expensive it is. Some managers believe that the historical average nursing cost per patient day is so inaccurate that an RVU-based system is a tremendous improvement, even with the problems cited here.

We have used a hospital as an example. The same principles apply whether the cost determination is for nursing care delivered in the hospital, nursing home, outpatient setting, or patient's home. However, in home care the costing is simplified by the fact that patient records explicitly indicate the level of staff that provided the care.

PRODUCT-LINE COSTING AND BUDGETING

One result of the work done on costing nursing services is that it is possible to group all patients of one type and find an average cost for that type of patient. In other words, *product-line* costing is feasible with this method. A product line is a group of patients with some commonality that allows them to be grouped together, such as a common diagnosis. In a similar approach, it is now common for organizations to focus on one disease, so-called disease management. Often an organization cannot eliminate one product in a product line without eliminating the entire product line. For example, if a hospital sells its bypass pump because it is losing money on bypass surgery, it will no longer be able to do heart valve surgery. They are both part of the open-heart surgery product line.

Many people believe that managers should be given hospital-wide responsibility for both the revenues and expenses related to specific patient product lines. For example, a manager might be responsible for the revenues related to the obstetrics product line. The manager is accountable for both the variance in the number of discharges and the revenue per discharge. Of course the manager would be responsible for the budgeted and actual costs of the product line as well.

Before one takes the step of costing by product line or budgeting by product line, it is necessary to question what the information will be used for. In terms of running a nursing unit, will knowledge of the cost for all patients in a given DRG be useful? The answer to that question depends a great deal on the types of decisions that a manager or organization faces.

Suppose that a hospital is trying to decide whether to accept a group of cardiac patients from an HMO at a discounted price. Knowing the costs for that type of patient would certainly be advantageous in the negotiating process. Often, product-line calculations include nursing costs simply as part of the overall per diem cost. The organization can have much better information about different types of patients if it relies on the costing procedures discussed above, in doing product-line calculations.

Direct Care Hours

The direct care hours approach to product-line budgeting consists of dividing the patients for a given nursing unit into product lines, determining the number of hours of care required for each product line, and aggregating that information to find the total hours of care needed in the budget. This is a straightforward approach to using product-line information to improve budgeting capability. It represents an alternative to using acuity adjusted patient days for determining nurse staff requirements.

Consider calculation of direct care costs for a hospital product-line. In this approach, the first step is to separate all patients for a unit into specific groups. These groups, or product lines, could conform to DRGs but do not have to. The next step is to determine how many patients are expected in the coming period in each group. This information can be generated using the forecasting techniques discussed in Chapter 6. Using historical information, forecasting can also be used to predict the average length of stay of the patients in each group.

Once the manager has predictions of the number of patient days in each group and the average length of stay, those two numbers can be multiplied to determine the total number of patient days expected in each product line. The number of patient days can be multiplied by the expected average direct care hours per patient day (HPPD) for patients in the product line to generate the total hours of direct care needed for each specific product line. The total direct care hours for each product line can then be aggregated to determine the total direct care hours needed for the unit for the coming year. Based on this information, the unit's budget for staff can be prepared. Table 16–1 presents a simplified example of this process. In this example, sufficient staff must be budgeted to provide 24,300 direct care hours. The benefit of this process is that it has the potential to provide accurate information on the resources needed by the unit.

The major difficulty with this process is determining an accurate measure of average direct care hours per patient day by product line. If this information is inaccurate, the resulting total direct care hours needed will be inaccurate as well. Gaining information on the actual average direct care hours per patient day can be accomplished using any of a number of the costing methods discussed in this chapter. If an accurate forecast of patient days by patient classification level cannot be generated, then planning the budget based on a forecast of the number of patients in each product line may be extremely helpful.

TABLE 16–1. *Product-Line Budgeting for Direct Care Hours*

	Forecast Volume of Patients	Forecast Average Length of Stay	Expected Patient Days	Expected Hours per Patient Day	Total Hours of Direct Care
Product Line 1	200	3	600	5	3,000
Product Line 2	50	5	250	6	1,500
Product Line 3	100	4	400	3	1,200
Product Line 4	300	7	2,100	6	12,600
Product Line 5	500	3	1,500	4	6,000
					24,300

Total Nursing Cost by Product Line

The discussion of direct care hours focuses on product-line budgeting primarily to help in preparing a budget for the amount of nursing staff needed for a unit. It is possible to think of product-line budgeting as a more complete approach to budgeting all the costs for a nursing unit or department. Such an approach is also more helpful for providing the organization with information on the total costs for nursing care for patients in each product line.

This approach to product-line costing has already been discussed earlier in this chapter, when the hypothetical costs for a DRG 128 patient were calculated. Using the RVU approach to patient costing, it was demonstrated in the example that the average costs for a patient in this product line would be $1,810.41. In the example, it was assumed that the actual total costs of the unit were known. Based on these total costs, the cost of having provided care to a DRG 128 patient was calculated.

If one were to use budgeted costs instead of actual costs, then one could project the budgeted or anticipated costs for treating a patient in each given DRG or product line. Such information would be useful for a wide variety of managerial decisions, such as whether or not to expand capacity for treating patients in a particular product line.

Standard Treatment Protocols

A central article on product-line costing established an even more far-reaching approach to the topic.[3] This approach centers on the idea that hospitals treat patients by providing them with a large number of intermediate products. By carefully examining each department, one can make a list of the various intermediate products produced by that department. For example, a laboratory department produces different types of lab tests. Based on this approach, the set of intermediate products consumed by the average patient in a specific product line can be used to determine the costs of that product line. The set of intermediate products consumed by a patient in each product line is referred to as the Standard Treatment Protocol (STP) for that product line.

In this system, each intermediate product is called a Service Unit (SU). A chest x-ray would be one type of service unit produced by the radiology department. A patient who has three chest x-rays receives three of this service unit. A Standard Cost Profile (SCP) must be established for each SU. This profile indicates the cost of producing that service unit.

Conceptually, this seems straightforward. The patient care provided by each department is broken down into intermediate products called Service Units. The cost of each SU is determined. The average number of each SU from each department is found for each product line. Then the SUs consumed for a product

---

[3]William O. Cleverley: "Product-Costing for Health Care Firms." *Health Care Management Review,* Vol. 12, No. 4, Fall 1987, pp. 39–48.

line are multiplied by their cost to determine the total costs for patients in that product line.

A difficulty with the approach is determining SUs for nursing units. One could try to break down nursing care into the various specific activities and then relate those to SUs. Administering a medication could be an SU. Taking a patient's vital signs could be an SU. Charting information about a patient could be an SU. At some point, when hospital computer information systems are adequately sophisticated, it would be possible to disaggregate nursing care and assign it to patients in this manner. It would then be possible to determine the average number of vital signs taken for a patient in a specific product line. For most hospitals, such a detailed level of information is not currently cost-effective to collect. However, nursing SUs could be based on patient classification. Thus, a patient day at level 3 could be an SU. A day at level 4 would be a different SU. When the STP is established, it would consider which nursing SUs are typically consumed and how many of each. The costs for those SUs could be determined using the RVU method discussed earlier.

This method is an ambitious approach to product-costing and budgeting. It is used in more health care organizations each year. It creates an ability to have detailed information from all parts of the organization, including nursing, about each product line. The management implications of such information are significant. By examining all the SUs consumed in each department, a team of clinicians might be able to find ways to more efficiently provide care. SUs with a lower SCP might be substituted for more expensive ones. Ways might be found to reduce the number of SUs in various departments. If one considers product-line costing broadly, as a tool to use in managing the organization's product lines, the potential benefits of product-line costing and budgeting are significant.

SUMMARY AND IMPLICATIONS FOR NURSE MANAGERS

Improving the costing of nursing services has become important to nurse managers for several primary reasons. One reason is that improved cost information can be used to get an improved understanding of the contribution that nursing makes to the organization as a whole. A second reason is that the information generated by improved costing can be used to help managers make effective decisions and better control the costs of providing nursing services. Thirdly, periodic nursing shortages make it more important to understand the nursing resources needed by patients. Costing information is also useful for examining changes in the way nursing care is provided. For example, the cost impact of primary versus team nursing or of using different levels of staff can be examined.

The most accurate costing system requires continuous observation of all nurses by data collectors. The cost of such highly accurate costing is prohibitive. However, one can think of a continuum of costing methods. Less expensive methods provide less accurate data; more expensive methods provide more accurate data.

Over time, bedside computerization may become inexpensive enough to be introduced to most hospitals. Also over time, software programs will be developed and perfected to make using the computers easy and efficient. At the time of the writing of this book, however, the majority of hospitals did not have such systems in place. On the other hand, many hospitals are experimenting with such systems. If demonstration projects can show the bedside computer to be a cost-effective tool for nursing, it will not be long before costing can be done routinely at the bedside and nurses' stations.

In the meantime, patient classification systems can be used to improve substantially the assignment of nursing costs to patients in an economical way. Combining classification with an RVU system is relatively simple. Once this has been done, all nursing costs can be allocated based on the RVU system or some costs can be allocated using RVUs while other costs are assigned to patients based on patient days or some other approach. Each hospital must decide how much refinement to the RVU approach is worthwhile. Other health care organizations are likely to follow hospital advancements. However, some may decide to leapfrog directly to sophisticated computerized costing systems.

It is important to stress that the RVU approach suggested here is not perfect. It has a number of limitations and weaknesses. However, the nurse manager must decide whether these weaknesses are so significant that the method should not be used, in light of the fact that the costs generated, while not perfectly accurate, are likely to be a substantial improvement over costing methods that have historically been used.

Costing out nursing services provides a tool that is extremely useful for product-line costing and budgeting. Information about product-line costs can show management where profits are being made and where losses are accruing. Product-line information can aide managers substantially in understanding which patients place the greatest burden on the unit and in helping the organization make appropriate decisions regarding changes in the organization's mix of patients.

SUGGESTED READINGS

Barfield, J., et al. (1997). *Cost Accounting: Tradition and Innovations.* Minneapolis: West Publishing.

Doyle, J.J. (1996, October). Full cost determination of different levels of care in the intensive care unit: An activity-based costing approach. *PharmacoEconomics.* 10(4), 395–408.

Ervin, N., Chang, W., and White, J. (1988). A cost analysis of a nursing center's services. *Nursing Economic$.* 16(6), 307–312.

Finkler, S.A., and Ward, D.R. (1999). *Cost Accounting for Health Care Organizations: Concepts and Applications,* Second edition. Gaithersburg, MD: Aspen Publishers.

Gardner, K., Tobin, J., Kamm, J., and Allhusen, J. (1997, July–August). Determining the cost of care through clinical pathways. *Nursing Economic$.* 15(4), 213–217.

Hansen, D., and Mowen, M. (1997). *Cost Management,* Second edition. Cincinnati: South-Western Publishing.

Heshmat, S. (1997, Winter). Managed care and the relevant costs for pricing. *Health Care Management Review.* 22(1), 82–85.

Jegers, M. (1997, June). Cost accounting in ICUs: Beneficial for management and research. *Clinical Therapeutics.* 19(3), 570–581.

Jones, K.R. (1995, September). Standard cost accounting. *Seminars for Nurse Managers.* 3(3), 111–112.

Kocakulah, M., Hagenow, N., and Cope, F. (1990, December). The true costs of nursing care. A simple approach provides more accurate accounting of nursing services. *Health Progress.* 71(10), 48–51.

Swindle, R.W., et al. (1996, March). The quality of cost data: A caution from the department of veterans affairs experience. *Medical Care.* 34(3), 83–90.

West, D.A., West, T.D., Balas, E.A., and Mcks, L.L. (1996, May–June). Profitable capitation requires accurate costing. *Nursing Economic$.* 14(3), 150, 162–170.

Additional Suggested Readings

Abbey, D.C. (1996). *The Ambulatory Patient Group Operations Manual.* Chicago: Irwin.

Abbey, D.C. (1998). *Outpatient Services.* New York: Healthcare Financial Management Association Educational Foundation—McGraw Hill.

Allen, J.E. (1997). *Nursing Home Administration.* New York: Springer.

Benson, J.A., Michelman, J.E., and Radjenovic D. (1996, December). Using information technology strategically in home care. *Home Healthcare Nursing.* 14(12), 977–983.

Emery, D.R., Finnerty, J.D., and Stowe, J.D. (1998). *Principles of Financial Management.* Upper Saddle River, NJ: Prentice Hall.

Ervin, N., Chang, W., and White, J. (1998). A cost analysis of a nursing center's services. *Nursing Economic$.* 16(6), 307–312.

Finkler, S.A. (1996). *Finance & Accounting for Nonfinancial Managers,* Revised and expanded edition. Upper Saddle River, NJ: Prentice Hall.

Finkler, S.A., and Kovner, C.T. (2000). *Financial Management for Nurse Managers and Executives,* Second edition. Philadelphia: W.B. Saunders.

Folland, S., Goodman, A.C., and Stano, M. (1996). *The Economics of Health and Health Care.* Upper Saddle River, NJ: Prentice Hall.

Getzen, T. (1996). *Health Economics: Fundamentals and Flow of Funds.* New York: John Wiley & Sons.

Holman, E.J., and Branstetter, E. (1997, September–October). An academic nursing clinic's financial survival. *Nursing Economic$.* 15(5), 248–252.

Horngren, C.T., and Sundem, G.L. (1998). *Introduction to Financial Accounting,* Seventh edition. Upper Saddle River, NJ: Prentice Hall.

Hunter, J.K., Ventura, M.R., and Kearns, P.A. (1999, January/February). Cost analysis of a nursing center for the homeless. *Nursing Economic$.* 17(1), 20–28.

Karr, J., and Fisher, R. (1997). A patient classification system for ambulatory care. *Nursing Management.* 28(9), 27–29.

McKeon, T. (1996). *Home Health Financial Management.* Gaithersburg, MD: Aspen Publishers.

Mitty, E.L. (1998). *Handbook for Directors of Nursing in Long-Term Care.* Albany: Delmar.

Spitzer-Lehmann, R. (1994). *Nursing Management Desk Reference: Concepts, Skills & Strategies.* Philadelphia: W.B. Saunders.

Glossary

activity based costing (ABC) An approach to determining the cost of products or product lines using allocation bases that relate to the activities that generate overhead costs.

activity statement See *operating statement.*

acuity A measurement of patient severity of illness related to the amount of nursing care resources required to care for the patient.

acuity subcategory Represents the amount that would have been budgeted for the actual output level if the actual acuity level had been correctly forecast.

acuity variance The variance resulting from the difference between the actual acuity level and the budgeted level; the difference between the flexible budget and the value of the acuity subcategory (see Chapter 14).

ADC See *average daily census.*

administration Management.

allowances Discounts from the amount normally charged for patient care services. These discounts are sometimes negotiated (e.g., with HMOs or Blue Cross) and other times mandated by law (e.g., with Medicare and Medicaid).

ALOS See *average length of stay.*

annuity A series of payments or receipts each in the same amount and spaced at even time periods. For example: $127.48 paid monthly for 3 years.

asset A resource owned by the organization.

average daily census The average number of inpatients on any given day; patient days in a given time period divided by the number of days in the time period.

average length of stay The average number of patient days for each patient discharged; the number of patient days in a given time period divided by the number of discharges in that time period.

bad debts Amounts that are charged to patients who are expected to pay but that are not collected because of a failure by the patients to pay.

balance sheet A financial statement that lists all the assets and liabilities of the organization.

benchmarking A technique that organizations use to find the best practices in an industry and to incorporate those practices within the organization.

Blue Cross A major provider of hospitalization insurance to both individuals and groups.

break-even analysis A technique for determining the minimum volume of output (patients) necessary in order for a program or service to be financially self-sufficient.

budget A plan that provides a formal, quantitative expression of management's plans and intentions or expectations.

budget foundations Environmental scan; statement of goals, objectives and policies; list of organization-wide assumptions; specification of program priorities; and set of specific, measurable objectives.

budgeting A process whereby plans are made and then an effort is made to meet or exceed the goals of the plans.

business plan A detailed plan for a proposed program, project, or service, including information to be used to assess the venture's financial feasibility.

capital acquisitions See *capital assets.*

capital assets Buildings or equipment with useful lives extending beyond the year in which they are purchased or put into service. Also referred to as long-term investments, capital items, capital investments, or capital acquisitions.

capital budget A plan for the acquisition of buildings and equipment that will be used by the organization for 1 or more years beyond the year of acquisition. Often there is a minimum dollar cutoff that must be exceeded for an item to be included in the capital budget.

capital budgeting The process of proposing the purchase of capital assets, analyzing the proposed purchases for economic or other justification, and encompassing the financial implications of accepted capital items into the master budget.

capital equipment Equipment with an expected life beyond the year of purchase. Such equipment must generally be included in the capital budget.

capital investments See *capital assets.*

capital items See *capital assets.*

capitation Payment of a fixed amount per person for health services regardless of the actual number or nature of services provided.

carve out An arrangement whereby coverage for a specific category of services is excluded from a broader contract for services.

case-mix The mix of different types of patients treated by a health care organization.

case-mix index A measurement of the average complexity or severity of illness of patients treated by a health care organization.

cash budget A plan for the cash receipts and cash disbursements of the organization.

cash budgeting The process of planning the cash budget.

cash disbursement The outflow of cash from the organization.

cash flow A measure of the amount of cash received or disbursed for a period of time, as opposed to revenues or income that frequently are recorded at a time other than when the actual cash receipt or payment occurs.

cash flow statement See *statement of cash flows.*

cash management An active process of planning for borrowing and repayment of cash, or investment of excess cash on hand.

cash payment See *cash disbursement.*

cash receipt The inflow of cash into the organization.

census The number of patients occupying a bed at a specific time of day (usually midnight).

charges The amount a health care organization charges for its services; its prices. Often it collects less than its charges due to contractual allowances, charity care, and bad debts.

charity care The portion of the organization's charges that are not paid because an uninsured patient cannot afford to pay.

chart of accounts An accounting document that assigns an identifying number to each cost center and each type of revenue or expense. These code numbers are assigned to all financial transactions. By looking at any code number and referring to the chart of accounts, one would know exactly which cost center was involved and the specific type of revenue or expense.

chief nurse executive The highest level nurse manager in the organization.

contractual allowances The difference between the organization's charges for patient care services and the amount actually paid by the government (Medicare or Medicaid) or by a third-party payer, such as an HMO that has contracted with the organization for a price discount.

compound interest A method of calculating interest that recognizes interest not only on the amount of the original investment but also on the interest earned in interim periods of time.

constant dollars Dollar amounts that have been adjusted for the impact of inflation.

contingency An event that may occur, although it is either unintended or relatively unlikely.

continuous budgeting A system in which a budget is prepared each month for a month 1 year in the future. For example, once the actual results for this January are known, a budget for January of the next year is prepared.

continuous quality improvement (CQI) A philosophy concerning the production of an organization's goods and services that proposes that there should be a constant focus on improvement of the quality of the goods or services.

contribution from operations The contribution margin from the routine annual operations of the organization.

contribution margin The amount by which the price exceeds the variable cost. If the contribution margin is positive, it means that each extra unit of activity makes the organization better off by that amount.

control An attempt to assure that actual results come as closely to planned results as possible.

controllable Those items over which a manager can exercise a degree of control.

co-payment The portion of a health care invoice that is the responsibility of an insured patient (after the deductible has been met). For example, an insurer bears a portion of the cost (often 80%) and the insured individual bears the remainder (usually 20%). (See also *deductible.*)

cost-based Charges for services that are determined based on the cost of providing care.

cost-benefit analysis Measurement of the relative costs and benefits associated with a particular project or task.

cost center A unit or department in an organization for which a manager is assigned responsibility for costs.

cost driver An activity that causes costs to be incurred.

cost effective An approach that provides care as good as any other approach, but at a lower cost, or an approach that provides the best possible care for a given level of cost.

cost-effectiveness analysis Assessment of whether an alternative provides outcomes that are at least as good as another alternative but for a lower cost.

cost estimation The process of using historical cost information to segregate mixed costs into their fixed and variable components, and then using that information to estimate future costs.

cost pass-through A payment by a third party that reimburses the health care organization for the amount of costs it incurred in providing care to patients.

cost reimbursement A system in which the amount paid for services received is derived directly from the costs of the services provided.

CPM See *critical path method.*

Critical Path Method (CPM) A program technique that indicates the cost and time for each element of a complex project and indicates cost/time trade-offs where applicable.

curvilinear Using curved lines.

decision package A zero-based budgeting term referring to a package of all the information to be used in ranking alternatives and making a final decision.

deductible An amount that must first be paid by an insured individual before the insurance covers any costs. Usually the first $100 or $200 per year for health insurance.

deductions from revenue Amounts that are subtracted from the organization's charges for reasons such as contractual discounts given to managed care organizations.

deficit An excess of expenses over revenues. This term sometimes is used to refer to the current year or budgeted year and sometimes to refer to the deficit accumulated over a period of years.

delphi A forecasting technique in which an expert group (which never meets) makes forecasts in writing. All forecasts are distributed to all members of the group, along with the reasoning behind them. This process is repeated several times, and eventually a group decision is made.

demographics The characteristics of the human population, including age, sex, growth, density, distribution, and other vital statistics.

dependent variable The item whose value is being predicted.

depreciation Allocation of a portion of the cost of a capital asset into each of the years of the item's expected useful life.

Diagnosis Related Groups (DRGs) A system that categorizes patients into specific groups based on their diagnosis, as well as other characteristics, such as age and type of surgery, if any. Currently used by Medicare and some other hospital payers as a basis for payment.

direct expenses Those expenses that can be specifically and exclusively related to the activity within the cost center.

disbursement Cash payment.

discount rate The interest rate used in discounting.

discounted cash flow A method that allows comparisons of amounts of money paid at different points of time by discounting all amounts to the present.

discounting The reverse of compound interest; a process in which interest that could be earned over time is deducted from a future payment to determine how much the future payment is worth in the present time.

discretionary costs Costs for which there is no clear-cut relationship between inputs and outputs. The treatment of more patients would not necessarily require more of this input; use of more of this input would not necessarily allow for treatment of more patients.

dividend A distribution of profits to owners of the organization.

DRGs See *Diagnosis Related Groups.*

employee benefits Compensation provided to employees in addition to their base salary (for example, health insurance, life insurance, vacation, and holidays).

employees per occupied bed The total number of paid FTEs divided by the average daily census.

EPOB See *employees per occupied bed.*

equity (a) Fairness. (b) Ownership (e.g., the share of a house that is owned by the homeowner free and clear of any mortgage obligations is the homeowner's equity in the house).

exception report A list of only those individual variances that exceed a specified limit.

expenditure Payment. Often used interchangeably with expense.

expense center Unit or department in an organization for which a manager is assigned responsibility for costs.

expenses The costs of services provided.

factor evaluation instruments An approach to patient classification that selects elements of care—critical indicators—that are the most likely predictors of nursing care needs. Individual patients are then assessed for the presence or absence of these critical indicators and based on this are assigned to a category.

favorable variance A variance in which less was spent than the budgeted amount.

fee-for-service A system in which there is an additional charge for each additional service provided (as opposed to a prepaid system in which all services are included, in exchange for one flat payment).

feedback Using information about actual results to shape future plans, in order to avoid repeating past mistakes and improve future plans.

financial statements Financial summaries that indicate the financial position of the organization at a particular time, as well as the financial results of the organization's activities for a period of time.

fiscal Financial.

fiscal year A 1-year period defined for financial purposes. A fiscal year may start at any point during the calendar year and finish 1 year later. For example, "fiscal year 2003 with a June 30 year-end" refers to the period from July 1, 2002, through June 30, 2003.

fixed costs Costs that do not change in total as volume changes.

flexible budget The amount that would have been budgeted had the actual workload level been accurately predicted. The flexible budget is the budgeted quantity of inputs, multiplied by the budgeted price of inputs, multiplied by the actual quantity of output.

flexible budget variance The difference between actual results and the flexible budget.

flexible budgeting A process of developing a budget based on different workload levels. Often used after the fact to calculate the amount that would have been budgeted for the actual workload levels attained. Depends heavily on the existence of variable costs.

for-profit An organization whose mission includes earning a profit that may be distributed to its owners.

forecast A prediction of some future value, such as patient days, chest tubes used, or nursing care hours per patient day.

forecasting The process of making forecasts.

free care See *charity care.*

fringe benefits See *employee benefits.*

FTE See *full-time equivalent.*

full-time equivalent (FTE) The equivalent of 1 full-time employee working for 1 year. This is generally calculated as 40 hours per week for 52 weeks, or a total of 2,080 paid hours. This includes both productive and nonproductive (vacation, sick, holiday, education, etc.) time. Two employees each working half time for 1 year would be the same as one FTE.

fund balance The residual value when liabilities are subtracted from assets. This represents the portion of the organization's total resources owned by the organization itself (not-for-profit organizations). See also *owner's equity.*

goal congruence Bringing together the goals, desires, and needs of the organization with those of its employees.

goal divergence The natural differences between the goals, desires, and needs of the organization and those of its employees.

GRASP A patient classification system "that measures, uses, and tracks the required care hours that are specific to each patient, as opposed to using an average hour figure for all patients within a broad category, or level of care" (Diane Meyer: "Costing Nursing Care with the GRASP System," in *Costing Out Nursing: Pricing Our Product,* Franklin A. Shaffer, ed., National League For Nursing, New York, 1985, p. 56).

hardware Computers and related equipment.

Hawthorne Effect The psychological effect that causes productivity of workers to improve when they receive attention.

health maintenance organization (HMO) An organization that provides nurse, physician, and hospital services to individuals or groups in exchange for a flat monthly payment.

HMO See *health maintenance organization.*

hours per patient day Paid hours divided by patient days.

HPPD See *hours per patient day.*

income statement See *operating statement.*

incremental costs The additional costs that will be incurred if a decision is made, which would not otherwise be incurred by the organization.

independent variable The causal variable used to predict the dependent variable.

indexation for inflation A process that adjusts a dollar value for the impact of inflation over a period of time by using a price index, such as the Consumer Price Index (CPI).

indigent care See *charity care.*

indirect expenses Expenses, such as administration or heating and lighting, that are shared by all departments. These expenses are not incurred within the cost center.

inputs Resources used for treating patients or otherwise producing output. Examples of inputs include paid nursing hours, chest tubes, and IV solutions.

internal rate of return (IRR) A discounted cash flow technique that calculates the rate of return earned on a specific project or program.

IRR See *internal rate of return.*

justification The argument used in defending a proposed budget or in explaining variances that have occurred.

lease An agreement providing for the use of an asset in exchange for rental payments.

length of stay (LOS) The number of days a patient is an inpatient. This is generally measured by the number of times the patient is an inpatient at midnight. (See also *average length of stay.*)

liability Legal financial obligation of the organization.

line item Any resource that is listed separately on a budget. For example, all nursing labor for a unit may appear in aggregate (one line item), or nurse manager costs may appear separately from RN costs and from LPN costs (resulting in 3 line items). Further subdivisions of nursing cost would create additional line items.

long-range budget A plan that covers a period of time longer than 1 year—typically 3, 5, or 10 years.

long-range planning The process of developing plans for a period of 3 to 5 years to achieve the general objectives of the organization.

long-term A period longer than 1 year.

long-term assets See *capital assets.*

long-term investment See *capital assets.*

LOS See *length of stay.*

managed care A system that integrates the financing and delivery of health care services, often using financial incentives to reduce provision of unnecessary care.

managed care organizations (MCOs) Insurance and provider organizations that adhere to the principles of managed care. (See *managed care.*)

Management by Objectives (MBO) A technique in which supervising managers and their subordinate managers agree on a common set of objectives against which performance will be measured.

margin At the edge. Usually refers to the impact of adding 1 more patient.

marginal costs See *incremental costs.*

market-based price A price set based on the prevailing price for a service that is charged by other providers in the community.

market share A percent of the total demand or volume for a product or service.

mark-up based price A price set based on the cost plus a predetermined percentage of cost.

master budget A set of all the major budgets in the organization. It generally includes the operating budget, long-range budget, programs budgets, capital budget, and cash budget.

MBO See *Management by Objectives.*

Medicaid A program funded jointly by the federal and state governments that pays for medical care for eligible low-income people.

Medicare A federal program under the Social Security Administration that pays for medical care for the aged and disabled.

mission The organization's set of primary goals that justify its existence, such as providing high-quality hospital care to the surrounding community or providing research and education.

mission statement Statement of the purpose or reason for existence of the organization, department, or unit. This statement provides direction regarding the types of activities that should be undertaken.

mixed costs A cost that contains an element of fixed costs and an element of variable costs, such as electricity. A unit or department budget as a whole represents a mixed cost.

moving-average A method of averaging out the roughness caused by random variation in a historical series of data points.

net assets Residual value when liabilities are subtracted from assets. This represents the portion of the organization's total resources owned by the organization itself (not-for-profit organizations). Sometimes called fund balance.

net cash flow The net difference between cash receipts and cash payments.

net patient revenue Charges, less contractual allowances, charity care, and bad debts; the ultimate amount the organization receives for its patient care services.

net present cost The aggregate present value of a series of payments to be made in the future.

net present value (NPV) The present value of a series of receipts, less the present value of a series of payments.

net revenue The organization's charges for services provided, less *deductions from revenue.*

nominal group technique A forecasting technique in which a group of individuals are brought together in a structured meeting and arrive at a group consensus forecast.

noncontrollable Those items that a manager does not have the authority or ability to control.

non-operating revenues Revenues that are not derived from the routine operations of the organization related to providing its goods or services.

nonproductive time Sick, vacation, holiday, and other paid nonworked time.

non-revenue-producing Departments, such as housekeeping, that do not directly charge patients for their services.

not-for-profit An organization whose mission does not include earning a profit for distribution to owners. A not-for-profit organization may earn a profit, but such profit must be reinvested for replacing facilities and equipment or for expanding services offered. Often referred to as nonprofit.

NPV See *net present value.*

NRGs See *Nursing Resource Groupings.*

Nursing Resource Groupings (NRGs) Classifications of patients into homogeneous groups based on nursing care consumed. Any patient in one NRG would consume a similar set of nursing resources as any other patient in that NRG.

objectives Specific targets that must be attained to achieve the organization's goals.

one-shot A budget that is prepared only once, rather than on a regular periodic basis such as monthly or annually.

operating Related to the normal routine activities of the organization in providing its goods or services.

operating budget The plan for the day-in and day-out operating revenues and expenses of the organization. It is generally prepared for a period of 1 year.

operating expenses The costs of the organization related to its general operations.

operating revenues Revenues earned in the normal course of providing the organization's goods or services.

operating statement A financial statement that subtracts expenses from revenues to determine the organization's profit or loss. Sometimes called the activity statement or income statement.

operations The routine activities of the organization related to its mission and the provision of goods or services.

out-of-pocket costs See *incremental costs.*

outcomes budget See *performance budget.*

outputs The product being produced (e.g., patients, patient days, visits, operations).

overhead Indirect costs that are allocated to a unit or department from elsewhere in the organization.

owner's equity The residual value when liabilities are subtracted from assets. This represents the portion of the organization's total resources owned by the owners of the organization (for-profit organizations). See also *fund balance* and *net assets.*

pass-through costs See *cost pass-through.*

patient classification A system for distinguishing among different patients based on their functional ability and resource needs.

patient day One patient occupying 1 bed for 1 day.

patient revenue Revenue derived from providing care to patients, in contrast to such things as gift shop revenue or contributions.

payback A capital budgeting approach that calculates how many years it takes for a project's cash inflows to equal or exceed its cash outflows.

per diem Daily charge.

performance budget A plan that relates the various objectives of a cost center with the planned costs of accomplishing those activities.

performance budgeting A process for evaluating the activities of a cost center in terms of the various objectives the center accomplishes and the costs of that accomplishment.

personnel Persons employed by the organization.

PERT See *Program Evaluation and Review Techniques.*

planning programming budgeting systems A program budgeting technique that seeks to integrate planning and budgeting into the process of evaluating programs.

position One person working 1 job, regardless of the number of hours that the person works.

PPO See *preferred provider organization.*

preferred provider organization (PPO) A health care provider organization that is recommended by an insurer or employer as being a preferred provider of services. PPOs generally offer the insurer or employer discounts. Employees or insured individuals who use the PPO generally pay a lower co-payment for their medical care than if they do not use the PPO.

prepaid group plan See *health maintenance organization.*

present costs See *net present costs.*

present value The value of future receipts or payments discounted to the present.

price index A tool that indicates year-to-year changes in the level of prices.

price variance The portion of the total variance for any line item that is caused by spending a different amount per unit of resource than had been anticipated (e.g., higher or lower salary rates, or higher or lower supply prices).

private insurers Insurance companies that are not related to the government.

pro forma A set of financial statements that present a prediction of what the financial statements for the organization or for a specific project or program will look like at some point in the future.

product line A group of patients that have some commonality that allows them to be grouped together, such as a common diagnosis.

productive time Straight time and overtime worked.

productivity The resources or inputs required to produce services or outputs.

profit The amount by which an organization's revenues exceed its expenses.

profit center A unit or department that is responsible for both revenues and expenses. Health care organizations have referred to profit centers as revenue centers, emphasizing the fact that a specific charge for such centers will appear on patient bills.

program budget A plan that looks at all aspects of a program across departments and over the long term.

Program Evaluation and Review Techniques (PERT) A multibranch programming technique designed to predict total project completion time for large-scale projects and to identify paths that have available slack.

programming A total organizational review with a focus on where the organization is headed.

proprietary See *for-profit*.

prospective patient classification Categorization of patients into a patient classification based on the anticipated nursing care requirements.

prospective payment Payment based on a predetermined price for any particular category of patient (such as a particular DRG), as opposed to reimbursement based on the costs of care provided to the patient.

prototype instruments An approach to patient classification that describes the characteristics of patients in each category and then assigns patients to the category that most closely reflects their nursing care requirements.

quantity variance The portion of the total variance for any line item, which is caused by using more input per unit of output (e.g., patient day) than had been budgeted.

rate-setting The process of determining the prices the organization charges for its services.

rate variance A price variance that relates to labor resources. In such cases, it is typically the hourly rate that has varied from expectations. See *price variance*.

regression analysis A statistical model that measures the average change in a dependent variable associated with a 1 unit change in one or more independent variables.

relative value unit (RVU) scale An arbitrary unit scale in which each patient is assigned a number of relative value units based on the relative costs of different types of patients. For example, if nursing care costs twice as much for Type A patients as for Type B patients, then Type A patients will be assigned a number of relative value units that is twice as high as that assigned to Type B patients.

relevant costs Only those costs that are subject to change as a result of a decision.

relevant range That range of activity that might reasonably be expected to occur in the budget period.

reliability of patient classification system A measure of the consistency of rating across different observers.

responsibility center Cost center; term used to emphasize the manager's control and accountability for the cost center.

retrospective patient classification Categorization of patients into a patient classification based on the nursing care needs that were met.

revenue Amounts of money that the organization has received or is entitled to receive in exchange for goods and/or services that it has provided.

revenue center A unit or department that is responsible and accountable for not only costs of providing services, but also for the revenues generated by those services.

revenue producing Departments, such as the operating room, that directly charge patients for the services they provide.

risk pool A pool of money established by withholding part of the payments otherwise due to a variety of different health care providers. The pool is used to pay for certain costs of providing health care services resulting from utilization in excess of an agreed-upon level.

risk sharing Situation in which the risk of high costs associated with high utilization of health care services are shared by more than 1 person or organization.

RVU See *relative value unit scale.*

satisfice The acceptance of a satisfactory or adequate result. This is in contrast to the effort required to reach an optimal result.

seasonality A predictable pattern of monthly, quarterly, or other periodic variation in historical data within each year.

seasonalization Adjustment of the annual budget for month-to-month seasonality.

self-pay patients Patients who are responsible for the payment of their own health care bills because they do not have private insurance and are not covered by either Medicare or Medicaid.

semivariable See *step-fixed.*

sensitivity analysis A technique in which the assumptions underlying a forecast are altered to see the impact of varying assumptions on the predicted result.

service unit A basic measure of the item being produced by the organization, such as patient days, home care visits, or hours of operations; when used in conjunction with standard treatment profiles, it refers to the intermediate products produced by each department of a health care organization.

simple linear regression Regression analysis that uses 1 dependent and 1 independent variable and that produces a prediction along a straight line.

software A computer program or programs that instruct the computer on what to do and how to do it.

special-purpose budget Any plan that does not fall into one of the other specific budget categories.

standard cost profile The average cost of a specific service unit.

standard treatment protocol The set of intermediate products consumed by the average patient in a specific product line.

statement of cash flows A financial statement that examines the organization's sources and uses of cash.

statement of financial position Financial report that indicates the financial position of the organization at a point in time. Often called a balance sheet.

step-fixed A cost that is fixed over short ranges of volume but varies within the relevant range (sometimes referred to as step-variable).

step-variable See *step-fixed.*

strategic management Process of setting goals and objectives for the organization, determining the resources to be allocated to achieving those goals and objectives, and establishing policies concerning getting and using those resources.

strategic planning 1. Process of setting long-term goals and designing a plan to achieve those goals; sometimes called long-term plan. 2. The process of developing a strategy for accomplishing the mission of the organization.

strategy The primary approach an organization uses to achieve its mission.

subcategory A device to allow separation of the flexible budget variance into the price variance and the quantity variance. The actual quantity of input per unit of output, multiplied by the budgeted price of the input, times the actual output level.

surplus See *profit*.

third-party payer An organization such as the government or an insurance company that is responsible for a portion of a patient's bill.

time-series analysis Use of historical values of a variable to predict future values for that variable without the use of any other variable, other than the passage of time.

time value of money Recognition of the fact that money can earn compounded interest, and therefore a given amount of money paid at different points in time has a different value—the further into the future an amount is paid, the less valuable it is.

total quality management (TQM) A philosophy that prevention of defects is cheaper than cure. TQM focuses on process improvements to improve quality and avoid errors.

total variance The sum of the price, quantity, and volume variances; the difference between the actual results and original budgeted amount.

trend A general tendency in a given direction, such as an upward or downward trend.

uncontrollable See *noncontrollable*.

unfavorable variance A variance in which more was spent than the budgeted amount.

unit-costing An approach for measuring productivity that measures the cost per unit of service provided, rather than focusing on units of resources consumed, such as hours or FTEs.

unit of service A measurement that describes the activity of the organization or a part of the organization (for example, visit, patient day, or procedure).

use variance Another name for the quantity variance. So-called because the quantity variance focuses on how much of a resource has been *used*. See *quantity variance*.

validity of patient classification A measure of the degree to which the system actually measures what it intends to measure.

variable billing A system in which the amount billed to each patient for nursing care per patient day varies based on the differing resource consumption of different patients.

variable budget See *flexible budget*.

variable budgeting See *flexible budgeting*.

variable costs Costs that vary in direct proportion with volume.

variance The difference between the budget and the actual results.

variance analysis A comparison of actual results as compared with the budget, followed by investigation to determine why the variance(s) occurred.

variance report A report of all differences between budget and actual results.

vendor Supplier; someone who sells things to the organization.

volume variance The amount of the variance in any line item that is caused simply by the fact that the workload level has changed.

Winters' exponential smoothing A curvilinear forecasting approach that works extremely well for seasonal data.

workload The volume of work for a unit or department; note that there should be a direct relationship between the workload and the amount of resources needed. Therefore, a workload measure such as patient days is inferior to one such as patient days adjusted for average patient acuity.

year-to-date The sum of the budget and/or actual values for all months from the beginning of the year through the most recent period for which data is available.

ZBB See *Zero-Base Budgeting.*

Zero-Base Budgeting (ZBB) A program budgeting approach that requires an examination and justification of all costs rather than just the incremental costs, and that requires examination of alternatives rather than just one approach.

APPENDIX

Sample Budget Forms and Instructions

APPENDIX CONTENTS

Guide to Abbreviations Used Above in Form Numbers

BD	Budget Detail
C	Capital
F	FTE
NS	Nonsalary
P	Personnel
PCU	Patient Care Unit
RE	Revenue and Expense
S	Salary
V	Volume
W	Workload

GENERAL INSTRUCTIONS

All budget worksheets are to be completed and returned to the Budget Office. Use N/A to indicate any worksheets or areas of worksheets that do not apply to your area of responsibility. Each individual sheet must be:

- identified by responsibility center number and name
- identified with the fiscal year for which the budget is projected
- signed and dated by the manager completing the worksheet

VOLUME, REVENUE, AND WORKLOAD

A. Patient Day Volume/Revenue (BD/V1)

This worksheet is used for calculating patient day revenue by type of accommodation. Total budgeted patient days for individual patient care units are determined jointly by the Budget Office, the Admitting Department, and the Nursing Department. FOR YOUR INFORMATION ONLY, the following data appears on this worksheet:

- 7-Month YTD Budget—budgeted volume for this type for the period July 1 through January 31.
- 7-Month YTD Actual—actual volume for this type for the period July 1 through January 31.
- Annual Budget—total budgeted volume for this type for this fiscal year.
- Projected Actual—straight-line volume projection for this year based on this year's actual through April, calculated as follows:

$$\frac{\text{7-month YTD Actual}}{7} \times 12$$

Note that these projections are simply the result of arithmetic calculations and are intended only to assist you in making your own projections. Your judgment and knowledge of your department must determine the appropriate budget projections for your area of responsibility.

1. Label and fill in the column FY _____ Budget with your projection for the coming year.
2. Fill in the column Charge per Day using the most current hospital rate book to identify the correct charge.
3. Calculate the Total Revenue by multiplying the FY _____ Budget by the Charge per Day.
4. Add the totals to calculate the Total Revenue for the cost center.

B. Other Volume/Revenue (BD/V2)

This worksheet is used for calculating revenue generated by supplies or services that are charged in addition to room revenue. FOR YOUR INFORMATION ONLY, the following data appears on this worksheet:

- 7-Month YTD Budget—budgeted volume for this type for the period July 1 through January 31.
- 7-Month YTD Actual—actual volume for this type for the period July 1 through January 31.
- Annual Budget—total budgeted volume for this type for this fiscal year.
- Projected Actual—straight-line volume projection for this year based on this year's actual through April, calculated as follows:

$$\frac{\text{7-month YTD Actual}}{7} \times 12$$

Note that these projections are simply the result of arithmetic calculations and are intended only to assist you in making your own projections. Your judgment and knowledge of your department must determine the appropriate budget projections for your area of responsibility.

1. Label and fill in the column FY _____ Budget with your projection for the coming year.
2. Fill in the column Charge per Unit using the most current hospital rate book to identify the correct charge.
3. Calculate the Total Revenue by multiplying the FY _____ Budget by the Charge per Day.
4. Add any line items to your cost center that you anticipate will occur in the coming year but that are not on this report.
5. Delete any line items that currently show actual or budget volume but that you do not expect to occur in the coming year.
6. Add the totals to calculate the Total Revenue for the cost center.
7. Explain briefly at the bottom of the page or on the reverse side your rationale for adding or deleting any line items.

C. Workload (PCU/W1)

This worksheet is used to calculate nursing workload on the inpatient units using the existing patient classification system.

1. Complete Current ADC using the most recent year-to-date patient classification data for this cost center.
2. Complete the Projected Change column based on your analysis of trend data and identification of anticipated changes in your patient population.

3. Calculate Revised ADC as Current ADC +/− Projected Change.
4. Calculate Projected Workload as Revised ADC times Relative Value.
5. Total all columns as indicated and calculate Average Acuity using formula on worksheet.
6. Include a brief discussion of the factors that led to the determination of the Projected Change.

BD/V1   PATIENT DAY VOLUME / REVENUE BUDGET WORKSHEET

FY _____

RESPONSIBILITY CENTER: 611 GENERAL SURGERY   BUDGETED DAYS _____

TYPE	7-MONTH YTD BUDGET	7-MONTH YTD ACTUAL	ANNUAL BUDGET	PROJECTED ACTUAL	FY BUDGET	CHARGE PER DAY	TOTAL REVENUE
Semiprivate	4,473	4,918	7,702	8,431			
Private	1,378	2,371	1,635	954			
Isolation	170	292	146	85			
TOTAL	6,021	5,957	10,365	10,212			

BD/V2   OTHER VOLUME / REVENUE BUDGET WORKSHEET

RESPONSIBILITY CENTER: 611 GENERAL SURGERY

FY _____

TYPE	7-MONTH YTD BUDGET	7-MONTH YTD ACTUAL	ANNUAL BUDGET	PROJECTED ACTUAL	FY ____ BUDGET	CHARGE PER DAY	TOTAL REVENUE
Discharge Visit	438	497	750	852			
ECG Portable	262	222	450	381			
Standby Equip	204	197	350	338			
				TOTAL			

PCU/W1

WORKLOAD BUDGET WORKSHEET

FY _____

RESPONSIBILITY CENTER: _____

PATIENT TYPE	CURRENT ADC	PROJECTED CHANGE	REVISED ADC	RELATIVE VALUE	PROJECTED WORKLOAD
1	_____	_____	_____	0.4	_____
2	_____	_____	_____	1.0	_____
3	_____	_____	_____	2.0	_____
4	_____	_____	_____	4.4	_____
Total	_____	_____	_____		_____

Workload_____   ADC_____   Average Acuity_____

Discussion:

FTEs AND SALARY EXPENSE

NOTE: Description of the method for determining FTEs requested must accompany the budget worksheets for FTEs and salary expense. Format for this description may vary by department and division. For the inpatient nursing units using the existing patient classification system, the Personnel Budget Worksheets (PCU/P1 and PCU/P2) will be completed for each responsibility center. In all calculations, an FTE is equal to 2,080 hours.

A. Position/Hours/FTE (BD/F1)

This worksheet is used to identify by specific position title the number of positions and the related hours and FTEs, both straight time (S/T) and overtime (O/T) to be budgeted for each cost center. The worksheet represents the current authorized budget for this cost center (including any adjustments that were approved during the current fiscal year):

- Curr Auth Positions—number of positions currently authorized in this position category.
- Position Title—description of position as it appears in the personnel position files.
- ST Hours—straight-time hours authorized for this position.
- ST FTE—straight-time FTEs authorized for this position, calculated by dividing ST hours by 2,080.
- OT Hours—overtime hours authorized for this position.
- OT FTE—overtime FTEs authorized for this position, calculated by dividing OT hours by 2,080.
- Total Hours—straight time plus overtime hours.
- Total FTEs—straight time plus overtime FTEs.

All columns are totaled, and the calculations for converting authorized hours to FTEs are shown at the bottom of the form.

1. Identify positions, hours, and FTEs to be requested for the cost center for the coming fiscal year (descriptions to accompany this worksheet).
2. Compare requests by position with current authorized and change authorized positions, hours, and FTEs to reflect requests.
3. If a position is requested that does not appear on the worksheet, it can be added on any available blank line. Positions that are no longer required should be crossed out.
4. Total all columns and complete calculations labeled Projected at bottom of form.

B. Base Salary (BD/S1)

This worksheet is used to calculate the base salaries generated by the FTEs described in the previous worksheet. There is a separate worksheet for each position title, and additional blank worksheets are available if a position that is new to the cost center is to be added. The worksheet lists by name all staff currently employed in that position category and in that cost center, and also includes:

- FTE—the portion of a full-time equivalent that the employee fills.
- Shift—the usual shift that the employee is scheduled to work.
- Base Hourly Rate—the rate at which the employee is currently being paid; does not include any increases that are scheduled for this fiscal year but that have not yet been added to the employee's salary.
- Base Annual Salary—base hourly rate times 2,080 hours times FTE.

Totals for the position category appear at the bottom of the worksheet.

1. Correct the data for current employees to reflect what will actually be in effect at the end of this fiscal year:

   - Correct FTE and shift designations if necessary.
   - Change Base Hourly Rate and Base Annual Salary for any employee who will receive a salary increase.
   - Delete any employees who will terminate or transfer out.
   - Add any employees who will be hired or transferred in.

2. Add as Vacant (Current) any positions that are currently vacant and include the FTE, Shift, Base Hourly Rate, and Base Annual Rate anticipated for those positions.
3. Add as Vacant (New) any additional positions that are being requested and include the FTE, Shift, Base Hourly Rate, and Base Annual Rate anticipated for those positions.
4. Correct the totals for the position category. *Totals in each position category must correspond with the S/T totals for the position listed on the Position/ Hours/FTE Budget Worksheet (BD/F).*

C. Differential Budget Worksheet (BD/S2)

This worksheet is used to identify the expenses for those differentials paid to employees for working particular shifts, such as evenings, nights, weekends, or holidays, or under special conditions, such as on call. Refer to the Personnel Manual for the policy on payment of differentials and to the current Wage and Salary Guidelines for the differential rates.

1. Calculate differentials for each position category individually (exception:

differentials may be combined for full-time and part-time staff with the same position title—e.g., Unit Aide FT and Unit Aide PT).

2. For evenings, nights, weekends, and on call, calculate from staffing patterns the required number of Hours/Week. Multiply by 52 to determine the Annual Hours.

3. Enter the Rate for each differential type, and multiply by Annual Hours to determine the Total $$$.

4. For Holiday, calculate the number of staffed hours required for each of the recognized organizational holidays, and enter under Annual Hours.

5. Since the holiday differential rate is 50% of base rate, it is necessary to determine the average base rate for the position category. This is calculated using the totals for the position category determined on the Base Salary Budget Worksheet, using the following formula:

$$\frac{\text{Total base salary}}{(\text{FTEs} \times 2,080)} = \text{Average hourly salary}$$

$$\text{Average hourly salary} \times 0.5 = \text{Holiday differential rate}$$

6. Enter the Rate for Holiday and multiply by Annual Hours to determine the Total $$$.

7. Sum all Total $$$ amounts to determine Total This Position.

D. Overtime (BD/S3)

This worksheet is used to determine the overtime expenses corresponding to the hours and FTEs identified on the Position/Hours/FTE Budget Worksheet (BD/F1). Overtime expense is calculated separately for each position title. Overtime is paid at 50% above combined (base + differential) hourly rate. Budget calculations must therefore include both of these types of dollars. The formulas for calculating overtime are detailed on the worksheet and use the following data for the individual position category:

- Overtime Hours—from Position/Hours/FTE Budget Worksheet (BD/F1).
- Total S/T FTE—from Position/Hours/FTE Budget Worksheet (BD/F1).
- Total Base Salary—from Base Salary Budget Worksheet (BD/S1).
- Total Differential—from Differential Budget Worksheet (BD/S2).

E. Salary Expense (BD/S4)

This worksheet is used to total the salary expenses by position category for the cost center. Each position title represented on the Position/Hours/FTE Budget Worksheet (BD/F1) must be represented. For each position category, enter the following:

- Base Salary—from Base Salary Budget Worksheet (BD/S1).
- Differential—from Differential Budget Worksheet (BD/S2).
- Overtime—from Overtime Budget Worksheet (BD/S3).

Sum the amounts across each line for the Total for the individual position category. Sum the columns for the Total for each expense type and for the cost center. Leave all salaries at this year's rates. The Budget Office will adjust for raises once the percentages have been determined.

PCU/P1

PERSONNEL BUDGET WORKSHEET Page 1

FY _____

RESPONSIBILITY CENTER: _____

Bed Complement _____ Total Patient Days _____ % Occupancy _____

ADC _____ Average Acuity _____ Average Workload _____

Average Workload _____ Target HPW _____ Hours/24 Hours_____

Hours/24 Hours_____ 8 Shifts/24 Hours _____

DAILY STAFFING PATTERN
Variable Staff (Preliminary):

SHIFT DISTRIBUTION		_____%	_____%	_____%	
Mix	Position	7–3	3–11	11–7	Total
%	Staff Nurse				
%	LPN/LVN				
%	Patient Care Technician				
%	Nursing Asst				
	Total				

Variable Staff (Adjusted):

SHIFT DISTRIBUTION		_____%	_____%	_____%	
Mix	Position	7–3	3–11	11–7	Total
%	Staff Nurse				
%	LPN/LVN				
%	Patient Care Technician				
%	Nursing Asst				
	Total				

Support Staff:

Position	7–3	3–11	11–7	Total
Secretary				
Unit Aide (M–F)				
Total				

Fixed Staff: Nurse Manager _____ Clinical Specialist_____

PCU/P2

PERSONNEL BUDGET WORKSHEET   Page 2

FY _____

CALCULATION OF NONPRODUCTIVE TIME

Factor for days off and nonproductive time:

YTD as of _____

(a) Total paid hours _____

(b) Total paid nonproductive hours _____ (sick   vacation   holiday
     other paid nonworked)

(c) Total paid productive hours (a)   (b) _____

(d) % paid nonproductive (b)   (c) _____(convert % to decimal)

(e) Factor   1   1.4   1(d)   1   1.4   _____   _____

CALCULATION OF TOTAL REQUIRED FTEs

CATEGORY	SHIFT/24 HOUR	FACTOR (e)	TOTAL FTEs REQUIRED	BUDGET FTE	
				ST	OT
Nurse Manager					
Clinical Specialist					
Staff Nurse					
LPN/LVN					
Patient Care Technician					
Nursing Assistant					
Secretary					
Unit Aide (M–F)					
Total					

BD/F1

POSITION/HOURS/FTE BUDGET

FY _____

RESPONSIBILITY CENTER: 611 GENERAL SURGERY

CURR AUTH POSITIONS	POSITION TITLE	ST HOURS	ST FTE	OT HOURS	OT FTE	TOTAL HOURS	TOTAL FTE
1	Nurse Manager	2,080	1.0	—	—	2,080	1.0
1	Clin Specialist	2,080	1.0	—	—	2,080	1.0
13	Staff Nurse FT	27,040	13.0	1,040	0.5	28,080	13.5
8	Staff Nurse PT	8,320	4.0	—	—	8,320	4.0
3	LPN/LVN FT	6,240	3.0	208	0.1	6,448	3.1
1	LPN/LVN PT	832	0.4	—	—	832	0.4
3	Nsg Asst FT	6,240	3.0	624	0.3	6,864	3.3
3	Nsg Asst PT	1,248	0.6	—	—	1,248	0.6
4	Secretary FT	8,320	4.0	208	0.1	8,528	4.1
2	Secretary PT	1,664	0.8	—	—	1,664	0.8
2	Unit Aide FT	4,160	2.0	—	—	4,160	2.0
1	Unit Aide PT	832	0.4	—	—	832	0.4
42	Total	69,056	33.2	2,080	1.0	71,136	34.2

CURRENTLY AUTHORIZED		PROJECTED	
ST FTE	$\frac{69056}{2080}$ 33.2	ST FTE	$\frac{}{2080}$
OT FTE	$\frac{2080}{2080}$ 1.0	OT FTE	$\frac{}{2080}$
TOTAL FTE	$\frac{71136}{2080}$ 34.2	TOTAL FTE	$\frac{}{2080}$

BD/S1

BASE SALARY BUDGET WORKSHEET

FY _____   Page ___ of ___

RESPONSIBILITY CENTER: 611 GENERAL SURGERY
POSITION CATEGORY: STAFF NURSE PART TIME

NAME	FTE	SHIFT	BASE HOURLY RATE	BASE ANNUAL SALARY
Briggs, Martha	0.2	3–11	$17.99	$ 7,484
Coram, Amy	0.5	11–7	17.73	18,439
Douglas, Ida	0.5	7–3	21.44	22,298
Francis, Jamie	0.5	7–3	15.21	15,818
Howells, Robert	0.5	3–11	19.37	20,145
Martins, Mary	0.8	3–11	22.85	38,022
Ridley, George	0.5	7–3	18.22	18,949
Westbury, Vickie	0.5	11–7	16.24	16,890

Total This Position Category:

Positions   8

FTEs   4.0   Base Salary $158,045

BD/S2

DIFFERENTIAL BUDGET WORKSHEET

FY _____

RESPONSIBILITY CENTER: _____ Page ____ of ____

Position Title: _____

DIFFERENTIAL TYPE	HOURS/WEEK	ANNUAL HOURS	RATE	TOTAL $$$
Evening				
Night				
Weekend				
Holiday				
On Call				
			Total This Position: $	

Position Title: _____

DIFFERENTIAL TYPE	HOURS/WEEK	ANNUAL HOURS	RATE	TOTAL $$$
Evening				
Night				
Weekend				
Holiday				
On Call				
			Total This Position: $	

BD/S3

OVERTIME BUDGET WORKSHEET

FY _____

RESPONSIBILITY CENTER: _____   Page ____ of ____

Position Title _____ Overtime Hours _____

Total S/T FTE _____ 2,080 hours _____Total Hours

Total Base Salary _____ Total Differential _____

_____ Combined Total

Combined Total _____ Total Hours _____

_____ Combined Hourly Rate

Combined Hourly Rate _____ 1.5 Overtime Hours _____

_____ Overtime Total

Position Title _____ Overtime Hours _____

Total S/T FTE _____ 2,080 hours _____Total Hours

Total Base Salary _____ Total Differential _____

_____ Combined Total

Combined Total _____ Total Hours _____

_____ Combined Hourly Rate

Combined Hourly Rate _____ 1.5 Overtime Hours _____

_____ Overtime Total

BD/S4

SALARY EXPENSE BUDGET WORKSHEET

FY _____

RESPONSIBILITY CENTER: _____

POSITION TITLE	BASE SALARY	DIFFERENTIAL	OVERTIME	TOTAL
TOTAL				

NONSALARY EXPENSE

This portion of your budget packet is used to describe the anticipated nonsalary expenses for the coming year. These include all of the 611. (Supply) and 911. (Interdepartmental) expense accounts that appear on your monthly responsibility center revenue and expense statements. The Revenue and Expense Budget Worksheet (BD/RE1) can be used to identify the accounts in which you have incurred expenses for the current year and in which you may wish to budget expenses for the coming year. FOR YOUR INFORMATION ONLY, the following data appears on this worksheet:

- 7-Month YTD Actual—actual expense for this account for the year-to-date (YTD) period July 1 through January 31.
- Annual Budget—total budgeted expense for this account for this fiscal year.
- 12-Month Projection—straight-line expense projection for this year based on this year's actual through April, calculated as follows:

$$\frac{\text{7-month YTD Actual}}{7} \times 12$$

Note that these projections are simply the result of arithmetic calculations and are intended only to assist you in making your own projections. Your judgment and knowledge of your department must determine the appropriate budget projections for your area of responsibility.

A. Revenue and Expense (BD/RE1)

This worksheet summarizes the projected revenue and expense in all categories for the next fiscal year.

1. Revenue
   - Enter total from Patient Day Volume/Revenue Budget Worksheet (BD/V1) on account line 010 Routine.
   - Enter total from Other Volume/Revenue Budget Worksheet (BD/V2) on account line 020 Other.
2. Salary Expense—from Salary Expense Budget Worksheet (BD/S4), enter:
   - Base Salary Total on account line 010 Salaries—Regular;
   - Overtime Total on account line 020 Salaries—Overtime; and
   - Differential Total on account line 030 Salaries—Differentials.
   Leave other expense lines blank; Budget Office will calculate other fringe benefit amounts.
3. Supply Expense—enter appropriate amount for each account line; this must be consistent with the total expense calculated on the corresponding Nonsalary Expense Budget Worksheet (BD/NS1).
4. Interdepartment Expense—enter appropriate amount for each account line; this must be consistent with the total expense calculated on the corresponding Nonsalary Expense Budget Worksheet (BD/NS1).

5. Budget Office will calculate totals and contributions when all expenses have been identified.

B. Nonsalary Expense (BD/NS1)

This worksheet is used to describe the elements included in the budget projections for each type of expense. A separate sheet is used for each nonsalary (supply or interdepartmental) account that is budgeted for more than $500.

For some nonsalary accounts, the amount to be budgeted may be determined by volume and related to volume changes from this year. For this type of expense, budget may be calculated using the formula:

$$\frac{\text{This Year YTD \$\$\$ Expense}}{\text{This Year's Volume}} \times \text{Next Year's Volume} = \text{Next Year's Expense}$$

If so, then the formula with the appropriate numbers are entered on the worksheet. Any adjustments that must be made to this result should be clearly explained. For other accounts, it may be more appropriate to list out on the specific items or activities that will generate the expense (e.g., in the Equipment or Seminar/Meetings accounts). A brief narrative is also acceptable for those accounts that are not clearly described by either of the above methods.

Budget all nonsalary accounts in this year's dollars. The Budget Office will adjust for inflation as needed when these rates are determined.

BD/RE1

REVENUE AND EXPENSE BUDGET WORKSHEET

FY _____

RESPONSIBILITY CENTER: 611 GENERAL SURGERY

ACCOUNT NUMBER/ DESCRIPTION	FY 01 7-MONTH YTD ACTUAL	FY 01 ANNUAL BUDGET	FY 01 PROJECTED ACTUAL	FY 02 BUDGET PROJECTION
311. Revenue				
010 Routine	($3,244,410)	($5,556,030)	($5,561,846)	
020 Other	(27,590)	(47,893)	(47,297)	
Total Operating Revenue	($3,272,000)	($5,603,923)	($5,609,143)	
411. Salary Expense				
010 Salaries - Regular	$730,881	$1,292,966	$1,252,939	
020 Salaries - Per Diem	2,758	0	4,728	
030 Salaries - Overtime	40,128	62,288	68,791	
040 Salaries - Differentials	97,995	170,419	167,991	
050 FICA	61,285	107,316	105,060	
060 Health Insurance	62,125	111,842	106,500	
070 Pension	19,855	35,816	34,037	
090 Other	17,228	29,092	29,534	
Total Salary Expense	$1,032,255	$1,809,738	$1,769,580	
611. Supply Expense				
010 Patient Care Supplies	$41,692	$62,023	$71,472	
020 Office Supplies	1,907	3,070	3,269	
030 Forms	3,111	5,560	5,333	
040 Supplies Purchased	1,210	1,935	2,074	
050 Equipment	1,553	2,903	2,662	
060 Seminars/Meetings	1,163	2,258	1,994	
070 Books	145	258	249	
080 Equipment Rental	385	1,703	660	
090 Miscellaneous	388	968	665	
Total Supply Expense	$51,554	$80,677	$88,378	
911. Interdepartmental Expense				
010 Central Supply	$7,828	$13,995	$13,419	
020 Pharmacy	9,527	17,019	16,332	
030 Linen/Laundry	16,046	28,678	27,507	
040 Maintenance	977	4,515	1,675	
060 Telephone	1,962	3,225	3,363	
070 Photocopy	124	323	213	
090 Miscellaneous	165	194	283	
Total Interdepartmental Expense	$36,629	$67,948	$62,793	
Total Operating Expense	$1,120,438	$1,958,363	$1,920,751	

BD/NS1

NONSALARY EXPENSE BUDGET WORKSHEET

FY _____

RESPONSIBILITY CENTER _____   Page ____ of ____

Account Number _____ Description _____

Current Year Budget $_____ Projected Actual $_____

Calculation/itemization for budget request:

Total budget request $_____

CAPITAL EQUIPMENT AND CONSTRUCTION

The capital budget identifies those requested items that are capitalized and charged to depreciation rather than to regular operational accounts. Items that must be capitalized include:

- Individual items (equipment, furniture, etc.) with a unit cost of $500 or more (including installation costs) and a life expectancy of 2 years or more;
- Items purchased in bulk with a total cost of $500 or more and a life expectancy of 2 years or more (even if the cost of the individual item is less than $500);
- Construction, maintenance, and renovations in excess of $2,500; and
- Computer software products with a cost of $20,000 or more (including installation costs).

All capital budget requests are to be listed on the Capital Budget Worksheet (BD/C1). In addition, any capital requests with a total cost of $2,500 or greater will require a separate Capital Justification Worksheet (BD/C2).

A. Capital Budget (BD/C1)

List each item on this form, completing the information required in each column:

1. Priority—assign a priority number to each request, using 1 for the highest priority number. Items do not need to be listed in priority order as long as the priorities are clearly identified.
2. Type—enter one of the following codes:
    - CR—construction or remodeling;
    - RE—item that replaces an existing item in the department;
    - RU—item that replaces and upgrades an existing item in the department;
    - AS—item that is in addition to similar items already available within the department; and
    - AN—item that is an addition and not currently available in the department.
3. Equipment Quantity—identify how many of this item are requested.
4. Description—provide simple description of the item or project, including relevant model numbers, etc.
5. Unit Cost—enter the price of a single one of this item, or the total cost of the project.
6. Extended Cost—calculate unit cost × equipment quantity.
7. Comments—include any additional information that will be useful in evaluating the request.

B. Capital Justification (BD/C2)

This form must be completed for each priority on the Capital Budget Worksheet (BD/C1) whose extended cost is $2,500 or greater. Attach additional pages if necessary, and identify them clearly with the responsibility center and priority number.

1. Description—include a brief but complete description of the item or project, including the proposed location.
2. Justification—provide a thorough justification for the item or project, including implications if funding is not made available.
3. Construction Costs—these should be reviewed with the Planning and Engineering Departments, as well as with any other affected services; enter date of cost estimates and name and title of individual providing this estimate.
4. Equipment Costs—include both purchase price and installation costs; attach vendors proposal if available.
5. Impact on Operational Costs—describe and quantify as much as possible the incremental costs associated with this item or project, including salaries, fringes, maintenance contracts, utilities, supplies, or interdepartmental expenses.
6. Impact on Revenue—describe and quantify as much as possible the incremental revenue that could be generated as a result of this item or project.

BD/C1

CAPITAL BUDGET WORKSHEET

FY _____

RESPONSIBILITY CENTER _____

PRIOR. #	TYPE CR/RE/RU AS/AN	EQUIP. QTY	DESCRIPTION	UNIT COST	EXTENDED COST	COMMENTS

BD/C2

CAPITAL JUSTIFICATION FORM

FY _____

RESPONSIBILITY CENTER _____   PRIORITY ITEM # _____

Description of Item or Project:

Justification:

Construction Costs: **Equipment Costs:**

Fees   _____   Purchase Price   _____

Construction   _____   Installation   _____

Contingency   _____

  Total   _____

Date of Estimate _____   By _____

Impact on Operational Expenses:

Impact on Revenues:

Index

Note: Page numbers in *italics* refer to illustrations; page numbers followed by a t refer to tables.